The Complete Guide to Soun

© 2013 David Gibson

Table of Contents

Foreward

The term Sound Healing is used throughout this book because it has become the accepted buzzword in the field. However, Sound Healing is only a small part of how sound can be used, or how it affects us. Sound does much more than heal. Sound can soothe, sound can raise our consciousness, and sound can take us into other realms of reality. Sounds can entrain our brains into a full range of states of consciousness. Healing is often thought of as fixing something that is wrong. Sound can harmonize everything that is right – beauty, harmony, love, and Spirit.

Acknowledgments

I have learned information, techniques and skills from so many people in this diverse field of Sound Healing – not to mention all the ancients that are no longer in the physical body. Ultimately, none of it came from me – I am just the vehicle through which it has come. However, I do take credit for the organization of all the material.

I would say that my primary mentor and helper has been Randy Masters. Randy has not only provided some information for this book, he has inspired me as to how to help others without ego. He has helped me to see a clear template of our birthright of divinity on this planet in this Universe. For that, I am forever grateful.

I am grateful for all my instructors from which I have gained many tidbits and gems: Silvina Vergara, Craig Godfrey, Richard Feather Anderson, James Word, Janis Arch, Suzanne Sterling, Matt Kramer, Erik Larson, Don Estes, Elizabeth Grambsch, Susanne Runion, Rabbi Steven Fisdel, Judy Cole, and Steven Halpern.

There are many past instructors that have also inspired me: Lisa Rafel, Jan Cercone, Amber Liev, Evelie Delfino Sales Posch, Maestro Curtis, Amrita Cottrell, Clare Hedin, Joshua Leads, Silvia Nakkach, Alex Theory, Karl Maret, Mark Deutsch, and Stuart Grace Greene.

There are so many in the field that I have drawn from in my own Sound Healing development: Tom Kenyon, Jeffrey Thompson, Jonathan Goldman, William at Crystal Tones, Fabien Maman, Jill Purce, Joel Andrews, Kae Thompson-Liu, Barbara Hero, Gary Schwartz, Harry Massey, Beverly Ann Wilson, and Don Campbell (May he rest in peace).

There are also all the editors that have worked on the book – Alexander Momirov (main editor), Ben Brown, Susanne Runion, Cour Barone, Kala Perkins, Dana Planetta, and Edith Sorrell. Thank you, thank you, thank you.

I also want to acknowledge my brothers, Bill and Jim Gibson, who whether they know it or not have inspired me to make this book less "woo-woo" and more scientific and accessible for the mainstream.

But most importantly, I want to thank all of my students. They have come up with so many creative ways of seeing things, and ways of doing things with sound and have challenged and inspired me to go ever more for the highest good of all.

INTRODUCTION
Peace on the Inside, Flowing on the Outside

We call this book "The Complete Guide to Sound Healing" because currently it is the first book to give such a wide perspective on the whole field of Sound Healing and Sound Therapy and all that it encompasses. Currently all the other books in the field focus only on specific areas of the field and they often focus on those specific areas quite well.

Because I own a California State approved College I strive to provide a full perspective so that students can then focus on whatever information, techniques and skills they are most interested in. Because I have over 20 instructors, and because I have put on 3 major Sound Healing conferences I have been blessed to be able learn and experience a very large portion of everything going on in the field, therefore developing this unique and wide ranging perspective.

Adding to this over the last 10 years I have taken the full range of techniques I have come across and have practiced them, experimented, researched and listened to my own intuition and what Source has chosen to share with me. This book is the culmination of all of this experience and information.

However, of all the information that is known in the field, we seem to know hardly anything. Not only is there very little definitive research, Spirit has not provided us with a manual on how it all works. Source gives us pieces here and there, and some get detailed downloads…However, it seems that these downloads often only apply to that one person or a group of people on the planet. Therefore, it seems that you cannot trust that their information is necessarily true for you.

In fact, it seems,
what we know about the whole Universe
is just a spec
compared to the vastness of information that we don't understand.

Therefore, to us
it seems much like mystery and magic
and from our perspective
that's exactly what it is.

Knowing how little we know about how it all works, I come at this from a complete attitude of humility. However, I have been doing my best to figure it all out based on the information that is available. And we have a lot of information now!

Therefore, throughout the book (and in my classes and in public), I am very careful to not say, "This is the way it is!!!" Often, I can say that this information means that "this seems to be true," but the mystery is always looming behind ready to show a whole new perspective.

In fact, there are many well-known people in the field of healing and consciousness that often say, "This is the way that it is!!!" and they say it so confidently that they develop huge followings. Often, much of their information makes complete sense; then there is another portion of their information that is based on conjecture and belief. However, that information gets thrown in as if it is "The way it is!!!" also.

Throughout the book you will see that I am very careful about saying "This is the truth!!!" I might say that I believe really strongly based on the available information. And, sometimes I might point out that I believe something <u>really</u> strongly because of the available information and my experiences. However, when it comes down to it, who really knows for sure?

In the field of Sound Healing, I have therefore become extremely skeptical when someone says that this frequency is **it!!!** For example, that a certain frequency opens the heart or changes your life. Especially, when no one else has come up with that frequency independently and there is no definitive (or clinical) research that is repeatable to back it up. It may be true for that person or even a large group of people, but it doesn't necessarily mean it is true for you or me.

However, and very importantly…based on the fact that we know so little compared to Source, I do not want to throw out any babies (with the bath water, that is). That frequency that a psychic downloaded just might be the exact thing I need to heal my kidneys, or transform my consciousness into a whole other level where my life is changed forever. Therefore, throughout the book I will be sharing information that is not proven scientifically.

On the other hand, I do provide the scientific basis behind how sound affects us – particularly physically and mentally. In these two areas the science is very definitive.

The science of Sound Healing is critical in order to bring it into the mainstream – hospitals and homes. And, science is important to help weed out the "woo-woo" that can actually hurt people – if not, just their pocketbooks. Because of this, we have set up the Sound Healing Research Association to help pin down things more definitively.

However, again, let us not throw out any babies. In fact, ancient traditions such as Sanskrit and ancient Egypt have already figured out much of how it all works – back in times when people were more tuned in and were still enough to receive even more detailed information from Source. We have also included this type of information.

For the beginners, the book provides many guidelines on how to proceed. However, now that Sound Healing has caught on and so many are working with such a wide range of techniques, perhaps you have already come across techniques that are consistently creating miracles. For those of you who are already working with the amazing power of sound there is always room to expand on what you do, and we will surely provide many avenues for expansion.

Much of the book is simply about using sound to raise your consciousness so you can once again hear the secrets of the Universe.

To simplify it all, there are two general directions that sound can take us: Up and Down; more activated and high or more calm and peaceful.

We often get more activated and high from music, especially when toning, chanting and repeating mantras for extended periods of time.

We get calm and peaceful from instruments that have consistent tones or rhythms, and most importantly from those that fade out smoothly and slowly to perfect silence. It is in this stillness that portals to other dimensions of consciousness open up...particularly connections to our Soul and Source itself – where we are one with everything and everyone in the Universe. Also, it is in this stillness that we are sometimes given the keys – whether it is a key to resolving a physical, mental or emotional issue, or in the extreme case, the key to powers beyond our imagination. Some say that the huge granite blocks of the Great Pyramid in Egypt were lifted with sound. Sai Baba was said to use sound to manifest all types of things in his hands including rings and special healing powders. They had been given the keys by expanding their consciousness from a place of complete stillness.

The more still we are
the more we can hear
the subtleties of our Soul and Spirit.
They whisper so softly.

"Surely again, to heal men's wounds by music's spell."
- Euripides, Medea (480-406 BC)

The basis of this whole book is actually quite scientific.

We know that everything is vibration
based on science and our own intuition.

"Everything is Vibrating, Everything is Frequency – Hum along."

"In ancient times music was the foundation of all the sciences.
Education was begun with music."
Cicero (106-43 BC)

The beauty of looking at everything as frequency is that there is no judgment – it is just what it is. And, as you will see, there are certain laws that govern how one frequency affects another. These laws of physics are relevant not only in our 3D world, but also seem to be the same in the quantum world of intention, and the world of Spirit.

In this book we are providing two basic avenues for healing: change and transformation. There are sections that give specific techniques for how to work with specific issues. There are also specific sections that explain how it all works (as far as we know at this point).

First, we provide a large number of specific techniques for the following:
1. Physical healing and dealing with pain.
2. Emotional stress relief, releasing stuck emotions and negative beliefs that are holding us back.
3. Mental brainwave entrainment for issues such as sleep deprivation, ADD, ADHD, more presence of mind, creativity enhancement and reconnecting to Source.
4. Spiritual advancement including resonating higher emotions such as gratitude, compassion, love and joy; and, resonating deeper connections to your Soul and Source.

However, the second healing avenue is certainly the most important. That is, techniques for raising your consciousness to higher levels. This means bringing you into states of consciousness where you have more access to information on how to live your life more fully with less stress and more blissful peace. It also means bringing more love and light into your relationships and work. Transformation is about learning to live your life in a way where you are given more and more keys. Ultimately, it is about returning to the place of knowing that we are all one – the illusion of separation in which we live is just silly!

Therefore, this book in its essence is more than just a bunch of techniques. It is an overall guide for how to transform your life – how to use the secrets of sound to expand your life into a state of peaceful bliss – a higher state of consciousness, so to speak. By obtaining as many of the pieces as possible as to how it all works, it is my hope and intention that you may be transported into that higher state of consciousness where you can receive all the answers you need on your own.

SECTION I – Healing and Transformation Frameworks and Paradigms

Introduction – Allopathic versus Health Models

*"The famous Greek physician Hippocrates administered musical treatments
to his patients in 400 B.C. Although this type of treatment did not originate with him,
it found in him an exponent of the highest order. With the increasing materialism
of Western civilization, the major tenants of ancient musical therapy
have been either forgotten or discarded."*
- Corinne Heline (1882-1975)

*"Eventually, musical therapists will compose prescriptions
after the manner of a pharmacist…"*
- Dr. Ira Altschuler (of the Eloise State Hospital) (1942)

There are two models of how to approach health and healing.

1. Allopathic Model – Focus on What is Wrong (though not all bad)
2. The Resonant Health Model – Focus on What is Right

<u>The Allopathic Model</u>
This model is the traditional medical model. It has two different approaches:

1. Warfare Model - Seek and Destroy – Once you find what is wrong – kill, kill, kill.
This is the model for dealing with cancer and many other diseases. It is the approach for
the majority of modern medicine. If you can't kill it with a drug, cut it out.

Surprisingly enough, this is also a common model used in Sound Healing. There are
many ways to use sounds to break up stuck energy, blockages and even to explode cells.
When you find the natural resonant frequency of a cell and play its frequency (voice,
instrument, or technology), you can feed the cell energy when playing the sound at lower
volumes. If you turn the volume up, you can explode the cells. Using ultrasound on
kidney stones is the prime example, but many in the field have been exploring how to
find the resonant frequency of a disease in order to then turn up the volume and ka-pooey
– the cancer is gone – **without affecting any of the surrounding cells that have a
different resonant frequency.**

However, the underlying problem that caused the cancer in the first place is still yet to be
resolved. And…the body doesn't necessarily go for the warfare method. It is murderous.

Some say that you can actually create karma
by destroying living things such as cells.

Others say that you can create karma by
actually taking away a person's opportunity
to learn the lesson that the physical issue is a result of.

However, I must admit, if I had cancer I would be trying every possible technique I know with sound to destroy the cancer cells. Bring on the big sound guns. One of our previous instructors used sound on her breast cancer and the tumor has now been gone for over 7 years.

2. Transformation Model – In this model we still focus on what is wrong, but we then use sound and vibration to transform the offending cells or incoherent vibrations into more coherent vibrations.

There are two general approaches. One is to match the vibration of the issue and then slowly transform that vibration into a more harmonious vibration. This is called the "iso-principle," where you lock onto the original vibration and slowly lead it into a different vibration.

The second approach is to find the resonant frequency of a healthy cell or tissue and simply play that frequency back to the cell in order to vibrate it back into harmony. Nutri-Energetics does this with their technology. They do an assessment to find where the problems are, and then they resonate the field back into harmony.

The Resonant Health Model
This is the new paradigm of healing. In this model we don't focus on what is wrong at all, but simply resonate what is right in a person. People in the field approach this from a wide range of perspectives. Some focus on resonating higher emotions such as gratitude, compassion, love and joy. Some focus on resonating a person's Soul or signature frequency. Some resonate direct connections to Spirit or Source. Some get more detailed and focus on resonating harmony in particular systems in the body. For example, acupuncture is all about creating flow in the meridians. The elementals in Homeopathy (a small portion of the overall Homeopathy approach) are focused on resonating what is right and boosting that frequency.

Any approach that focuses on relaxation, releasing stress, boosting the immune system or simply making people feel good in any way is using this model.

Many people I know believe this is the main medicine of the future – Resonating more and more harmony so that issues and diseases simply fall away.

Ultimately, we will discover how to find a person's
Divine Template
then use sound and music
to resonate a person back into their natural perfect healthy harmony.

We will be discussing specific techniques based on each of these models in detail later in the book.

Chapter 1 – Four Levels of How Sound Affects Us Physically, Mentally, Emotionally and Spiritually

There are four main areas of our system where sound has been proven to be effective. Obviously these areas often overlap. An emotional release can make a physical pain go away, or a Spiritual breakthrough can clear the mind like nothing before.

Physically

When it comes to how sound affects matter, the science is extremely definitive. Physics explains how sound affects matter in detail. Once we know the resonant frequency of something, there are several proven ways that sound can be used to cause changes in the matter. We'll be exploring these techniques in detail throughout the book.

Physics completely dispels the notion that Sound Healing is superstitious (or "woo-woo") and lacking scientific basis. This is really important, because if someone doesn't believe in a healing modality, it is way less likely to work. If someone does believe in the modality, it will normally work (this has even been proven to be the case with something as physically based as chemotherapy).

This is not to say that Sound Healing is all about the placebo effect. The science is definitive. However, belief systems can override physical reality – and commonly do. However, the problem is we still do not know the resonant frequencies of many cells and parts of the body. There are many charts of frequencies that have been published, but very few of them actually have real research backing them.

We know that everything naturally vibrates to its own innate resonant frequency. When we find that resonate frequency and play a sound that matches, it actually feeds energy into the object. This could be a cell, an organ, or any part of the body. Also, when we use vibration to trigger a natural resonance in something, we are effectively massaging it – loosening it up and causing more flow. This can be extremely effective for an organ like the heart, or for relaxing muscles.

However, if you play a sound that matches a resonant frequency, and turn up the volume, you can explode the object. You can also use this technique to break up stuck energy or blockages in the body. In this way parts of the body can be entrained back into health by resonating their natural healthy frequency.

Sound can also be used to get rid of pain. Pain receptors can only handle so much information, so when you fill them up with sound they can no longer transmit pain impulses. Later we'll discuss how to make the sound of a pain. In just about every case, the pain goes away.

There are many tools for creating physical changes in the body: Voice, Crystal Bowls, Tuning Forks, and Tone Generators to name a few. Tuning forks are also extremely effective for relieving pain. The Voice is incredibly effective when used directly on the body.

Probably the most effective tool is the use of Cyma frequencies.. These are frequencies that have been researched in detail. There are frequencies for just about every part of the body. Go to www.SoundHealingCenter.com/music.html to checkout the Cyma CDs that we offer.

Besides influencing specific cells or organs, these tools can be used to create an overall sense of wellbeing, causing the body's natural healing response to kick in. It has been proven that these instruments can dramatically boost the immune system. Often sound works to create a more harmonious flow in many of the systems in the body – these include the skeletal system, nervous, system, muscular system, digestive system, circulatory system, respiratory system, and endocrine system.

It has also been shown that you can actually create very specific vitamins and minerals in the body by resonating their frequency in the body. In one study, a frequency was shown to increase the oxygen content of the blood.

Besides musical instruments or voice, there is also the tool of Intention. When you hold an intention for a positive outcome (as in prayer), you are transmitting a frequency via the quantum field. Intention has been proven in many clinical studies. Lynn McTaggart covers all of these experiments in her book, "The Intention Experiment."

When intention is coupled with sound, it can have a profound effect on the Physical body. Additionally, when the energy of Love, Spirit or Source is incorporated into the sound, dramatic changes can happen to parts of the body or to the systems in the body as a whole. (Go to www.SoundHealingCenter.com/miracles.html to see many miracle stories).

Mentally
When it comes to brainwave entrainment, the science is also extremely definitive and proven in many clinical studies.

There has been extensive clinical research clearly proving that when we listen to frequencies within the range of a brainwave (beta, alpha, theta and delta) our brain will be entrained into that frequency within a few minutes. By hooking up an EEG unit to the brain you can actually see the brainwaves being entrained by sound.

"Binaural beats" are frequencies below the normal hearing range that entrain the brain into these various brainwave states. These states commonly help with a variety of issues including ADD, ADHD, posttraumatic stress, learning disabilities, and sleep disorders, as well as enhancing mental clarity, memory, and creativity. When we listen on headphones these frequencies also synchronize the left and right brain, which is our optimal state.

There is now research showing how to use these binaural beat frequencies to lead us into states of deep meditation, and higher emotions of love and joy. When our thoughts flow as smoothly as a beautiful song, we have less stress in our life, and better overall health.

Emotionally
Although there has been a huge amount of research on how music affects us emotionally, the exact science is still not completely understood – though quantum physics is getting closer to explaining the emotional world. So many people have now been working with sound to release and transform emotions that many extremely powerful techniques have emerged. People commonly report emotional relief that has led to complete transformation in their lives.

In the world of emotions the key is to get them flowing – just as music flows. Many in the field of healing believe that stuck emotions account for as much as 50% of the issues and diseases we manifest (our environment being another part). We already know how powerful music can be to transform our emotions. The emotions inside us are actually very similar to sound and music. As babies and children, we naturally made the sound of our emotions to release them. But we soon learned that this was not the mature way to deal with our emotions. The good news is that learning to express and release emotions with sound comes naturally to us, as we remember how we once did it so easily.
We will be sharing eight simple techniques on how to release emotions when in the thick of upsetting circumstances. Many can be done in the car and/or in a professional sound therapy setting.

Aside from our emotions, the other thing that prevents us from manifesting great relationships, health, and wealth in our lives is the frequency of our subconscious beliefs. The most common culprit is simply, "I am not good enough." Based on laws of resonance (which are the basis of the Law of Attraction) these deep resonant patterns keep attracting what we don't want or need. We will be covering a profound set of techniques for using sound and intention to completely transform these errant sounds and songs into those that aid in our happiness and expansion.

Spiritually

"The wonders of the music of the future will be of a higher & wider scale
and will introduce many sounds that the human ear is now incapable of hearing.
Among these new sounds will be the glorious music of angelic chorales. As men hear
these they will cease to consider Angels as figments of their imagination."
- Mozart (1756-1791)

Sound and music have been used since the beginning of time in all cultures to help bring us into a state of Spiritual healing, harmony and awakening. Science has done little to help us with understanding and resonating higher Spiritual realms. However, again, the study of quantum physics is on the leading edge of making sense of it all. But once again, in this realm understanding is not nearly as important as experiencing the unimaginable benefits.

Most people think of Spiritual healing as a process whereby we clear out negative emotions and belief systems, so that we can more clearly resonate love and light. Some people focus on techniques to gain more mental clarity, so that it doesn't lead us into roller coasters fraught with anxiety and dead end traps full of repetitive thoughts. We have already discussed how sound can help with both of these types of issues.

Sound can also be used to entrain us into harmony and a direct connection to our Soul, and to Spirit and Source.

Connecting to the Frequency of Your Soul

"A wise man seeks by music to strengthen his Soul:
the thoughtless one uses it to stifle his fears."
- Confucius (551-479 BC)

Many Spiritual teachings talk about returning to your Soul. Science has shown us that because everything is vibration, so even our Soul must be a frequency. Therefore, the key to connecting to your Soul, and all the information that comes with it, is to simply resonate its frequency – particularly the profound consistency and stillness of this Soul frequency.

Alice Bailey says that our Soul frequency is the same from lifetime to lifetime. This makes sense because something must carry our essence into each new life.

It stands to reason that our entire body at every level has a fundamental or root frequency. Every song has a home key. Every sound has a fundamental, and everything in the Universe has an overall resonant frequency. Because each of us is a symphony of frequencies, we must have a key or home note – a frequency that our entire system is based on. In fact, hospital research has shown that when the human body resonates its root frequency, all organs and systems in the body naturally go into a healthy alignment.

We will be explaining how to find this home note for you. We will then explain how you can use that frequency of your Soul to come home…to yourself…where you are at complete peace and connected to Source at the same time.

Connecting to Spirit and Source

Sound and music can also be used as an avenue to connect us to the higher energies of what many call Spirit, Source, or God. For those who already know how to connect to Spirit, the right sounds and music can enhance that connection and make it even stronger.

Certain frequencies can achieve this, but specific sounds (timbres) or passages in a song are often more effective. You can also do this energetically with intention. Connecting to Source, whole worlds of unfathomable healing power, and levels of consciousness that we have never imagined, open before us.

The brainwave state of theta has been used to access this state. We will explain how you can use this frequency and other brainwave states to also access Universal consciousness. There also seems to be a direct relationship between consistent sounds (pure vowel sounds) and the consistent energy of Spirit.

I always think of the frequency of God or Source as being all frequencies in the Universe. In fact, when people explain the experience of being one with Source and everything in the Universe, they say that it is not just one frequency in particular. Instead, it is as if they become all the frequencies in the Universe simultaneously.

Tuning into multiple sounds at once can bring you into the state of Oneness, particularly tuning into all of the frequencies of the Universe at once. In fact, each and every one of us contain within us all of the frequencies of the Universe. This is where we are all one. Some call this sound "The Cosmic OM." To merge with the cosmic OM is a profound experience. You normally return with a clear perspective that the illusion of separation we all live in is just silly.

We will share multiple techniques for doing this so that you can experience the ultimate state of bliss and healing – and know how to access it whenever you want.

Another Framework for Working with Sound – Physical Body, Chakras, Auras, Soul and Higher Self
Instead of looking at sound Physically, Mentally, Emotionally and Spiritually, some in the field look at it from a perspective that builds from cells to Soul.

Some sound healers focus on the physical body, looking at each part of the body. Some look at the flow one part of the body to another. Some focus on systems in the body such as circulatory system, respiratory system, skeletal system, muscular system, digestive system or endocrine system. Some get extremely detailed, down to the cellular level, and examine the healthy metabolism of cells. Some focus on the brainwaves on how they affect the rest of the system. Some actually focus on how different systems in the body are in or out of harmony with other systems in the body! At the Sound Healing Institute we found that, of the physical parts of the body, the endocrine glands and digestion are the most receptive to sound.

On the other hand, many believe that sound is the most effective on the energy bodies, which in turn affect the physical body and all of its parts.

Many sound healers focus on Chakras. The general consensus is that the energy of the Chakras affects particular endocrine glands in the body, which then branch out and affect all of the organs and their components, down to the cellular level. Many have developed their whole practice around using sound on Chakras. From personal experience I know this technique to be extremely effective. In the past I used to have panic attacks, and I found that I was able to completely stop the panic attack with a sound Chakra treatment. This was so major – particularly to be able to get rid of the fear of losing control (and possibly dying), and to not only stop it, but to be able to **go to** a complete state of bliss.

Others believe that you should only focus on the auras or subtle bodies that surround the body. They say that sound is particularly effective on the auras.

The general consensus here is that the auric fields affect the chakras, which in turn affect the endocrine glands and the rest of the body. Barbara Brennan says that all disease actually begins in the auras as energetic distortions. Some say that diseases actually occur in an aura for years before it manifests as a disease in the body. Many psychics who see auras report almost immediate changes with the use of sound, music and intention. Sound seems to be the ideal tool for harmonizing these distortions back into complete harmony.

As mentioned, many in the field believe that it is best to focus on the core Soul or signature frequency since this then resonates the rest of the system into harmony. There has been some good research in hospitals to back up this theory.

It seems that the ideal is to approach the system from a holistic perspective. We are dealing with an entire hologram that is the body, mind and Soul. When we focus on any one area we could be missing some important connections. In fact, I have always felt that it is best to work on as many areas as possible. As they say (transformed a bit),

**"The more ways you lead a horse to water,
the more chances that it will actually drink."**

Ultimately, when we can look at the forest and the trees simultaneously, we begin to see the human system as it really is – a complex system of energy flowing from one frequency to another throughout our entire system – creating, in essence, our Soul song.

Chapter 2 – One Resonant Frequency vs. A Full Range of Frequencies

*"The highest goal of music is to connect one's Soul to their Divine Nature,
not entertainment"*
- Pythagoras (569- 475 BC)

There are two basic schools of thought in the field of Sound Healing. The first is each person has a unique resonant frequency that is the core of who we are. When we resonate our Soul frequency (so to speak), we become more centered and grounded.

We have had huge success healing many symptoms at our Sound Healing Therapy Center with this technique. A dozen researchers in the field also subscribe to this concept in one form or another. A study, conducted by Dr. Jeffrey Thompson, who has done research at Scripps Hospital in San Diego, showed that when one finds and listens to their "central processing" frequency, the sympathetic and parasympathetic systems come into balance, and the rest of the systems come into a healthy alignment. The problem is that in the noisy and chaotic world we live in, it is easy to lose track of this still frequency within us.

The second school of thought is that we need a balance of all frequencies. This is the basis of the research done by Dr. Alfred Tomatis and for the dozen or so voice analysis companies that identify missing frequencies in the body's systems. The remedy is normally to then resonate these missing frequencies back into your system by either toning (singing) the note or by listening to a bowl, tuning fork or song in the key of the missing note. Research has shown that when a person is missing a certain pitch or note in their voice, they are actually missing essential nutrients that can affect organs in the body and create learning disabilities. Some research also points to missing frequencies as the cause of autism.

It's interesting that the people who hang out in various schools of thought don't normally get along. In fact, I've seen them argue quite adamantly for their perspectives. Sharry Edwards and I seem to be some of the few that feel we should all be able to get along.

It seems that the concept of replacing frequencies that are missing is more helpful for what is going on at a particular moment or time in your life. It is more about focusing on what is wrong, with the positive intention of balancing out all of the frequencies.

On the other hand, the concept of a central core frequency is more concerned with a general frequency that harmonizes your whole system. This is also the frequency that leads you into higher states of consciousness and ultimately to your own Soul purpose. It is about focusing on what is right and resonating that.

I strongly believe that both approaches are completely valid and useful and we'll be exploring both concepts in practices throughout the book.

Chapter 3 – Our Need to Come Home to the Home Note

We have a built-in need to return to the home note – whether it is in music, a sound or our Soul.

I have come to believe really strongly that home is a basic need when it comes to our whole being _and_ all of its parts. In music theory, the definition of the home note is the note where we are "at rest." It is the resolution; it is the note where we don't need to go anywhere else; it is where we are at peace.

Although you can mathematically figure out the home note in music, everyone knows when we are there – everyone can feel it. In music, the home note is the key of the song. Jazz musicians will often try and avoid the home note. In Sound Healing music, we go to the home note often. When you play an instrument that is only one note, like a crystal bowl, it automatically becomes the home note.

Most sounds have multiple frequencies in them called harmonics (which we'll discuss later). However, even though a single sound is made up of multiple notes, our brain focuses only on the home note. In sound, it is called the root or fundamental tone within the overall conglomeration of harmonics present in the sound. Even if the fundamental is missing in a sound (like with an oboe), our brain will actually make it up! So, again, we are very focused on the home note.

In Sound Healing, the home note is an important key to bringing us into a state of peace. In fact, it is the key to much of the physical, mental, emotional, and Spiritual healing process.

Physically, every single cell, organ and part of the body has a home note. In physics it is called the resonant frequency of the object. Research has shown that every cell in our body has its own home note; even our heart and every organ in the body have its own home note. When we are in tune with our own home note we feel more grounded.

When we go to the home note in our voice people believe we are sincere. And, when we are truly feeling and expressing love, most of us will go the home note of the key of our voice.

Emotionally, we are always trying to come back to the home note in our thoughts and emotions. In fact, the definition of a stuck emotion is a frequency that has never resolved to the home note.

Mentally, when the home note is apparent in our thoughts, they are much clearer. Our thoughts resolve to a place of peace instead of anxiety and stress.

Spiritually, when we are in touch with the ultimate home note – our Soul – we are at complete peace no matter what happens. When we are resonating with the home note of higher emotions like Unconditional Love, we feel tremendous amounts of peace and equanimity.

Stillness does not ensue from any of the other notes, like it does when we come home to our Soul frequency.

Chapter 4 – Consistency as Higher Consciousness
People often talk about "raising your vibration," in order to become more Spiritually oriented. However, the phrase is actually a little confusing. Otherwise, someday we might all be talking like the chipmunks.

If we are actually going to a higher frequency, what part of our system is going there?

When you look at higher consciousness from the reality of how frequencies actually work, we are not necessarily going higher, but rather becoming more consistent. Higher consciousness is more about having 100% clarity of focus and presence at all times. This means we are less affected by outside energies and are much better at focusing our attention.

It is a frequency that doesn't waver – just like the frequency of Love, Soul, Spirit and Source never waver – ever. They are all as pure and consistent as any vibration on earth and in the Universe. So when we resonate with them – we find the profound peace of this consistency and purity.

A higher vibration is simply a more consistent vibration,
one with fewer distortions and distractions.

This consistency manifests in slightly different ways Physically, Mentally, Emotionally, and Spiritually.

Physically, it is about having each part of the body resonating at its optimal frequency. From cells to organs, every part should resonate at its own natural frequency in order to contribute perfect harmony **to** all the instruments in the symphony that we are. In fact, the more in alignment with nature and Spirit we get, the more our cells and organs resonate at their natural healthy frequencies – no higher or lower.

Mentally, it has been discovered that when in high states of consciousness or deep states of meditation, our brainwaves are both really high and really low at the same time. We actually exhibit extremely slow brainwaves of sub-delta (less than .5 cycles per second), and extremely fast brainwaves of gamma (more than 30 cycles per second) simultaneously. Therefore, mentally higher consciousness is not just higher – it is higher and lower brainwave rates at the same time.

In the emotional world, consistency is just as important. The higher emotions of gratitude, compassion, love and joy are not technically "higher" in frequency than the lower emotions of anger, fear and anxiety. Whenever, I ask a person or group to express the sound of the higher emotions they always make vowel sounds. In fact, when asked to express the sound of compassion people often make a powerfully deep low sound. On the other hand, just think of the sound of fear, anxiety or anger. They are something like *"gxgxgx or ickckck or grurrrr"* – sounds that are grating and distorted. In fact, when you look at the actual waveforms created by these sounds, they randomly jump around from one frequency to another. On the other hand, if you ask someone to make the sound of any of the higher emotions such as gratitude, compassion, love and joy they always make a vowel sound (oo, oh, ah, eh, ee). Vowel sounds do not jump around at all. They are totally coherent and consistent tones, staying on the same note, and thus have no random distortion or noise. Therefore, higher emotions are distinguished more by purity and consistency than by higher or lower frequencies.

The best example of consistency from higher emotions is the feeling of being in love. It is the most consistently peaceful feeling imaginable, dwarfed only by the feeling of the consistency and stillness of Universal Divine Love.

Emotionally, we go from feeling and expressing irritating and annoying sounding negative emotions that are distorted and inconsistent, to feeling and expressing beautiful sounding positive emotions that are pure and consistent sounds, which support our health in every way. The higher emotions that include gratitude, compassion, love and joy are actually not higher sound frequencies at all. Therefore, at the emotional level, "Raising Your Vibration," is really about purity and consistency of frequency versus raising the frequency.

Spiritually, there could be something to raising our vibration. I do know people who talk about tuning into extremely high frequencies (above 10,000 hertz) in order to access higher states of consciousness. I still don't quite get how this works, but I remain open to the possibility that there is something in us Spiritually or at a Quantum Level that can be raised.

When I am one with Source (in the zone, so to speak) I feel the most incredibly consistent peace ever. Everyone seems to describe the same consistency when explaining his or her experience of oneness. I believe Source to be the most consistent collection of frequencies in the Universe.

I believe the Soul (which is always connected to Source) is also unwaveringly stable and consistent. The Soul never wobbles. I do believe it goes to higher levels of consciousness, however I don't believe that it rises in vibration. The Soul vibrates at the frequency that it is. The higher levels of consciousness are simply clearing out the distortions and distractions that separate us from a more and more consistent connection to Source.

Look at any spiritual leader – they are normally perfectly still. They are resonating the consistent vibration of Spirit. Their essence is all about consistency.

In a Vibrational World
the definition of Peace
is a
Frequency
Consistently Humming

Silence is not always peaceful. In fact, it is often uncomfortable. It is the consistent hum of a frequency on one's home note that is peaceful.

At all levels of reality, consistency is the key. When we resonate with any consistent sound we find the profound peace in its coherence.

Consistent Instruments

One of the primary keys to the effectiveness of most of the sounds and instruments used in Sound Healing is their consistency. Instruments that are able to naturally play sustained notes for long periods of time seem to resonate this consistency the most. Instruments like bowls, tuning forks, gongs, and didgeridoos naturally sustain. The most powerful instrument of all – the voice – creates sustained notes with vowel sounds. All of these instruments entrain us into consistency at all levels of our being.

However, instruments that naturally play short staccato sounds, including drums, can create consistency with consistent rhythms – rhythms that don't change tempo or density abruptly. Consonants are not considered consistent sounds unless they repeat themselves rhythmically as in many mantras.

Then there is the most powerful sound healer of all – nature. The sounds of nature bring us deep peace in more ways than we know. Nature demonstrates this consistency in the Fibonacci spiral that is found in all life: 1, 1, 2, 3, 5, 8, 13, 21, 34, 55, 89, 144, etc. Every number is a combination of the two previous numbers before it. This is the ultimate example of consistency.

The true essence of Nature and Spirit is consistency.

Ultimately, healing and health are about a consistent flow. The 3D level of normal day-to-day reality is also about resonating with patterns, and the flow of nature and Spirit, versus those of machines and the ego, which exhibit little consistency. Machines are practically defined by the fact that they ultimately break down.

The more we resonate with a consistent flow, and find that natural flow within us, the more we experience spiritual harmony – a state in which diseases and physical issues often fall away entirely, emotional issues sometimes resolve on their own, and mental clarity seems to ensue out of the blue.

Raising Your Consciousness

"Consciousness is somehow a by-product of the simultaneous, high frequency firing of neurons in different parts of the brain. It's the meshing of these frequencies that generates consciousness, just as tones from individual instruments produce the rich, complex, & seamless sounds of a symphony orchestra."
- Francis Crick (1916-2004), Molecular Biologist and Co-Discoverer of DNA and its significance for information transfer in living material.

Ultimately raising your consciousness is the same as raising your vibration. Many in the field define "raising your consciousness" as simply resonating higher emotions such as gratitude, compassion, love and joy. It is also about resonating more with our Soul, Spirit and Source – our true essence.

Alice Bailey talks about "initiations" that we go through on our path to enlightenment. The first main initiation is to actually get off the roller coaster of emotions – to become present in that place where you are still. The second initiation is about getting clear within the mental body – getting clear thoughts that are connected to Spirit. The third initiation is about going into the world of Spirit. There are several other initiations where we go into ever more and more subtle realms of direct connection to Source.

Consistency on the home note is the best of all.
It is the true essence of peace.

Consistency and Flow

Even though nature is consistent, it also breathes. Little in nature occurs in perfect mathematical patterns. Everything is based on perfect mathematical patterns but there is always an ebb and flow – a bit of chaos thrown in to make things breathe.

In fact, an electronic tone generator that is 100% consistent can actually be detrimental to the body's system in certain instances. Pure tones on a sound table have been shown to be irritating. The perfection of a mechanical drum rhythm machine can actually cause us stress.

Everything needs to breathe in and out of this perfection.

Love, Soul and Spirit all have the breath of life moving through them (chaos, that is), so technically they are *not* 100% consistent, but their energy is 100% consistent.

A crystal bowl, although it is playing one note consistently, goes up and down in volume ever so slightly as we play it. It breathes with a slight bit of unpredictable chaos. These natural variations help keep us awake.

Even though we like consistency, we also need sounds and music that breathe naturally.

Chapter 5 – Our Need for Harmony

Each celestial body, in fact each and every atom,
produces a particular sound on account of its movement, its rhythm or vibration.
All these sounds and vibrations form a universal harmony in which each element,
while having its own function and character, contributes to the whole.
- Pythagoras (569-475 BC)

I have an interesting relationship with the concept that all things should be in harmony. I remember reading a book when I was in college that claimed that non-harmonic sounds were the essence of evil. I remember actually taking pleasure in listening to "avant-garde" jazz that was actually a total cacophony of sounds rising and falling in energy.

And since then, I have come to believe that all frequencies in the Universe are part of Source – even to the extreme of those frequencies that make up an atom bomb or a horrible disease such as AIDS.

However, when it comes to living systems, if there is no harmony, there is no health. Our body is made up of about 70 trillion cells that must all work together harmoniously in order to get the job of life done. Since every cell has its own natural resonant frequency that means that every cell must be in musical harmony with every other cell.

At its simplest, harmony is when two or more notes sound good together. Dissonance or disharmony is when two or more notes do not sound good together. Rhythmical harmony is much the same...two or more rhythms that seem to be in time and work together.

You can think of any disease (whether physical or emotional) as disharmony that has entered into the system. It's like a member of the symphony of frequencies that make up the body is just playing out of time or out of pitch.

In fact, there is good science that shows that dissonance does break down our system more than harmony (also called consonance). Discordant sounds wear us out and can make us physically ill. There are technologies to help deal with noise in factories for this very reason.

Therefore, we can easily say that harmony is the essence of health in our system.

However, I would not describe dissonance and disharmony as evil. In fact, dissonant sounds can be just the thing you might need to break up stuck energy in a muscle or a deep-rooted emotional issue. Activating dissonance might be exactly what someone with depression needs to get energy moving again. Dissonance also teaches us to be more aware and tuned into our own frequency so we're not at the mercy of the outside world. We create our own happiness.

However, it seems clear that the normal healthy state of any living system (including that of the earth) is when everything is working together in harmony. We see such harmony from the atom to our solar system and beyond.

SECTION II – The Hierarchy of Sound, Music and Energy

"If you want to find the secrets of the Universe,
think in terms of energy, frequency and vibration."
- Nikolai Tesla

Introduction – Five Levels of Vibration

There are five primary levels of energy in the Universe when looking at it all from a frequency or vibration level – Frequencies, Tones or Timbres (combinations of frequencies), Musical Intervals and Chords (combinations of Tones or Timbres), Music (combinations of Tones, Timbres, Musical Intervals and Chords over time), and Energy. We'll first give a quick overview of each level, and then go into detail in the following chapters. As we go down the list each aspect becomes more and more powerful.

1. Pure Frequencies
Pure frequencies are individual tones. Pure frequencies manifest in tone generators, tuning forks, crystal bowls, and also as concert pitch and tuning systems. The typical frequency range is from 20 to 20,000 cycles per second. You can think of pure frequencies as atoms.

There are also some sounds that are not technically "frequencies." This is a whole set of sounds that are actually incomplete sounds. In physics, these sounds are called "noise." Noise includes white and pink noise, the ocean, rivers and streams, waterfalls, the wind, whispers, shakers, rattles and the breath. These "non-frequencies" are extremely powerful for breaking up stuck frequencies such as emotions or post-traumatic stress.

2. Tones or Timbres
A timbre or tone is a combination of pure frequencies. Different sounds have different combinations of frequencies, or harmonics, that makeup the sound. The particular array of harmonics account for all of the different instrument sounds, including vocal and nature sounds. Because tones and timbres are combinations of frequencies they are more powerful.

3. Musical Intervals and Chords
Combinations of frequencies and timbres create musical intervals, which create different states of consciousness. Multiple sounds (frequencies or timbres) create a chord, which creates even more complex states of consciousness. Musical intervals and chords are even more powerful than timbres because they are combinations of timbres.

4. Music
Music is pure frequencies and timbres changing over time. When we add time, we get rhythms, which have specific effects on the heart and brainwaves in particular. Most importantly, changing frequencies and timbres create a "musical flow." The musical flow is the most important aspect of music, and is especially effective when it matches

(or becomes) the same "flow" that is found in nature and Spirit. Music is even more powerful than intervals and chords because they do not move or change over time, and thus are not creating a flow.

5. Energy

One person can sing a song and it's cool. Another person can sing the same song and you are brought to tears, or you see God, and your whole life is transformed.

Energy is the most powerful of the whole hierarchy. It is that indescribable, invisible flow of energy that can only be described by quantum physics. Many people do energy healing without sound and commonly perform miracles. When energy is added to sound, it is extremely effective. Adding an "intention" or a prayer to a sound normally does this. However, the quality of a person's consciousness will drastically affect the energy that comes through their music. Just as with music, the quality of the flow of the energy is the most important aspect.

Here is a diagram showing the relationship of all five levels:

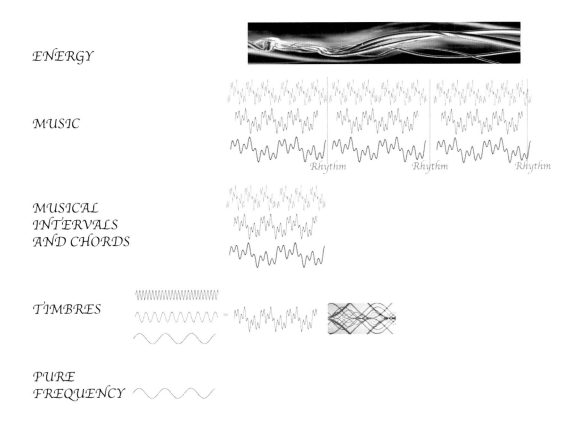

Notice that a timbre is simply a combination of multiple frequencies that make up a waveform. A musical interval is a combination of waveforms. And, music is changing frequencies, timbres, musical intervals and chords – which, then gives us rhythms that affect us on another level. Energy is like a higher octave, which contains each of the

27

other 4 levels of frequency.

It is important to focus on these five different areas of the hierarchy because each level will affect us differently physically, mentally, emotionally, and Spiritually. But more importantly…

**When each of the 5 aspects are "tuned" to the flow of nature and Source,
and all aspects are working in alignment together,
the effect can be powerful beyond belief.**

This is really the essence of the whole book.

Now, let's go into more detail on each of the five levels.

Chapter 6 – Pure Frequencies and Pitches

Frequency is the number of soundwaves that go by us (or into us) per second. Imagine standing in the ocean watching the waves go by. If one wave were to go by you every second, that would be described as 1 cycle per second or 1 hertz. In the ocean the waves do not normally change frequency (although they do come in sets). The lowest sound we can hear is 20 hertz. When listening to 20 hertz, 20 waves go by us every second. When listening to 20,000 hertz, 20,000 physical sound waves go by us every second. This means that a speaker is actually going in and out 20,000 times per second!!! It also means that your ear drum is going back and forth 20,000 times per second – and, every water molecule in your body is vibrating at 20,000 times per second.

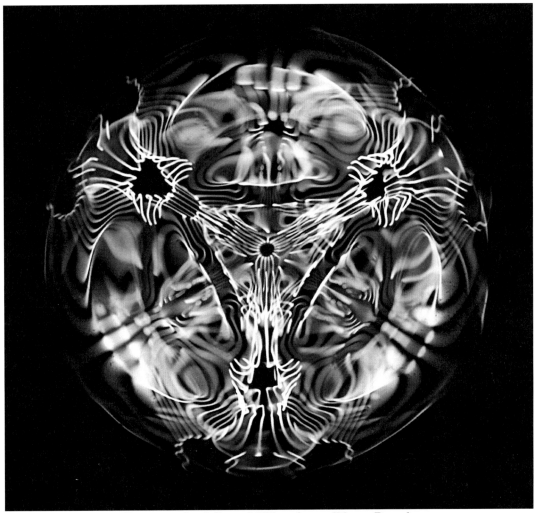

Photograph of Sound Vibrating a Water Droplet
(Thanks to Erik Larson for the image – www.Cymascope.com)

Who needs coffee?

In both the ocean and in airwaves the speed of the waves is quite consistent. Therefore, the way we get different frequencies is not by sound traveling faster through the air, but by the size of the wave – or the wavelength. If there are long waves you get fewer waves going by you every second. With short waves (the speed being the same) we have more waves per second going by us, simply because they are smaller – not faster.

The only difference between frequency and pitch is that frequencies are labeled with numbers, and pitches are labeled with letters. Pitches also repeat themselves, so you can have the same pitch at different octaves. Frequencies are more specific than pitches. A particular pitch can be many different frequencies. For example, the note A could be any frequency from 425 hertz all the way up to 455 hertz.

Appendix B online shows the relationship between frequencies and pitch.

Pure Frequencies

"All things are aggregations of atoms that dance & by their movement produce sound.
When the rhythm of the dance changes, the sound it produces also changes...
Each atom perpetually sings its song,
and the sound at every moment creates dense subtle forms."
- Alexandra David-Neel (1868-1969)

Many people these days are now focused on pure frequencies. Pure frequencies manifest in the world through Tuning Forks, Tone Generators, Flutes (not completely pure), Crystal Bowls (also not completely pure), Concert Pitch and Tuning Systems. You can also think of cells, atoms, and the elements as pure frequencies.

There are many pure frequencies that have been shown to create very specific effects on us physically, mentally, emotionally and Spiritually. For example, 45 hertz has been proven to regenerate bones. Many people use 136.102 hertz as the "OM" frequency in gongs and tuning forks because it is a frequency based on the spinning of the Earth.

Many people are now using the frequencies called the Solfeggio frequencies that were discovered by Joseph Paleo around 2000 (A.D. that is). They also have some unique numerological synchronicities – each of the frequencies add up to 3, 6, or 9 numerologically. For example, the numbers in 528 hertz add up to 15, and 1 plus 5 = 6. Many people don't believe in the importance of numerology, although others swear by it. Even if these frequencies were meaningless, many people are using them and it has therefore created a resonant field of positive energy that others can tap into.

Our brain vibrates at specific frequencies. Whenever we play frequencies that match one of the brainwave states of delta, theta, alpha and gamma, our brain is entrained into the corresponding brainwave state – normally within one minute. (We cover the full range of brainwave states in Section IX, "Mental Expansion with Sound".) There are also some general frequencies that seem to correspond to higher emotional states such as gratitude, compassion, love, and joy. Then there are frequencies that can open our hearts (covered in Chapter 45, The Sound of Love) or lead us into a direct connection with our Soul, Spirit, and Source (Chapter 47, Connecting to Spirit and Source with Sound). Later we provide techniques for finding the particular frequency of your Soul. I think of Source itself as all frequencies in the Universe.

Here is a chart of some very powerful archetypal frequencies.

You can listen to some of these frequencies at
www.SoundHealingCenter.com/frequency.html

200,000-500,000 Dolphins highest range

18,500	Highest frequency heard by average woman
17,500	Highest frequency heard by average man
15,700	High frequency that old televisions scream at
5k-8K	Treble control on a stereo
4096	Highest note on a piano
4096	Quartz crystal (786,432 hertz octavized down)
4000	The most irritating frequency (chainsaw frequency)
3000	Frequency that telephones are centered around (voice consonants)
852	Solfeggio Frequency LA – Returning to Spiritual Order
741	Solfeggio Frequency SOL – Awakening Intuition
639	Solfeggio Frequency FA – Connecting/Relationships
528	Solfeggio Frequency MI – Transformation and Miracles (DNA Repair) and Frequency of the Heart (Leonard Horowitz)
452.459	Venus (based on it's rotation around the Sun)
432	Frequency of average baby just out of the womb; Relates to the diameter of the Sun
417	Solfeggio Frequency RE – Undoing Situations and Facilitating Change
396	Solfeggio Frequency UT – Liberating Guilt and Fear
297	A frequency found in the Crop Circles
292	Nogier cell rejuvenation
268.8	Ali Akbar Khan's favorite
266	Good for Nervous System
256	Physical and Scientific mean - Philosopher's middle C
250	Main resonant frequency of the King's Chamber in Great Pyramid
250	Average Voice (Common to everyone)
144.72	Rotation of Mars around the Sun
144	Represents the code within the golden spiral of all the atoms
136.102	The OM frequency used in many tuning forks. Based on revolution of the Earth around Sun
117.1875	The Sarcophagus in the Kings Chamber
111	Good frequency for Cell Rejuvenation - Bob Beck – Brain tuner Mood Pacer
85	Beethoven's Fire frequency
73	Paul Nogier core healing frequency. Multiply by 2 to get the full array of frequencies.
64	C - Base of spine
50	Main harmonic of a kitty purr; Hummingbirds flap their wings 50 times per second.
45	Resonant frequency of bones
40	Thunder's key fundamental frequency
40	Key Gamma Brainwave frequency
40-60	Bass control on a stereo
32	Lowest C note on a piano (good for the nervous system)
25	Frequency at which cats purr
25	Stimulates mitochondria
25	Lowest frequency that most people can hear

16	Main low frequency put out by Whales (extremely on-pitch, in-tune)
12	Seemingly negative frequency from moon during full moon
12-20	Beta Brainwaves
11	Energy between pillars
10.666	Average ultrawave healing frequency (when healers are in the zone, they've measured it as brainwaves). Diameter of hydrogen molecule.
10.53	Brainwave frequency used in Silva Mind Control to get you in the zone.
8	Lowest frequency put out by Whales
7-12	Alpha Brainwaves
7.83	Schumann Resonance of the earth's atmosphere between the earth and the ionosphere
7.8125	Spherics controlling the weather
4-7	Theta Brainwaves
3-4	Lowest frequency put out by Elephants
1.45	A frequency that many sacred sites emit
1.2	Average Heart Rate
1.042	Very Healing Heart Rate
.5-4	Delta Brainwaves
<.5	Sub-Delta Brainwaves (deep meditation)
.1	Brainwaves when transmitting love (Heartmath)

Get the interactive version for detailed lists of healing frequencies (Appendix F).

Concert Pitch

Frequency also affects us as "concert pitch." Concert pitch is the "frequency" that the overall orchestra or band tunes to. Even though the orchestra plays the full range of frequencies this one "concert pitch" is the core frequency that every sound is based on.

This frequency has varied over the years, and has always varied from country to country. However, in the 30's it was set to A = 440 hertz. It is clear that different concert pitch frequencies affect us in different ways. Many people agree (with a bit scientific evidence to back it up) that frequencies such as 432 hertz and 444 hertz more effectively align with the body both physically and emotionally (and perhaps Spiritually). If you do a search on YouTube you will find over a hundred such videos where people are tuning to A432, and C528 (same as A444 hertz). Check them out and see if you can notice a difference.

As you can imagine, when these frequencies (432, etc.) are played by themselves – as with tone generators or tuning forks – they are more effective than when part of a whole song as concert pitch. However, listening to pure frequencies by themselves can be quite annoying to many people.

Tuning Systems

A Tuning System is the particular frequency of each of the 12 notes within an octave.

C	65.4060
B	61.3181
A#	57.2303
A	55.1863
G#	53.1424
G	49.0545
F#	47.0106
F	42.9227
E	40.8788
D#	38.8348
D	36.7909
C#	34.7469
C	32.7030

12 notes in an Octave with their frequencies

Tuning systems are actually quite a bit more important than concert pitch, because we're now talking about the frequency of 12 notes versus one note. Ancient tuning systems such as Just Intonation and Pythagorean tuning systems are based on the natural harmonics found throughout nature. However, all of the songs on the radio and most CDs are tuned to Equal Tempered Tuning, which has no relationship to anything in the natural world.

Because the actual frequencies are based on harmonics we will discuss tuning systems in more detail in the next chapter on Harmonics.

Pitches
A pitch is simply a frequency expressed in letters, however pitches repeat themselves as octaves. Technically, if you double or halve a frequency you will get the same pitch an octave above or below, respectively. Each of our 12 notes C, C#, D, D#, E, F, F#, G, G#, A, A# and B each has a certain "energy" to it, regardless of its octave.

For example, we can scientifically find the frequency of flower essences and essential oils, although they are in the millions of hertz. If we cut their frequencies in half many, many times, we finally get down to a frequency range that we can hear. Then we can tell what note it is. And, because we simply cut the frequency in half over and over, it is still the same note. As above, so below. If it's a B above, the B below will affect us in a similar way – there is a difference in hearing a pitch at a higher octave, but the energy of that pitch is the same in all octaves.

Everything in the Universe is vibrating at a particular frequency. Most things are made of multiple frequencies. For example, a molecule is made of a combination of atom frequencies. However, (and this is a really important concept) things with multiple frequencies always have a **home note,** in the same way that every song has a home key. The definition of a home note is the note where you are at rest. It is the note that takes you to a state of equilibrium and peace. For example, an organ has multiple types of cells and materials that make it up, and therefore multiple frequencies. But it also has one overall frequency, which is its home note.

Because it follows that since we are a symphony of frequencies, we must have a key, or home note. I have come to strongly believe that this is the most important frequency in our whole system. It is the frequency or pitch that we are tuned to. When we play this note, it can entrain us into that state of peace, where you are at rest.

Our home note is one of the most powerful frequencies or pitches within us. Some say this is the frequency or pitch of your Soul.

Even the earth, as complex as it is, has an overall frequency, although it is more noticeable when we look at our planet from outer space.

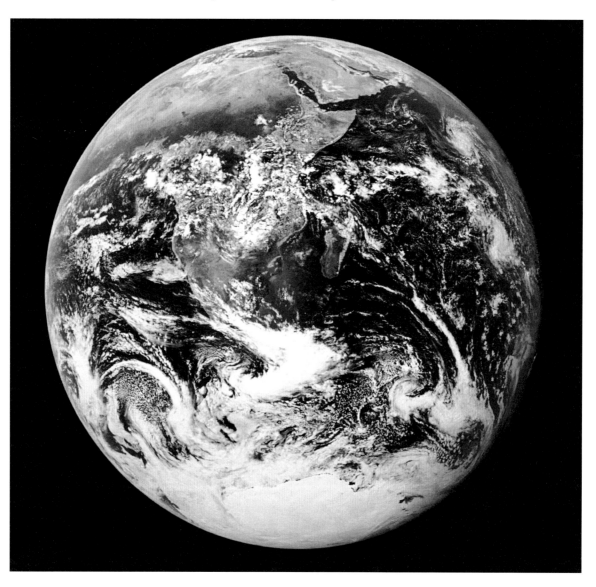

It is actually quite easy to be aware of the overall frequency of something. We already do it all of the time. We notice the "vibe" of a person. We commonly choose our mate based on their vibration. We even consider whether a particular food resonates with us when we look at a menu. We resonate with a plant, tree or flower. And, we choose the particular music we want to listen to based on its overall vibe.

As you see everything as vibration,
as it really is,
everything comes into focus.

Things become even clearer as we recognize both the overall frequency of something, and its complete frequency makeup (the forest and the trees). The more we tune into the complexity of the frequency makeup of something (or a person), the clearer we see its overall frequency. A perfect example is how you see someone when you first meet them, compared to the complexity that you become aware of after you have known them for years.

Finding and Using Pure Frequencies and Pitches
There are many, many charts of frequencies for the body, for diseases, psychological issues, and even higher emotions of compassion, love and joy. The problem is that no two people ever seem to come up with and agree on the same frequency for anything! And, worse, the charts have no reference as to how the frequency was discovered. If it is clinical research, we should know what type, how the research was performed, and on how many people. If not, we should know how else it was found. Did a psychic discover it, or did someone download it from the Universe, or what?

This isn't to say that many of these frequencies are ineffective. The lists are often a good place to start. Many people have gotten good results (sometimes miraculous results) from using the frequencies on these lists.

However, until there is more definitive research I prefer to find frequencies intuitively. At the Institute we have developed a range of techniques for doing just this – and the more you practice, the better you get. Sometimes, you can actually feel the vibration when you find a frequency; sometimes you have to trust your intuition. We'll be going into detail about these techniques later. There is also a wide range of technologies that can us help find frequencies.

When you find the frequency of something and vibrate it, the frequency feeds that thing energy and also provides a kind of massage. If you turn up the volume far enough, you can explode it – just like ultrasound breaks up kidney stones. This normally only happens on something as fragile as cells. Small things, like cells, are much more susceptible to frequency than large things (like organs, the body, or a planet) simply because they are so small relative to the size of soundwaves. The volume would have to be way louder than what we can make with the voice or an instrument to explode anything else. Although, some people say that loud music at a concert can actually drive your Spirit out of your body.

Therefore, you can use sound to break up or harmonize any part of the body.

Throughout the book, we discuss how to find and use frequencies. In Appendix A online, I provide a complete list of every way to find a frequency and what to do with it once you have found it.

Coherence - Consistency of Frequency
Once again,

**Peace is a frequency
consistently humming.**

A frequency that is jumping around creates instability. One that simply stays the same without variation instills stability in us. Vowel sounds, crystal bowls, Tibetan bowls, tuning forks and many other instruments create this consistency in us physically, mentally, emotionally and Spiritually.

Therefore, getting the perfect frequency for something is not nearly as important as consistent coherence! Even if the frequency is not exact, you will still get an extremely positive response from the consistency of the sound.

When you add a positive frequency of intention to a consistent frequency, the power can boggle the mind (and science).

If the frequency happens to be just the right positive frequency needed, then the effect is doubly effective.

So, don't worry so much if you happen to get the frequency wrong. It is really rare for a frequency on its own to create a negative effect. Let me repeat:

It is really rare for a pure frequency on its own to create a negative effect.

Frequency Tools
We will be going into detail on the most common Sound Healing instruments and tools in Section 5, "Your Sound Healing Toolbox;" however, I wanted to touch on each of the particular tools that use mostly pure frequencies.

Tuning Forks
Tuning Forks make almost pure frequencies. If they do have other frequencies in them, they are normally so low in volume that they are hardly noticeable. People use tuning forks with very specific frequencies for many issues. Many tuning fork systems (including Acutonics) use frequencies based on the rotation time of planets around the sun, or the time it takes to for a planet to complete its spin (the planetary day). However, you can use just about any of the frequencies on the lists as long as it is more than 40

hertz or less than 2,000 hertz (the frequency limits of tuning forks).

One of our instructors, Randy Masters, has complete systems of tuning forks that are tuned to very auspicious frequencies. You can review them at www.UniversalSong.net.

Tone Generators
Tone generators are electronic devices that create one frequency. Here's some links to get one:

Free online version (site that is selling Sound Healing Tinnitus treatment):
http://www.audionotch.com/app/tune/

Free software for Mac or PC (two week demo, then about $35)
http://www.nch.com.au/tonegen/index.html

Tone generators can be played right on specific parts of the body with headphones or small computer speakers. You can also use them to find a frequency, and then use your voice or an instrument to play it.

Tone generators are especially effective for creating Binaural Beats to entrain the brain into different brainwave states (see Section IX).

Pure Instrument Frequencies
Certain instruments tend to be more pure frequencies like Crystal Bowls, Flutes, and even Whistles. Tibetan bowls are not normally very pure frequencies.

When you buy a Crystal Bowl (Singing Bowl) they are commonly tuned to a specific pitch. You actually have to pay quite a bit more to get them tuned to specific frequencies. However, you can change the frequency of a bowl by putting water in it. The more water you put in, the lower the frequency becomes.

Flutes and Peruvian whistles are also very pure and can be used to focus on specific cells, organs or parts of the body.

The voice is normally not that pure although some female singers do have particularly pure voices in the high ranges (like Mariah Carey and Celine Dion). Whistles are very pure. However, when someone does overtone singing they can create extremely pure tones (more on this later).

Pure Nature Frequencies
Pure frequencies don't happen very often in nature, except in cells. Birds often do sing using very pure frequencies. Other animals and some insects also create pure notes, and the wind sometimes whistles through the trees. Even the plop of a drop of water going over a rock creates pure frequencies.
There are some very important pure frequencies that are created by the earth itself.

The frequency of 136.102 hertz is the most common frequency associated with the earth. It is often called the "Om" frequency and is a mathematical calculation based on the rotation of the earth around the sun.

The frequency of 194.18074 is based on the spinning of the earth.

The Schumann Resonance is an electromagnetic resonance in our atmosphere triggered by lightning that is vibrating at an average of 7.83 cycles per second, entraining every brain on the planet into a brainwave state around alpha and theta. It is so important for our health that astronauts are fed this vibration while in outer space. This frequency connects us to nature; however, it is obscured by electromagnetism in a city. Resonating with the Schumann Resonance or tuning music to it can return one to harmony with nature.

Although pure frequencies can be extremely powerful, in the overall hierarchy of sound, music, and energy, they are actually the least powerful. As you will see, Timbres are quite a bit more powerful.

Chapter 7 – Timbres (Tones or Harmonic Structures)

"I believe that from the earth emerges a musical poetry that is,
by the nature of its sources, tonal. I believe that these sources cause to exist
a phonology of music, which evolves from the universal,
and is known as the harmonic series."
- Leonard Bernstein (1918-1990)

Most sounds are not simply pure frequencies. Most sounds are made up of a combination of frequencies called harmonics, or overtones. It is the particular combination of harmonics that accounts for the differences in sound quality, or the timbre of the sound. Timbre is often referred to as tone, tonality, or harmonic structure of a sound. Every instrument's sound (including our voices and the sounds in nature) is simply a different combination of frequencies.

As mentioned, you can think of the elements and atoms as frequencies, and a molecule as a Timbre (a combination of frequencies). Flower essences and even food can actually be thought of as Timbres. Certain traditions from Tibet also speak of organs in the body as having very specific Timbres. In fact, the 70 trillion cell frequencies that makeup our whole body, also makeup the very specific Timbre that we are!

A particular timbre within an instrument or a voice is quite a bit more powerful and effective than single frequencies (although frequencies do matter). The primary reason that timbres are more effective is because they are not only a combination of frequencies (called harmonics); they also now include the effect of musical intervals – the relationship of one frequency to another within the sound itself. Different musical intervals create different states of consciousness (covered in the next chapter). Finally, the mathematical structure of the harmonics is the same as the mathematical structure of the Universe – that is, the distance between the planets, the weight of each vertebra, and the distance of electron shells around the nucleus of an atom (and some say the frequency of each aura). All of these have the exact same mathematical structure as the harmonics that make up almost all sounds – therefore, this combination of frequencies, which we call timbre, actually taps us into a higher level of consciousness and harmony found throughout nature.

The Beautiful Mathematical Structure of Sound

Most people believe that a single sound is comprised of only one frequency or pitch. In fact, when someone sings one note, to keep things simple, our brain focuses primarily on the fundamental or root frequency and practically ignores the rest of the harmonics. Even though we don't focus on the higher harmonic frequencies we do hear them. Harmonics or overtones account for the different tonalities in sounds. They are what make a clarinet sound different from a piano, bagpipes from a harp, or my voice from your voice. It is also what makes one guitar sound different from another of the same model guitar. Subtle differences in the construction create subtle differences in the harmonics that the guitar puts out.

Some harmonic structures are activating; others are calming. This is critical to be aware of when choosing a sound for a particular issue. It is also important to be aware of our own harmonic structure and how it affects others every time we speak.

MATH ALERT
For those of you that have been traumatized by your math teacher,
I assure you that we are not doing this math for nothing.
You will be rewarded in the end.

The truth is that sounds normally contain multiple frequencies that have very specific mathematical relationships to the fundamental pitch.

For example, here is the structure of the harmonics when we play the A string on a guitar or a violin. This mathematical structure is the same for just about all sounds.

Frequency	Harmonic	Pitch
7040	16th	A (4th Octave)
6600	15th	G#
1540	14th	G
1430	13th	F ¼ sharp
1320	12th	E
1210	11th	D ¼ sharp
1100	10th	C#
990	9th	B
880	8th	A (3rd Octave)
770	7th	G ¼ flat

660	6th	E
550	5th	C#
440	4th	A (2nd Octave)
330	3rd	E
220	2nd	A (Octave)
110	Root	A

If you play an "A" on a guitar most people will hear an "A." But the whole sound is actually: A, A, E, A, C#, E, G, B, C#, etc. In the guitar there are actually about 30 frequencies within one note. Each harmonic is only a single pure frequency.

Just about all sounds are made up of multiple pure frequencies.

Note that each of the harmonics is a multiple of the root frequency, 110 hertz. Mathematical multiples are 1x, 2x, 3x, 4x, 5x, etc. (note that this is a different formula than doubling the frequency).

This structure of mathematical multiples is found in almost every sound. and is found throughout nature.

The Four Aspects of the Harmonic Structure of Sound
There are 4 things about harmonics that make one tone sound different from another.

1. Which harmonics – Odd or Even

2. How many harmonics – Pure or Rich (Complex)

3. Volume of the harmonics

4. Phase or Timing of the harmonics

These are the key differences about how a sound affects us differently physically, mentally, emotionally, and Spiritually.

1. Which Harmonics – Odd (Activating) vs. Even (Calming)
Almost all sounds are made up of a combination of pure tones. Even someone screaming is made of many pure tones. But pure tones are not edgy-sounding, so the question is, "How do we get such sharp sounds from sweet sounds?" The answer is that certain combinations of harmonics create a dissonant chord. The best example of a dissonant chord is a car horn. If you play a bunch of notes that are not in key or in tune, they will sound quite edgy, which is irritating to some. In the field of Sound Healing we don't call them edgy or irritating; we call them "activating." The dissonance in these sounds is actually very effective at breaking up stuck energy at all levels: physically, mentally, emotionally and even Spiritually.

It just so happens that God has set it up so that the odd-numbered harmonics (1, 3, 5, 7 in the chart below) create these dissonant chords.

Frequency	Harmonic	Pitch
7040	16th	A (4th Octave)
6600	15th	G#
1540	14th	G
1430	13th	F ¼ sharp
1320	12th	E
1210	11th	D ¼ sharp
1100	10th	C#
990	9th	B
880	8th	A (3rd Octave)
770	7th	G ¼ flat
660	6th	E
550	5th	C#
440	4th	A (2nd Octave)
330	3rd	E
220	2nd	A (Octave)
110	Root	A

If you were to play the notes A, E, C#, G ¼ flat, B, D ¼ sharp, F ¼ sharp, and G# all together at the same time you would create a chord that is quite activating.

On the other hand, the even numbered harmonics A, A, A, E, A, C#, E, G, and all together you would create a chord that is quite warm and calming.

The best example of an odd harmonic sound is the sound of bagpipes. All reed instruments (clarinet, saxophone, oboe) are mostly made up of odd numbered harmonics. Also, things made of metal create more odd harmonics, such as Tibetan bowls. Distorted rock guitars are mostly odd harmonics. Even the sitar has a large preponderance of odd harmonics. The harmonium and shruti boxes that are commonly used in chanting put out mostly odd harmonics because they have reeds in them. People with odd harmonics in their voice include most heavy metal singers (Axyl Rose), Bob Dylan, Janis Joplin, Tiny Tim and the whiners on Saturday Night Live, and Fran Drescher in the TV show, "The Nanny."

Again, whether an instrument puts out odd or even harmonics is based on the construction of the instrument and how the sound is produced. Odd harmonics are created by rough textures (the throat of Janis Joplin), asymmetrical shapes, chaotic movement (hitting an object or the movement of a reed), and metal. Guitars with steel strings instead of nylon strings have more odd harmonics.

Also, when an instrument is played loudly, it will put out more odd harmonics. When someone screams, odd harmonics are what make their voice sound edgy. The sound of a drum being hit really hard contains more odd harmonics. A really loud guitar amp puts out more odd harmonics because both the electronics and the speaker are being stretched and pushed to their limits.

When using the voice, the vowel sound of "Eee" is mostly odd harmonics and therefore, the most activating.

Sounds that are mostly made up of even harmonics are warm sounding and include the harp and acoustic guitars with nylon strings (Classical or Flamenco style guitars). Even harmonics are created by smooth surfaces (including smooth skin in the throat and symmetrical shapes). Two good examples of singers with harmonic voices are Barry White and Nora Jones.

The vowel sound of "oo" (as in moo) is mostly even harmonics.

The progression in vowel sound from even to more and more odd harmonics is as follows:
uu (as in "moo") – mostly even
oh (as in "owe") – more even than odd
ah – good balance of odd and even
eh – more odd than even
eee – mostly odd

The violin and the cello are just about the perfect balance of odd and even harmonics.

Nature sounds run the full gamut. Animal sounds can be extremely calming, like a cat's purr, or activating, like a crow or raven. The roar of a lion is mostly odd and activating. A kitty cat purr is mostly even. Even though crickets produce mostly odd harmonics they still create a consistent sound that is soothing to most.

When choosing the sounds you are going to make with your voice, or the type of instrument you are going to play, or the type of music you put on – the amount of odd versus even harmonics is a huge deal because they can affect a person in dramatically different ways.

Odd harmonics are extremely beneficial and healing depending on the need. Dissonance is only negative if we think of it as negative.

First, odd harmonics can be used to gain our attention, as with car horns or the ring of a telephone. Probably the best example is the tone of the Emergency Broadcast System. Odd harmonics can be extremely effective in creating more alertness. They keep us awake. For someone who is depressed, odd harmonics are the deal. If you play even harmonics for someone who is depressed they may never get out of bed again. My CD for depression has way more odd harmonics than even harmonics. Also, sounds that are too warm could put you to sleep while driving.

Odd harmonics are also incredibly effective for breaking up stuck energy, and getting energy flowing again. If you have a frozen muscle or a blockage in an intestine, odd harmonics can be quite helpful. If you have an energetic blockage in any part of the body, or a mental or emotional block, odd harmonics can be way more effective than even ones to get the energy moving.

However, you do have to be careful with odd harmonics. People who are hypersensitive to sound can easily be irritated by these activating sounds. Odd harmonics are the last thing someone needs if they are having a panic attack. In fact, odd harmonics can trigger a panic attack in someone who is prone to them. Many of us have plenty of activation in the form of stress in our lives, so we don't need any more activation. When using sound to help someone sleep, you use mostly even harmonics. You don't need activation while trying to go to sleep. It is the same for someone who is dying. You don't need activation when dying!

On the other hand, we all need and want more energy. If we listened to totally calming sounds all the time we might become catatonic or bored. Someone who is depressed needs activation, but also someone who is overwhelmed and doesn't have enough energy to deal with the world, seriously needs activation. And someone with blocked energy in their muscles, meridians, or chakras needs activation to get the energy smoothly flowing through their system again.

Again, even harmonic sounds can be very calming. These warm sounds are good for a fragile nervous system or someone who is hypersensitive to sound. They are good for hospice work and those who are dying. However, they are not always appropriate. If someone is depressed, they might never get out of bed again if they heard only sounds with even harmonics.

At the risk of giving odd harmonics a bad rap, Love is always expressed with more even harmonics in the voice. You don't squeal, "I love you," you say it with warmth in your voice if you want it to sound credible. When you are more loving, your voice naturally resonates more even harmonic warmth.

The overall amount of odd activating harmonics versus the amount of even calming harmonics in a song is a huge deal. Generally, people prefer less activation in the morning when they first wake up and more calming at night (unless going dancing). Young people generally prefer more odd activation. Older people (to over-generalize) normally prefer less activation and more calming. Different people also prefer more or less based on their system's sensitivity to sound.

It is also helpful to notice the level of odd harmonic versus even harmonic sounds in your environment. TV is the most extreme example. Most sounds on TV tend to be extremely activating – including the tonality of most of the voices. It is only occasionally that you will find even harmonics (mostly within romantic shows). Commercials are the extreme case of odd harmonics – out to grab your attention.

Notice all of the sounds around you and how they entrain you into more activation or calming – particularly the timbre of people's voices. Notice how activating or warm the sounds of people's voices are that you encounter throughout the day. As you become aware of your sound environment you can take action to modify it, if it is affecting you negatively. Or, use some of the techniques we'll explain later to create your own inner sound environment that is more to your liking, and more healthy.

Most importantly, notice whether your own voice tends to be more odd or even. Of course, when we get upset or stressed we transmit more odd harmonics. As you become more aware of how your voice is affecting others, you can consciously adjust the level of activation or calming depending on the needs of a particular situation.

You can also think of the rest of the world in terms of odd or even harmonics. Certain combinations of colors create harmony. Others, like orange and green together, create more activation. Salty and spicy foods are more odd harmonics. A soft warm blanket is more even harmonics.

As you can see, when choosing the sounds to use on someone in a healing session, it is absolutely critical to be aware of whether the sounds or activating or calming – based on the type of issue you are working with. It is important in the types of sounds you make with your voice, the type of instruments that you choose to use, and even the music you choose to use on someone or the music you listen to – at different times of the day, and for different issues and intentions.

2. How Many Harmonics

Besides "which" harmonics are present, the number of harmonics also determines why one sound sounds different from another. Pure sounds have no or very few harmonics. Rich or complex sounds have large numbers of harmonics.

We have already discussed pure sounds and their effects. They can resonate very specific parts of the body. I often think of them as a laser poking you. Whereas a rich sound massages you with a whole spectrum of frequencies – kind of like scratching an itch. Rich sounds give the system a full range of frequencies to choose from. The intelligence of our system will normally choose which frequencies it needs from the full array.

Pure sounds include tuning forks, tone generators, flutes, crystal bowls and many bird songs. For the most part, women tend to have purer voices than men. This is for two reasons. First, women have smoother skin inside their throats that create fewer harmonics, and women speak at a higher octave. This means that women's harmonics go out of our hearing range quicker, so we end up hearing less of them.

Some women have extremely pure voices like Mariah Carey, Celine Dion, and the Irish singers in RiverDance especially in the high vocal ranges.

Men tend to have more harmonics, however when men sing or speak in falsetto they have fewer harmonics. Michael Jackson, Aaron Neville, and Barry Gibb of the Beegees are excellent examples.

Opera singers also have richer sounding voices (although they can make their voices very pure as well). The cello and violin have all the harmonics so are very rich sounding. Large instruments with many parts also have more harmonics – like the piano and sitar. Electric instruments like the electric guitar and electronic keyboards tend to have fewer harmonics than natural sounds and instruments.

I will often make my voice more rich and full (not necessarily loud) when I want to calm someone. I use pure, whistle like tones when I want to activate a chakra or a specific organ or part of the body. I commonly do overtone singing to activate the full range of charkas with the pure tone.

3. Volume of the Harmonics

The volume of each of the harmonics is also an important aspect of the differences between sounds. Here are examples of the volume of harmonics for some common sounds.

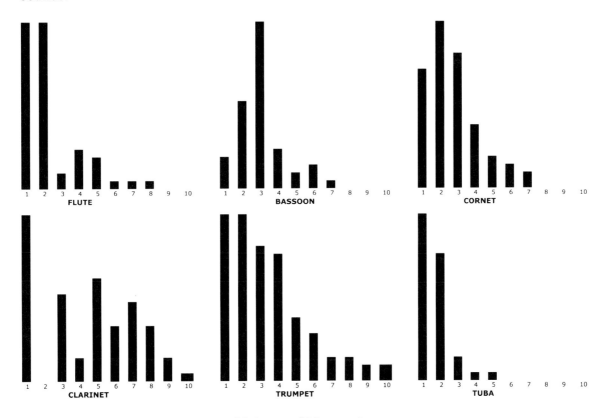

Volume of Harmonics

If the volume of the harmonics were altered these sounds would not sound right. In the recording studio we use an equalizer to turn up and down the harmonics. We also turn up and down the harmonics present in our voice, when we do overtone singing.

4. Phase (Timing) of the Harmonics

Another component of harmonics is the timing of the harmonics relative to each other. When we make a sound it comes directly out of our mouth. However, there are some sounds that bounce around inside our mouth cavity before they come out. They come out ever so slightly later than the sounds that come out directly from your vocal chords. Therefore, these harmonics are delayed by the time they reach our ear.

Both Volume and Phase of Harmonics may not seem that important, but they contribute to the overall harmonic structure of a sound – particularly that of the voice. They also carry information about our body and who we are every time we open our mouth.

Harmonics in Your Voice – The Map of Your Being

Every single thing about you –
your template of perfection, your template of health,
and all the distortions you have come up with in your life
are embedded in the harmonic structure of your voice.

Based on kinesiology, every single thing going on your system affects your muscles, and since your voice is created with your vocal muscles, everything about you is expressed through the harmonics of your voice.

There are about a dozen companies that have created Voice Analysis software to read and decipher the information carried in the harmonics of our voice. Some are so sophisticated that they can detect weaknesses in organs. Others show what is going on within you physically, mentally, emotionally and Spiritually. Some even show the past and present, and use frequencies to access your future potential.

I have met and talked with most of the owners of these companies to see how they decipher the information within the harmonic structure of our voice. I still think that we have not completely cracked the code (although many are well on the way). I believe we are on the threshold of a day when we will be able to see every distortion, blockage, stuck emotion and energy that is getting in the way of our perfect health. We will then be able to also create a harmonic structure that resonates the divine template of healthy perfection that we were born with.

On a similar level, research is now showing that dolphins actually transmit healing information within the harmonic structure of sound – more so, than in the melodies they sing. I have also now met several people who have received information from dolphins in one harmonic blast – as if in a hologram. In Hawaii, there is a birthing center where you can deliver your baby in the water with the dolphins and they send sound "information" into the baby when it is born. These babies are now consistently ending up as "indigo" or "crystal" children with amazing psychic powers and awareness.

In our classes on Quantum Mechanics, the instructor talks about the Quantum world (in which time is absent) being the harmonic world – in which our 3D world of time and space is the world of melody (which requires time to exist).

The Harmonic world is mathematically able to encode much more information than our simple melodic world.

Harmonics of the Universe
Now, let me take you to the next level (in case you aren't already there).

The mathematical structure that makes up all harmonics is that of mathematical multiples: 1x, 2x, 3x, 4x, etc. This same mathematical structure is found throughout nature! In fact, the distance between the planets is governed by almost the same proportions.

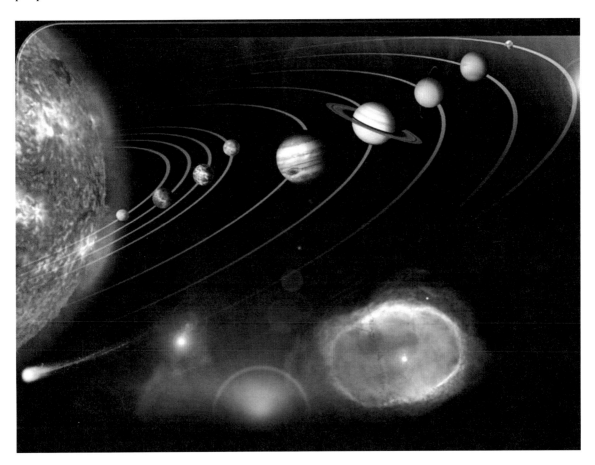

The distance from the Sun to Mercury is the root frequency. The distance from Mercury to Venus is twice that distance. Venus to Earth is 3 times the distance. Earth to Mars, 4. Mars to the Asteroid belt is 5 times the distance of the Sun to Mercury, and so forth.

The weight of each vertebra in our spine also has the same mathematical structure as the harmonic structure of sound. At the top of the spine vertebrae are lightest, then get heavier and as they go down.

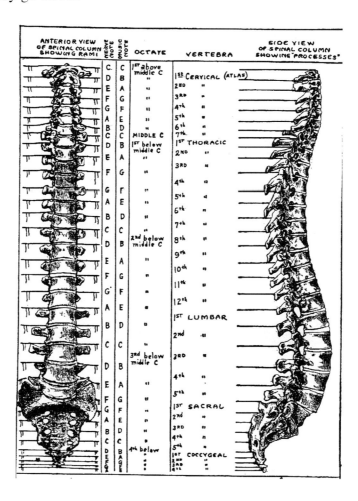

The distance between the electron shells in an atom also shares the same mathematical structure.

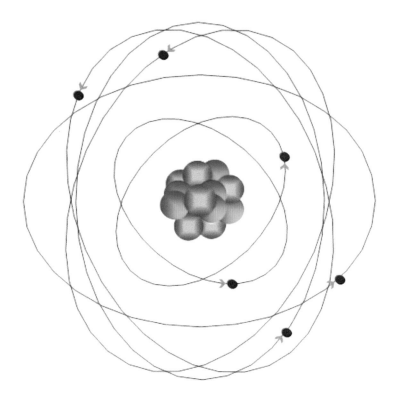

There are also those who believe the frequencies of our auras are based on the harmonic structure of sound.

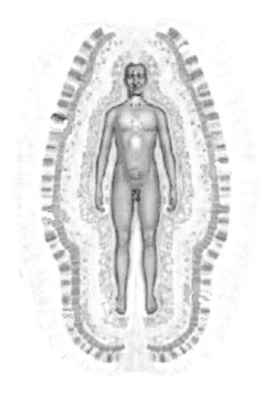

This accounts for the fact that acoustic sounds without amplification are better for us than electronic sounds or sounds that are amplified with a PA System (as they are at concerts) – because they massage our subtle bodies or organs more precisely and harmoniously. However, I would not stop going to concerts or only use acoustic instruments. With intention these instruments can be just as powerful (I saw God at a Pink Floyd concert with David Gilmore playing electric guitar).

It has also been discovered that in the quantum world matter jumps from one level of energy to another. These levels of energy are based precisely on the mathematical structure of sound. Science has now proven that we are all connected (or entangled) at the quantum level.

Whenever a mathematical system (such as multiples) is replicated at different levels of reality (such as sound and the atomic structure), a resonant connection exists.

**Whenever we work with sound,
particularly when we focus on the harmonics,
we are connecting to all the other levels
that share this same mathematical structure.**

**Therefore, when we make sound,
we are connecting the solar system that we are a part of,
the atomic structure and quantum mechanics that we are made of,
and the frequencies of our spine and auras.**

**Every sound we make
is resonating and affecting all these other levels.
In particular, when we make a sound (even while simply speaking)
we are resonating the mathematical structure of sound at the quantum level
where we are all connected by entanglement.**

**Therefore, every sound is affecting everyone else on the planet!!!
Even the sound of every breath we take.**

**Making a sound
comes with a huge sense of responsibility
(I don't know if I can handle it).
Resonating higher vibrations of gratitude, compassion, love, joy,
and a direct connection to our soul, Spirit and Source
are therefore helping to change the planet in a very real way.**

Tuning Systems
Now, let's revisit tuning systems.

A Tuning System is the particular frequency of each of the 12 notes within an octave. Ancient tuning systems based every frequency in an octave on the harmonic series found in nature. Doing so means that each of the notes played in a scale in a song are the same as the harmonics found in one string.

This not only means that the sounds are resonating with the distance between the planets and the entire Universe, but that every note played is also resonating with the inner and outer cosmos, so to speak. The notes are the notes of the spine, atoms, and levels of quantum energy. There is harmony at all levels.

Before the 1700's almost all cultures (including our own) used these ancient tuning systems based on the harmonics. However, musically, there is one small problem with these tuning systems – you can't go from key to key (as is often done in jazz). It sounds out of tune if you do. There are also certain chords that can't be played at the same time. It sounds completely out of tune.

Realizing this, Bach started using what is called the "equal tempered tuning system." In this system the distance between each note is exactly the same – something that you never find in nature! This is only found in the mind. However, it does give the advantage of changing key in the middle of the song, which does give us way more emotional options in music. The only problem is that we are now no longer in alignment with nature. We are no longer connected to the solar system and atom. We are disconnected.

Now, 99% of music on the radio and CDs that we listen to are in equal tempered tuning. Most classical music is still tuned to natural tunings, and accapella groups naturally sing in natural tunings. Also, there is not a bird or animal on the planet that sings in equal tempered tuning (except maybe a parrot that has lived with a professionally trained singer).

Therefore, many people in the field of Sound Healing are adamant about using these ancient tuning systems in music, tuning forks and crystal bowls. Particularly with sounds that are going to be applied to the body, it seems critical that you should use frequencies that are in alignment with nature instead of the mind. It just doesn't make sense to have tuning forks on chakras that are tuned to equal tempered tuning.

For more detail on these ancient tuning systems, Just Intonation and Pythagorean Tuning see Appendix E online on Tuning Systems. Just be aware, that the study of tuning systems gets really deep and mathematical quite quickly.

Chapter 8 – The Beauty and Power of Noise

Before, we continue with the hierarchy, let's take a look at the sounds that are <u>not</u> made up of frequencies. The term "noise" can mean many things – including something as general as "sounds we don't like." But in physics, noise is defined as an incomplete waveform, so it actually does not contain frequencies or harmonics.

Tone   Noise

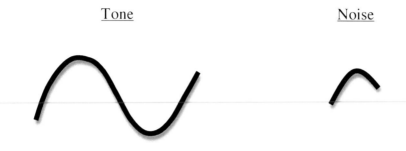

Complete Waveform   Incomplete Waveform

Without a complete waveform there is no way to know what the pitch of a sound is. Examples of noise are white noise, pink noise, the ocean, rivers and streams, waterfalls, the wind, shakers, rattles, whispers, and the most important noise of all – the breath!

Because noise is actually not a frequency at all, it is really good for breaking up stuck energy – whether it is a stuck emotion, a learning disability, or the frequency of grief over someone you have lost. Stuck energy is simply a frequency that is looping – repeating the same incongruent sound over and over and over and over and over and over, ad infinitum.

In fact, when we use EEG on a person with Post Traumatic Stress syndrome, we can see a frequency (theta) looping over and over in the brain. Because noise is random and is devoid of frequency, it breaks up the repeating frequency pattern of the stuck issue. All types of noise: white and pink noise, the ocean, waterfalls, rushing rivers, shakers, whispers, and the breath – can be used to breakup stuck frequencies found in emotions, post-traumatic stress, and learning disabilities.

Many people use white noise generators to help them sleep. White noise has a unique ability to obscure other sounds around us – such as traffic or neighbors. Not only do these "non-frequencies" help mask or hide other sounds around us, they also help mask our own chaotic thoughts.

(Pink noise is simply white noise that has a boost in the bass and treble to compensate for weaknesses in our hearing in those ranges. Therefore, we seem to hear all the "non-frequencies" of noise more evenly).

The ocean is mostly white noise coupled with a little bit of tone (harmonics). The tone happens when waves curl over creating parallel walls that resonate a particular frequency.

As the waves change size we get the familiar frequency sweep that a crashing wave makes. If you've had the opportunity, you know how a day at the beach immersed in white noise all day long seems to clear away all our stresses – in fact, all of our stuck emotional frequencies. We feel clear when we leave the beach.

However, we do feel somewhat tired also. Technically, noise is hundreds of incomplete waveforms hitting us every second all day long. This can wear out our ears and all of the cells in our body since they are surrounded by water. This accounts for that relaxed tired feeling we experience after having been at the beach all day. This also happens when we sleep through the night with a white noise generator. It may help us to get to sleep, but technically we are being hit by millions of incomplete waveforms throughout the night. For some, this results in a sleep that is not as deep. Others are grateful that they can sleep at all and use the white noise makers every night.

Streams, rivers, and waterfalls all are extremely effective noisemakers and are excellent for clearing out stuck frequencies within us. I remember hiking by a raging river for over an hour and then being able to hear my Soul frequency as clear as day. All of my "stuff" had been washed away by the noise of the river. Waterfalls are particularly powerful – especially large ones like those at Yosemite or Niagara Falls.

Shakers and Rattles have been used by many Native American and aboriginal cultures to clear out blockages in the body. Shaking a rattle over a blockage can be incredibly healing.

Whispers are amazingly powerful. There is nothing better than having someone whisper in your ear, "I love you." A soft whisper on a stressed out part of the body can be way more effective than a louder and more powerful sound.

One of the most powerful examples of noise is the breath. The sound of the breath is one of the most powerful sounds on the planet! Just the sound of a relaxed breath can relax our entire body, mind and soul. A sound of a sigh has the power to relax even a tiger.

Also, when music is created to the breath, it affects us much deeper physiologically and psychologically. Most music is not slow enough to breathe to. However, most chants are actually breathable. Often we find ourselves breathing in time to the music. Most of my music is also created to a really slow breath.

Even if your breath does not entrain to the breath in the music, it's like sitting next to someone who is meditating with a deep, soft and calm breath. Just being next to them is calming. The same applies to listening to music that is based on a deep, soft and calm breath.

We have now looked at pure frequencies and timbres, the voice and instruments used to create them, and how they affect us. Now let's look at one higher level – Musical Intervals and Chords.

Chapter 9 – Musical Intervals and Chords

A musical interval is simply the relationship between one frequency, pitch or timbre to another. When you learn what the relationship between two notes sounds like and **feels like**, you then have the key to understanding and **feeling** the relationship between all things in the Universe – because everything has a frequency. On a higher level, every musical interval relationship is associated with a particular state of consciousness. These states of consciousness can be used to describe the relationship between any two things in the world – two cells, two organs, two different plants, two different foods on your plate, two different colors you are wearing, two different planets that are affecting you today, the relationship between you and another person, or the relationship between you and me.

In music we have two types of musical intervals: Harmonic musical intervals where two sounds play at the same time, and melodic musical intervals where there is one sound after another. In both cases the relationship between two sounds puts us into a certain energy or state of consciousness – even if for a moment.

Here are some examples of the different feelings and emotions associated with some of the more common various musical intervals.

Archetypal Relationships of Musical Intervals

Unison (1:1)
Two identical pitches sounding together associated with primal cosmic union, which represents serenity and perfect peace. Very comfortable interval. There is a "sameness" about the sounds, as it is in complete harmony with the fundamental sound.

Musical Examples: C-C "Row, row, row your boat" "Happy Birthday"

Octave (1:2 or 2:1)
Generated by two sounds where one is two times the frequency of the other. The second Harmonic in the harmonic structure. This interval is restful, grounding, meditative, calming, also called the yin and yang interval. The lower tone is now representing the masculine energy and the higher note the feminine energy. Final resolution. Reaching for the higher self. Foundation for stability. Linking past to the present memory. Transformational. Home again, at a higher or lower level.

Musical Example: C-C^{8VA} "Somewhere over the Rainbow"
'Chestnuts…'from "Merry Christmas"

Perfect Fifth (3:2)
The 3rd Harmonic in the harmonic structure. This interval is comfortable, evoking feelings of opening, home, sturdiness, completeness, joy, and healing; it also stimulates power and movement. It can bring forth new life, creative

ideas and rebirth. A very nice interval that is pretty far off from the tonic. Awe-inspiring. This is also a pivot interval, which can bring you back to the one or lead to the octave creating a full circle. Creation, Actualization. Strong. Youthful. Bright, contemplative, full of light, heavenly or divine (when gentle). Passage of the inner to outer. Creative potential.

Musical Examples: C-G "Twinkle, Twinkle Little Star" "Born Free" "2001 Theme" "Flintstones Theme (descending)" "Star Spangled Banner" (descending). A major harmonic component in Tibetan and Crystal bowls.

Perfect Fourth (4:3)

A 4th is often called suspended. This interval is airy and evokes feelings of serenity, clarity, openness and light. It can also be like an ancient trumpet alarm. It creates the some tension harmonically. In certain contexts it is an unstable interval that likes to resolve to another note. Grand, Ta-da! bright, uplifting, joy. Awakening of the heart to control issues causing one to feel unpleasant. Associated with awakening. Paralyzing (on the negative). In Indian traditions it represents a return to the mother.

Musical Examples: C to F "Here Comes the Bride" "Hi ho, hi ho, it's off the work we go!" "Hi ho" "Amazing Grace" "Smells Like Teen Spirit"

Major Third (5:4)

This interval is considered to have or possess "great sweetness", manifesting auspicious possibilities. Three is also considered to be a number associated with perfection and divinity. It is often the next sweet step. Steady, calm, normal, comfortable, square and resolved, without a lot of character. Sense of beauty expressed in your external world. Pulls a bit at my heartstrings. Waiting for something else to happen, creating a little bit of stress.

Musical Examples: C to E. "When the Saints Come Marching In" "From the Halls of Montezuma" "Kumbaya" "Summertime" (descending). "Swing Low Sweet Chariot" (descending). Found frequently in church music, children's, folk, country, gospel, jazz, Baroque and many other styles.

Major Second (9:8)

The note is very unstable and wants to be resolved - especially when the notes are going down. Rousing, wakening, hopeful. Somewhat dissonant sounding. As a harmonic interval the Major 2nd can create discord and irritation. However, tends to promote growth and ultimate beauty. Building blocks of life. Patient steps toward larger goals. Connections between things. Complication of life.

Musical Examples: C-D "Do Re Mi" "Frere Jacques" "The First Noel".

Often used in melodies around the world.

Major Sixth (5:3)
Soft and sweet. Dreamy and full of possibility. Sad, sorrowful, weeping. Portal of total opening - feelings of offering oneself to the Universe. The flowers open to at dawn. It is the most etheric of intervals. No tension, no wait, no emotional heaviness, very pleasing. Ambitious. Associated with lullabies.

Musical Examples: C-A First two notes of "My Bonnie Lies Over the Ocean" "NBC theme" "It Came Upon a Midnight Clear" "Nobody Knows the Trouble I've Seen" (descending). It's in a lot of Gospel Music. 4th's, 5th's, and 6th's are in a lot of Scottish Music (bagpipe music).

Major Seventh (15:8)

It is called the "leading tone". There is a quality to its resonance that encourages resolution of a musical phrase towards the root tone above. Piercing, sensitive, ready to move. Provokes growth in consciousness. It has a profound influence on physical, musical, subtle, and etheric bodies. It calls for urgency to move into oneness. Very similar to the minor 2nd, it's inverse in some ways.

Musical Examples: C-B "Take on Me" "Bali-Hi".

Minor Seventh - Flatted, Dominant, Diminished Seventh
This is a bit dissonant, quite energizing and dark much of the time. There is certainly a fun quality to it when the energizing shade is amplified. Deeper emotional music.

Musical Examples: C-Bb "Star Trek Theme" Sacred music, gospel, country, R&B, Blues. Chinese healing and minor pentatonic music.

Minor Sixth (8:5)
Here is another interval with mixed applications. It can evoke sacredness, sadness, confusion, a bit of darkness or pending doom, emotional, loving or the feeling of lost love. The minor 6th, as a ratio, is closest to the golden mean (followed closely by the Major 6th). This can be used for natural, spiritual growth. Taking the next steps along in life. Doing one thing after another. Also waiting for something to happen.

Musical Examples: C to Ab "The Love Story" "Charlie Brown Theme" "In my Life" (guitar intro) "The Entertainer" (leap after intro). Chopin's music is filled with this interval in parallel motion.

Minor Third (6:5)

Alerts us to seriousness. Needs attention and needs to be resolved. Melancholy (not depression). State of mind that requires some immediate love. It can be pleasantly tense, requiring satisfying resolution - as in Brahms' Lullaby.

Musical Examples: C-Eb "Greensleeves" "So Long, Farewell" "Hey Jude" (descending). Slow and serious songs often have prominent minor 3^{rds}.

Minor Second (16:15)

This is definitely dissonant. It creates a tense and uneasy feeling that is expectant, anticipatory, busy and mysterious. Breaks up blockages or dense nodes of energy. Leads to inner emotions. When descending it can hold joy or release in the right context, partly through its resolution to the next tone.

Musical Examples: C-Db "Jaws" theme, "Joy to the World" (descending)

Diminished 5th or Augmented 4th (45:32) – "Tritone"

The "Inverse" or "Complimentary" Frequency

It is the most dissonant. This non-conformity creates critical and creative thinking – very energizing and uplifting. Stimulates the left and right sides of the brain. Considered VERY POWERFUL. Jazz players often refer to this as the 'blue' note.

According to archaic music theory, this interval is not to be used in music. In fact, it is called: Deabolics en Musica (The Devil in Music). Considered to be the devil's interval ... summoned demons.

Musical Examples: C-F# This interval is used frequently in horror films and is used in Leonard Bernstein's, "Maria" from "The West Side Story." The harmonics in the Tibetan bowls often have this interval. Hendrix "Purple Haze", Simpsons "Bop" in jazz.

A chord is more than two musical intervals – essentially creating a more complex state of consciousness. It is well known that different chords can take you into altered states and other dimensions of consciousness. The chord that is created by the relationship between the walls in the King's chamber has taken many into other realms – including myself.

Musical Intervals in a Timbre

A timbre is made up of multiple frequencies – all of which have a musical interval relationship to each other. This is why a timbre is quite a bit more powerful than a frequency because we now have musical intervals between each of the frequencies creating a complex chord. Furthermore, all of these different musical relationships add up to create one massive chord, or energy field.

Here are the musical intervals of the first 16 harmonics (in relation to the fundamental or root frequency). Again, this is the same in all tones on the planet.

Frequency	Harmonic	Pitch	Musical Interval
1760	16th	A (4th Octave)	4 Octaves
1650	15th	G#	3 Octaves + major 7th
1540	14th	G	3 Octaves + minor 7th
1430	13th	F ¼ sharp	3 Octaves + minor 6th
1320	12th	E	3 Octaves + 5th
1210	11th	D ¼ sharp	3 Octaves + 4th
1100	10th	C#	3 Octaves + 3rd
990	9th	B	3 Octaves + 2nd
880	8th	A (3rd Octave)	3 Octaves
770	7th	G ¼ flat	2 Octaves + 7th
660	6th	E	2 Octaves + 5th
550	5th	C#	2 Octaves + 3rd
440	4th	A (2nd Octave)	2 Octaves
330	3rd	E	Octave + 5th
220	2nd	A (Octave)	Octave
110	Root	A	

In fact, these musical intervals that are found in one sound

are the basis of all music on the planet.

Let us pause for a second to let this sink in.

Ahhhhooooooohhhhhmmmmmmmmmmmm.

Yes, this is where all musical intervals come from that make up all the music we know – from one sound! The musical intervals within one sound are like the codes that God gave us to then create all music.

Again, here is the quote from Leonard Bernstein:

"I believe that from the earth emerges a musical poetry that is,
by the nature of its sources, tonal. I believe that these sources cause to exist
a phonology of music, which evolves from the universal,
and is known as the harmonic series."
- Leonard Bernstein (1918-1990)

Chapter 10 – Music

"What makes us feel drawn to music is that our whole being is music: our mind and body, the nature in which we live, the nature which has made us, all that is beneath and around us, it is all music."
Hazrat Inyat Khan (Sufi Master) (1882-1927)

"Every illness is a musical problem – the healing, a musical solution..."
Novalis (1772-1801)

"If I were not a physicist, I would probably be a musician.
I often think in music. I live my daydreams in music.
I see my life in terms of music"
- Albert Einstein (1879-1955)

Next on the hierarchy is Music. As we know from experience, music is unbelievably powerful – bringing us into states of ecstatic joy, emotional bliss, heart opening tears, and perfectly divine peace and stillness.

Music is changing frequencies, musical intervals, and chords with rhythm.

Music is obviously quite a bit more powerful than musical intervals or chords by themselves. A full tree is much more powerful than one leaf (although beauty and source exist within the leaf itself).

Melody
Pitches and timbres moving up and down over time also create melodies, which also affect us in profound ways. A melody is a series of musical intervals with a rhythm. Melodies stimulate and entrain us into the flow of feelings and emotions. They can open our heart or take us into Spirit. In pop music the key is often to have a melody that is the perfect balance of simple and complex. This is still true in healing music, but it normally tends towards more simplicity. We create the complexity in the sounds themselves.

Melodies in nature are rarely extremely complex. In the body, you could say that there is melody created by the flow of energy from one part of the body to the next since every part of the body is a frequency or note.

Harmony
Harmony is simply two sounds happening at once. These two sounds create a musical interval that resonates certain feelings and emotions. Obviously harmony parts (particularly vocal harmonies) can be one of the most beautiful things on earth. Harmonies in music also resonate a need for harmony with nature and Spirit.

Rhythm
When we add time to frequencies, musical intervals, and chords, we get rhythm. Rhythms themselves have very specific and measurable effects on our heart rate, brainwave rhythms, breath, nervous system, cranial sacral rhythms, and our walking or dancing rhythm.

Technically, rhythm is simply a very slow frequency. In fact, every rhythm is actually a musical note – frequency and pitch. Therefore, the essence of a particular rhythm can be described in the same way that we explained pure frequencies. The difference is that rhythms match body rhythms in the body and affect them dramatically. Heart rates are affected almost immediately by any rhythm. Brainwaves are entrained within about 15 seconds (we explore rhythms on the brain in detail in Section IX). The time it takes to affect the breath depends on the person.

Here is an overall structure of rhythm.

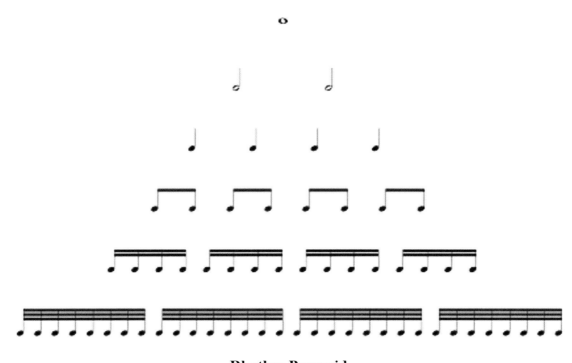

Rhythm Pyramid

On a higher level, rhythm ranges from the slowest rhythm of galaxies moving around each other to the fastest rhythmical vibrations within an atom. What is interesting is that a very slow rhythm seems very peaceful, and a very fast rhythm can also be very peaceful. Using heart rate monitors and galvanic skin response (which measures tension in the body), we have tested 100's of people and faster rhythms create just about the same amount of stability as slower ones.

The most stressful of all rhythms is "bad rhythm." When someone has really bad rhythm (God bless them), our whole system practically goes into fight or flight.

It is has also been shown that perfect rhythms, like a drum machine, create stress in the body. However, the stress often goes away when an instrument played by a real human is played on top of the stable rhythm of the drum machine. One of the key aspects to a healing rhythm is one that breathes, changing ever so slightly. Natural rhythms in nature are never perfectly stable (except for those in radiation). The ebb and flow of a human rhythm, or a rhythm in nature is nurturing to all of our body rhythms.

Another key aspect of rhythm is the way we go in and out of rhythm. The most interesting and sometimes the most stressful times in our day-to-day existence are the moments when we are transitioning from one rhythm to another. It has been shown that this moment of transformation is really chaotic and disorienting. However, it is a necessary aspect of moving from one state of consciousness to another.

It is important to be aware of all of the rhythms that we encounter throughout the day: In our body these include our breath, heartbeat, tempo of our walk, menstrual cycles, our cranio-sacral fluid, biorhythms, and the cycle of life, growing older, and death. We also have many rhythms around us – motors, motors and more motors. And those in nature: the sun, the moon, the stars, the seasons, life and death spans of animals and insects.

Of course, the more we are aware of the natural rhythms around us and we tune into them, the more we seem to find harmony in our life.

The Flow

The movement of musical intervals and chordal progressions create a powerful flow of energy that taps into our system very deeply – physically, mentally, emotionally and Spiritually. We can look at the flow on a micro or macro level. We can notice the flow from one note to another, one musical interval to the next, or the overall flow of a section of the song, or the overall flow of the entire song.

In my top selling book on audio recording, "The Art of Mixing," I cover all of the components that make up a good song. But over 30 years of writing, recording, mixing and producing music I've come to understand and believe that the "quality of the flow" of the music is the most important aspect of music by far (however, a particular frequency or timbre that is not in alignment can inhibit the flow). It is a flow that can take you many places. It can transport you into the world of Spirit and it can heal you physically, mentally, emotionally and Spiritually.

The quality of flow for healing music specifically includes:

1. The smoothness of the flow. A smooth flow has minimal amounts of stress. Like the flow of a river – it naturally follows a path of least resistance. It is without sharp turns.

2. The consistency of the flow over long periods of time. No disconnection, no loss of awareness as to the direction. A flow that is unbroken and void of scatteredness is more in alignment with Spirit, our Soul, and Source.

I believe consistency is the most important component of flow. I first noticed this at a Pink Floyd concert. I heard the music flowing consistently in the same direction, either up or down, over a long period of time. Up for over 5 minutes, sometimes as long as 15 minutes, or down in the same manner. This aspect of flow is an extremely consistent energy that is ever so slowly moving in a specific direction – similar to the flow of making love when *in love*. An beautiful energy that is powerful beyond words.

3. A flow that taps into the flow of nature and Spirit. In fact, this slow consistent flow in certain music seems to tap into the same slow smooth flow often found in nature. It reminds me of the movement of the planets, or even the movement of the sun around the Milky Way every 23,000 years. It reminds me of many natural long-term biorhythms of nature.

It is a movement that we seem to recognize at a deep level of Soul and Spirit that seems to be the flow of Source. It is a special manner in which the flow resonates with mathematical patterns of flow in nature and Spirit. We know that nature and Spirit often create particular mathematical and geometric patterns (such as Fibonacci sequences or Golden Mean Ratios) when they are unaffected by man or machinery.

4. Flows that mimic or align with flows within the body. These include emotions, heart variability, breath changes, and the flow of energy through the meridians.

When the flow in the music is right, we know it and feel it as if the music is a living being. It is the natural flow of life.

As we'll discuss later in Chapter 12,

The quality of health in any living system is directly related to the quality of flow in the system.

This is true whether we are looking at an amoeba, a human being, the earth, or the entire Universe.

Healing systems that deal with flow tend to be more powerful than those that only deal with static frequencies. The medical field is a perfect example. Much of the medical field simply focuses on one part of the body – as if it is somewhat disconnected from the rest of the systems in the body – with little regard as to how the whole interacts and creates an overall flow of energy in the body.

Chapter 11 – Energy - Consciousness and Intention in the Music

Energy is the most important and powerful level of vibration we know of. A song sung by one person can be nice, while the same song sung by another person can completely blow your mind, give you chills and tears, and sometimes completely transform a life.

Energy healers often perform miracles without the use of audible sound. Loving energy often creates miracle healings on its own – and often is transformative for the receiver in major ways.

Sometimes people refer to the effect of energy as "the placebo effect," although energy healing has now been proven scientifically in multiple controlled studies. There have been many detailed experiments that have proven the effects of energy healing. Lynne McTaggart talks about a very detailed experiment at California Pacific Medical Center where they proved that simply having a positive healing intention towards someone actually creates a positive physiological effect – even over a long distance, and when the person is not even aware of the energy being transmitted. A similar controlled experiment at the Institute of Noetic Sciences in Northern California revealed the same findings. Lynne's book, "The Intention Experiment," covers a wide range of scientific experiments proving energy healing.

Compared to Frequencies, Timbres, Musical Intervals or Music on their own, Energy is the most powerful. However, there is nothing more powerful than bringing energy through a person with sound and music. When you combine all of these components together you can obtain a level of power that most people could never have imagined.

Now, you have both the physical healing energy of the soundwaves _and_ the healing power of energy itself. When energy is coupled with sound and music the effect is amplified.

Even further, when energy is infused into sound and then recorded, the energy has the same effect as when it is performed live. Even if it is a bad recording, the energy is transmitted completely intact. Technically, a live session is still better because of the interactivity that happens between the musician/healer and the receiver. Also, the electromagnetic fields that are transmitted by way of the heart and brain do not get recorded. However, the energy component is the same.

Just as with music, the quality of the flow of the energy seems to be the most important component. The ideal energetic flow seems to be one that smoothly flows unimpeded and taps into the blessed flow of higher powers of nature, Spirit or Source. Universal Love is one of the best examples of such a powerful energetic flow.

Energy is encoded in the sound and music in two ways – consciousness and intention.

Quality of Consciousness of the Composers and Musicians
Energy in music and sound manifests as the quality of the consciousness of the person that is creating the music. It seems very clear that the more conscious a person is the more we can feel it in the music. Beethoven's consciousness came through his music very clearly. The more that someone is capable of tapping into higher levels of consciousness including gratitude, compassion, love, joy, a direct connection to Spirit, a direct connection to their own Soul, or a merging with Cosmic Consciousness or Source, where we are all one – the more these energies come through the music, lighting us up.

Also, the more proficient one is at navigating higher dimensions of consciousness with awareness, grace and lack of ego or glamour, the higher they are able to bring us energetically.

Sometimes people do have moments of inspiration where their music reaches heights way beyond their normal waking state of consciousness. This often happens when the rapture of angels or pure Spirit or Source takes people away.

Intention

A key component to the effectiveness of any healing work is a clear focus of attention without distraction. Just as important as a person's consciousness, is how consistently the musician and recording engineer hold a clear intention while playing, recording and mixing the music. When holding an intention with 100% focus, it is as though you are in a trance. This is difficult for many people. We are so easily distracted by wayward thoughts. The secret is that the sound can help you hold this 100% focus.

The key is to see the sound itself as the intention.

Because intention is a frequency, you can make a sound with your voice that personifies the energy of the intention. First, tune into the intention. Then, listen for a sound that seems to resonate the energy of the particular intention. Don't worry, you can't get it wrong. Play with it and you will find a sound that works. You can do the same thing with an instrument. Just set your intention that "the sounds coming out of the instrument are the intention" (you can even do this when playing back a CD). Then, the sound or music actually helps you stay focused on the intention. All you have to do is simply focus on the sound and music to bring your focus back to the intention.

Let's do a little interactive experiment. Set your intention to "heal the planet" – the earth, water, and everyone on the planet. No small intention (thought we would start big – no use fooling around). Now, chant an "OM" and bring that intention into the sound of the "OM." Tone "OM" with the intention of "healing the planet" for about 1 minute (you can even do this silently so you have no excuse to not do it now). Now, go.

When done, check in and ask yourself what percentage of time you were consistently holding the intention. 100%, 70-100%, 50-70%, less than 50%? Notice what the distracting thoughts were.

The key is to be able to do this with 100% focus without distraction. When there is 100% focus the intention is incredibly powerful (just like a really focused prayer). And…when you get a roomful of people holding an intention without distraction, it is unbelievably powerful. You might be able to heal someone of cancer. Ultimately, if you get a large percentage of people on the planet doing this at one time, planetary transformation can happen!

Now try this exercise again. However, this time tone the "OM" for at least 5 minutes. You can also choose another intention. You could focus on healing or harmonizing whatever you have going on physically, mentally, emotionally or Spiritually. Or, you could focus on healing or harmonizing one of these areas for someone else (although some believe that you must first get permission – at least from their higher self). Come back when you are done.

Because everything is vibration, even intention is a frequency. In fact, a complex intention can hold more than one frequency – as if it were a timbre. If we hold an intention of love it is a simple and pure frequency. If we hold love for the planet, it is a little more complex than simply holding the energy of love. If we hold the intention of love, forgiveness and compassion we are holding multiple frequencies. An intention can even include the flow of music. We can also hold an intention of a flow of energy. For example, imagine for everyone on the planet an intention of Spirit coming into the top of our head, Earth energy coming up through our feet, with both of them meeting at the heart and emanating out into the world. Or imagine everyone on the planet transmitting and receiving love at the same time. The whole focus is on flow now.

The quality of the particular intention itself is also really important. Very specific intentions (such as healing a specific disease in a particular person) can be incredibly effective, however it seems to me that Intentions that address the whole of the planet or humanity on a global level seem to bring more power with them.

Prayer
Intention and prayer are very similar. Just like intention, the power of the prayer has to do with the clarity and purity of the focus of the prayer without distraction. However, there is one big difference. Prayer generally involves a third party – God or Source (funny to call Source a third party, huh?). With prayer you are transmitting a frequency of intention to someone through Source. In one way, this is more powerful, because Source, we assume, has its own intentions for the person…your intention is filtered through a much smarter, higher power, so that there is no way to create harm.

Also, Source has a way it seems, of amplifying the frequency of intention to make it even more powerful.

People commonly get focused on one of the 5 levels or another of frequencies, pitches, timbres, musical intervals, chords, or music. Some people say that 528 hertz or the Solfeggio frequencies are the whole deal. Some say the pitches of each of the chakras are what it's all about. Others say that the sound of a tuning fork, crystal bowl, or a harp is the most healing. Music therapists, for the most part, only focus on the musical component. Others are just energy healers and feel that sound is the purest way to go.

However, when all the components of music – frequencies, pitches, timbres, musical intervals, chords, rhythms, melodies, harmonies and flow – come into harmony, an energy that is greater than the whole can emerge.

**We are carried on a multi-level wave of energy
that is more than the sum of the parts...
just as in nature and Spirit.**

Chapter 12 – The Hierarchy of Sound, Music and Energy in Living Systems

Now let's take a look at living systems and see how they work in relation to the five levels – frequencies, timbres, musical intervals, flowing music, and flowing energy. In particular, we'll look at the human system (including the realm of Soul, Source, and Spirit), the earth's eco-system, and the Universe (as we know it).

We will then look at different healing systems and how they use these five levels of vibration.

The Human System
The body is made of pure frequencies, timbres, intervals, chords, music, and energy.

We have separated out all the components of frequency, timbre, music and energy within the body in order to discuss them; however, all of the systems within the body work together as a whole within a healthy human organism. Ultimately any healing system must work with the system as a whole (traditional medical approaches do not honor this fact). It doesn't mean that we don't focus on individual parts of the body (frequencies and timbres), but that we also see how they are contributing to the overall harmony of the human symphony.

The key is to see the forest and the trees at the same time.

Let's take a look at how frequencies, music and energy manifest at each level of the human system.

You can think of the cells as pure frequencies, and organs and other body parts as timbres. The relationships between the cells, organs and other parts are musical intervals and chords. There are many flowing systems in the body, from blood flow, to electrical flow, to the flow of food and water, and on to the flow of our movement. Then there is the energy flow that encompasses our whole system, whether it is emotions, Soul, or Spirit.

**In any living system
energy flow
is the most important aspect.**

A body that is dead still has frequencies and timbres – the whole symphony is still there, but without the flow through the system there is no life. If we focus on any particular component without considering its part in the overall flow of the system, we are in danger of interrupting the flow.

The core frequencies would be the cells that make up the body. There are over 70 trillion cells in the body. What a symphony!!!

(Technically, every cell is actually a timbre because there are various parts to the cell. In fact, the molecules that make up the cells are timbres, and even the atoms are timbres that are made up of even smaller parts. So that we don't end up getting lost down the rabbit hole, we'll think of the cells as the main core frequencies that make up the body.)

You can then think of each part of the body as a timbre made of many individual cell frequencies. The organs, bones, tendons, ligaments, blood, skin, etc. are each a complex combination of pure frequencies. However, every one of these parts of the body has its own overall resonant frequency. For example, the kidneys might have a dozen main frequencies within them – the material that makes up the kidneys, the blood vessels, the blood, and every cell type within the kidneys; however, the kidney as a unit has its own fundamental frequency.

Then we look at the music within the body. Every part of the body is interacting with every other part of the body. Therefore, there are musical intervals between the different parts of the body that are resonating certain states of consciousness. Multiple parts of the body make up particular chords. It seems that the chords are most important within particular systems of the body – skeletal system, nervous system, digestive system, muscular system, and endocrine system (or meridian system). For example, if each organ has an overall frequency, all of the organs working together <u>must</u> create a musical chord.

**It seems obvious that in a healthy person,
all of the musical intervals and chords within the body
<u>must</u> be harmonious.**

It just wouldn't make sense that one part of the body is creating dissonance or tension with another part of the body in a healthy person.

Then there is the music within the body consisting of rhythms, changing frequencies, intervals, and musical flow.

First, there are many rhythms throughout the body – the heart being the key conductor. Our breath is another critical rhythm within the song of our body. Our cranial sacral fluids have a rhythm that is also tied into the rhythm of our blood flow and our nervous system. Even our walking rhythm and tempo are tied into all of our other body rhythms.

Just as with intervals and chords…

**it seems obvious that
all rhythms in the body <u>must</u> be in sync in a healthy person.**

But most importantly, there is the flow of the music in the body. Again, the quality of the flow through the system is very important. Tension and stress constrict this flow. We do exercise, yoga and dance to help things flow.

We see flow in each of the systems within the body – some more than others.

In the digestive system flow is a really big deal. Constipation or other disruptions in flow are a major cause of many health issues. In the circulatory system, if you don't have good blood flow to all parts of the body and all the cells, you are in trouble. The skeletal system and particularly the muscular system support good flow of movement. Professional or very fluid dancers demonstrate a beautiful expression of this flowing energy through the body. The nervous system also is all about flow – especially electrical flow.

There is also the vital flow through the meridians. This is a unique system when it comes to frequency, timbre and music. Various books have now identified the frequency of each acupuncture point in the body. It follows that there are specific musical intervals between any two acupuncture points – particularly those that are next to each other on a particular meridian. But more importantly, you can think of the energy flowing from one acupuncture point to another as an actual song being played through the meridians. The **quality of the flow** through the meridians of this song is very important. It is the core essence of the goal of all acupuncture. Acupressure has the same goal – flow. And, when you use tuning forks on these acupuncture points the goal is exactly the same.

One acupuncturist I've spoken with said
that the musical flow of energy through each of the acupuncture points
is your particular "Soul Song."

Many people now focus on finding the particular song of your Soul – the **core** musical
tone or melody that lights you up and brings you into harmony with yourself.
Wouldn't it be amazing if it were true that this song is actually pulsing through your
meridians as we speak (or read)?

I would say the health of every system in the body is primarily based on the **quality of the flow** through the system. Nutrients, including all food, minerals and vitamins support the individual frequencies and timbres of cells and organs to allow them to function harmoniously within this musical flow within all the systems in the body. And, at one level higher, all of the systems in the body have an interactive musical flow between them. For example, the nervous system is interacting in perfect harmony with the muscular system and the digestive system in a healthy person. You can think of it as sections of the symphony interacting with each other – the violin section with the horn section, and so forth – again, all in perfect musical harmony with each other.

Even more importantly than the frequencies, timbres and music within the body is the energy within the body. Again, the essence of healthy energy is also about the quality of the flow.

The essence of Spirit is about flow. A corpse is only a complex timbre made up frequencies with no enlivening flow at all.

Besides the enlivening energy of Spirit, there are many other energies that we can run through our system. There is the energy of gratitude, compassion, love and joy. All of these can facilitate smooth energetic flow through the system. There is also the flow of energy that comes when in direct contact with your Soul essence. This also helps the flow of healing and inspirational energies to move smoothly through the body. And, whenever energy flows through the body energetically it lubricates the flow of energy throughout all of the systems within the human system!

This is why energy healing on its own seems to be one of the most effective healing modalities in many cases. It facilitates flow.

Healthy emotions are also about flow. Resistance to the flow of emotions is the biggest problem. Stuck emotions and deep emotional issues are stagnant. As we'll cover in detail in the chapter on how to release stuck emotions, sound is an incredible catalyst in creating the necessary flow in emotions.

When our thoughts don't flow freely our health also breaks down. Thoughts can get stuck at dead ends, where we don't have a solution, can't figure it out, and have no where to go – all of which cause stress. We can also have thoughts that are flowing like a bumpy ride – often with stops and starts and lots of tension along the way. Flowing thoughts flow as freely as a river flowing around obstacles big or small.

The big question is, "Who is the conductor of this symphony?"

**If I had to guess, I would say
it is a combination of our Soul and Source –
Our own essence of our own frequency,
and how it ties into the whole Universe
where there is ultimate flow.**

**When you find the frequency of the conductor
and resonate it
all is in harmony.**

Healing Systems
Various healing systems focus on one or more of the five levels – frequency, timbre, musical interval, music, and energy. I believe the systems that focus on healing at an energetic level are more effective than the others. However, systems that focus on all five levels are most powerful of all.

Let's take a look at how common healing systems focus on one or more of the four levels. First, we'll provide a brief explanation of the healing system, and then explain how it uses frequency, timbres, music or energy as its primary modality. Specialists in these areas might see the essence of the modality quite differently than how I explain it. Also, many people take a modality and modify it based on their own understanding of healing – so a particular person might well be using all four levels of healing within the modality.

If you are working within any of these modalities, you might consider expanding the treatment to include all five levels.

Acupuncture and Acupressure - Fine needles are inserted at specific points to stimulate, disperse, and regulate the flow of vital energy, and restore a healthy energy balance. In addition to pain relief, acupuncture is also used to improve well-being and treat acute, chronic, and degenerative conditions in children and adults. Acupressure is similar to acupuncture, but using finger pressure rather than fine needles on specific points along the body to treat ailments such as tension and stress, aches and pains, menstrual cramps, arthritis.

It seems that this modality focuses on all 5 areas – frequency, timbres, musical intervals, music and energy. I especially like the fact that it is focused on flow through the system. However, practitioners do not normally focus on sending energetic intention through themselves to the client. I do know a few practitioners who do add this component to their work. When using tuning forks on acupuncture points, the treatment is much more powerful if you add an intention or send loving energy at the same time.

Herbalism - An ancient form of healing still widely used in much of the world, herbalism uses natural plants or plant-based substances to treat a range of illnesses and to enhance the functioning of the body's systems. Herbs are simply frequencies and timbres that are brought into the body to resonate specific frequencies and timbres of organs into their natural harmony so that they can resume their healthy functioning within the overall flow of the system.

Vitamin Therapy - A complementary therapy of vitamin usage is combined with other treatments to address a range of illnesses and to enhance the functioning of the body's systems. It is commonly used to assist the immune system in combating diseases such as Chronic Fatigue Syndrome and HIV/AIDS.

Vitamin Therapy is basically the same as Herbalism in that it brings in frequency nutrients to resonate parts of the body into their natural, healthy state.

Aromatherapy - Using "essential oils" distilled from plants, aromatherapy treats emotional disorders such as stress and anxiety as well as a wide range of other ailments. Oils are massaged into the skin in diluted form, inhaled, or placed in baths.

This system is mostly about timbre. Each "essential oil" is a combination of various frequencies (there might be a few that are very pure frequencies, but I haven't come across any). They are incredibly powerful because they resonate with the frequencies inside your system. Through experimentation or working with someone who is intuitive it is easy to find a timbre that helps your system. I'm sure there are many practitioners who do look at how a particular essence or timbre affects the overall flow of the system.

Bach Flower Remedies - A system of herbal remedies devised by Edward Bach, these floral remedies can supposedly alter the disharmonies of personality and emotional state that trouble us all from time to time. These remedies are mostly aimed at curing emotional states rather than physical ones. As in aromatherapy, this system also uses timbres to focus on creating emotional flow.

Gem Therapy - Involves the use of specific gems to treat specific ailments. It seems that Gem Therapy is almost the same as flower essences. However, the gems can be very pure frequencies (like gold or diamonds), or they can be a nice combination or timbre.

Chromotherapy or Color Therapy - The use of color (usually in the form of colored light) to produce beneficial or healing effects.

I see this treatment as being very similar to Aromatherapy, Bach Flower Remedies, and Gem Therapy in that it focuses on resonating specific frequencies or timbres in the body. It seems a bit different in that certain colors can be extremely pure, which would be more akin to pure frequencies. Some colors are actually a combination of colors, which makes them timbres.

Naturopathic Medicine - Naturopathic physicians work to restore and support the body's own healing abilities using a variety of modalities including nutrition, herbal medicine, homeopathic medicine, and oriental medicine. This primary health-care system emphasizes the curative power of nature, treating both acute and chronic illnesses. It is often about finding specific frequency and timbre remedies to help the body unlock its natural healing response and flow.

Astrology - Astrology is a humanistic attempt at trying to understand the cycles that we share with the forces in the Universe. The planets have corresponding rulership to certain vitamins, minerals, cell salts, herbs, metals, colors and parts of the body. Through the chart, one can look to see what natal health conditions exist. Through these precepts, we can then look at the present and into the future to see what areas of our lives are being affected and potentially how we can head off ill health and promote wellness.

Astrology can be an incredible system to show you the frequencies, timbres and musical flow of your own system. Each planet is a frequency, and the relationships between the planets are timbres. The changing transits are all about flow. The highest astrologers do see the celestial bodies as a flowing system – a perfect mirror of our own system. I have met some astrologers who also bring in energy work, but not many.

Holotropic Breathwork - It is a simple yet powerful technique for self-exploration and healing, based on combined insights from modern consciousness research, depth psychology, and perennial spiritual practices. The method activates non-ordinary states of consciousness, which mobilize the spontaneous healing potential of the psyche. Sustained effective breathing, evocative music, focused energy work and mandala drawing are components of this subjective journey. 'Holotropic' literally means 'moving towards wholeness'.

I really like this system because it focuses so much on flow. The core of the technique is the quality of the flow in the music of the breath. It also reaches higher levels of consciousness, so it is holistically accessing energy flow.

Chiropractic - The chiropractic system views the spine as the backbone of human health: misalignments of the vertebrae caused by poor posture or trauma cause pressure on the spinal nerve roots, leading to diminished function and illness. Through spinal manipulation or adjustment, treatment seeks to analyze and correct these misalignments.

The nice part about chiropractic is that it focuses on getting energy moving through the spine. There are some chiropractors who find the resonant frequency of vertebrae. When resonating, the vertebrae will begin to "float," and an adjustment can be done by barely touching the vertebrae. Sound tables are also really powerful to help relax the muscles around the spine so that an adjustment can be done with very little effort.

I have also known some chiropractors who couple their work with energy healing.

Network Chiropractic - This refers to an association of independent chiropractic offices that use Network Spinal Analysis, a method characterized by the sequential application of a number of gentle, specific adjusting techniques. Care progresses through a series of levels that parallel spinal and quality-of-life changes.

I have performed this technique and it seems to be very focused on getting a wave of energetic musical flow moving up and down the spine. Much of the technique seems to be about being present with this natural flow within the body.

Osteopathic Medicine - Osteopathic physicians provide comprehensive medical care, including preventive medicine, diagnosis, surgery, prescription medications, and hospital referrals. In diagnosis and treatment, they pay particular attention to the joints, bones, muscles, and nerves and are specially trained in osteopathic manipulative treatments that rely on using the hands to help diagnose, treat, and prevent illness. It is very similar to chiropractic therapy in creating flow through the system.

Craniosacral Therapy - This is a manual therapeutic procedure for remedying distortions in the structure and function of the craniosacral mechanism - the brain and spinal cord, the bones of the skull, the sacrum, and interconnected membranes. It is used to treat chronic pain, migraine headaches, TMJ, and a range of other conditions.

As with chiropractic therapy, this system is about removing energetic blockages in the system that interrupt flow – particularly the smooth rhythmical flow of the craniosacral fluids.

Counseling/Psychotherapy - This broad category covers a range of practitioners, from career counselors to psychotherapists who treat depression, stress, addiction, and emotional issues. Formats can vary from individual counseling to group therapy.

This modality is focused primarily on creating flow within the mind. Most of the issues within the mind are about stuckness: dead-end thoughts, incomplete thoughts and emotions, and stressful grating thought processes. A healthy mind and emotional body have good flow, without stress.

Dance/Movement Therapies - Dance and/or movement therapy uses expressive movement as a therapeutic tool for both personal expression and psychological or emotional healing. Practitioners work with people who have physical disabilities, addiction issues, sexual abuse histories, eating disorders, and other concerns. There is nothing more focused on musical flow within the body than dance.

Feng Shui – This is an ancient Chinese practice of arranging the home or work environment to promote health, happiness, and prosperity. Consultants may recommend changes in the surroundings – from color selection to furniture placement – in order to promote a health flow of chi, or vital energy.

It seems that Feng Shui is the essence of all four levels in one's physical environment. Think of the furniture and things in the room as the frequencies, which create an overall timbre in the environment, and so their placement determines the flow of energy. It seems that this system completely connects to all four levels.

Homoeopathy - A medical system that uses infinitesimal doses of natural substances – called remedies – to stimulate a person's immune and defense system. A remedy is individually chosen for a sick person based on its capacity to cause, if given in overdose, physical and psychological symptoms similar to those a patient is experiencing. Common conditions addressed by homeopathy are infant and childhood diseases, infections, fatigue, allergies, and chronic illnesses such as arthritis.

Homeopathy is using specific frequencies or timbres to resonate the particular issue or symptoms so that the body recognizes its imbalance, and therefore kicks in and restores balance. Some homeopathic remedies, known as the "elementals", actually focus on resonating what is right instead of what is wrong in order to induce flow in the body.

Hypnotherapy - A means of bypassing the conscious mind and accessing the subconscious, where suppressed memories, repressed emotions, and forgotten events may remain recorded. Hypnosis may facilitate behavioral, emotional, or attitudinal changes to support such goals as weight loss or smoking cessation. It is also used to treat phobias, stress, and as an adjunct in the treatment of illness.

Hypnotherapy is a unique system that uses just about all levels of vibration. First, it commonly uses frequencies in the theta brainwave range (whether by the practitioners voice or by sound and music) to bring a person into the realm of the subconscious. The practitioner then looks for stuck energy, and creates an alternative resonant flow to replace the stuck system of flow in the mind. As with all work in the mind, flow and stress relief often cause physical symptoms to go away.

Therapeutic Massage – This is a general term for a range of therapeutic approaches that have roots in both Eastern and Western cultures. It involves the practice of manipulating a person's muscles and other soft tissue with the intent of improving a person's well-being or health, and may include, but not be limited to, effleurage, deep tissue, percussion, vibration, and joint movement.

Massage can also access all levels of vibration. First, the way in which the massage practitioner is connected to his or her own soul frequency and is therefore grounded affects the quality of the massage given. This grounded energy comes across as confidence. Second, the quality of the flow that the practitioner creates when moving across the body is critical. A great massage practitioner has a flowing movement similar to a great dancer – therefore, creating flow in the body. Some massage practitioners also use intention and/or run energy through a person's body during the massage, which takes the massage to a whole new level. The quality of the music that is played during the massage can be as effective as the massage itself in creating flowing energy in the body, and energetic flow throughout a person's Soul and Sprit.

Radionics - A therapy that has grown up around the ability of the human being to use radioesthesia together with simple instruments to help in the diagnosis of disease in animals, plants and humans and then to treat the disease at a distance without the presence of the patient.

This technique is basically the same as Sound Healing in that it uses frequencies and timbres to help trigger the body's natural healing response or flow. It uses electromagnetic energy frequencies instead of sound.

Reiki - Practitioners of this ancient Tibetan healing system use light hand placements to channel healing energies to the recipient. While practitioners may vary widely in technique and philosophy, Reiki is commonly used to treat emotional and mental distress as well as chronic and acute physical problems, and to assist the recipient in achieving spiritual focus and clarity. This system is focused primarily on energy, and bringing energetic flow into the body.

Yoga Therapy - Yoga is used to address mental and physical problems by integrating body, mind and movement.

Yoga is completely about creating flowing flexible energy within the body – particularly when in stressful situations or predicaments. It is also about resonating a frequency of stillness and peace. Most yoga brings in the energetics of a Spiritual life. Often yoga also uses sound and music to enhance the energetic and Spiritual aspects.
Music Therapy - Music Therapy is primarily focused on musical components for

healing. It generally does not focus on frequencies. Even though it doesn't get into the structure of the sound or harmonics, music therapy does talk about using specific instruments for certain issues and situations. I would bet that some music therapists secretly do use intention and energy in their work, but traditional music therapy does not focus on these areas.

As mentioned, depending on how it is administered, Sound Healing and Music can focus on **one of the five levels of vibration,** or on all of them.

Again, if you are working within any of these modalities, you might consider expanding the treatment to include all five levels – frequency, timbre, intervals, musical flow and energetic flow. If you are not including energetic flow as part of your healing modality – now is the time!

Now, whenever you come across any healing system you can look at which of the five levels it is addressing – in order to help gauge its possible effectiveness for whatever you might have going on. It is often difficult to decide whether we want to invest the time and energy in embarking on any healing modality – especially since there are so many out there these days. Recommendations are helpful, but you can also look at how holistic the system is at all levels of vibration.

Eco-Systems – Our Planet and Universe
Every living system including the Earth is made of pure frequencies, timbres, music and energy.

There are frequencies everywhere on the earth. The core frequencies are the atoms that create everything. At another higher level there are the timbres of the elements – earth, air, fire and water. All of these timbres are flowing around and through the earth – wind, rivers, streams and ocean, fires, and even movement of the earth's tectonic plates. The quality of the musical flow of the systems on the earth is the key indicator of the health of the environment.

Currently pollution, global warming, and environmental toxins are disrupting the frequencies and timbres that contribute to the nature flow of these systems on the earth.

Then there is the energy of the earth. Some call if "Gaia." It is the living essence of the earth energy. It is the Spirit of the Earth, or the Soul of the Earth as a living entity.

Just as healing a human system requires seeing the trees (frequencies, timbres) and the forest (music and energy) at the same time, so must the ideal modalities for helping to heal our planet be focused on the eco-system from an interrelated perspective. Fortunately, most ecologists do look at the way eco-systems are interrelated. Unfortunately, politicians don't normally look at it this way. They look at how to create a better economy without considering the harm being done to the planet.

The planet is a bit different from the human system in that it always has plenty of food – the sun! Both the Earth and the body have a natural feedback system that naturally heals itself (so to speak). In the body we often think of this as the body's natural healing response. When left alone, the earth does the same. It is only when we inject discordant frequencies into its system that the natural flow gets thrown off. We do this through pollutants, whether physical or emotional. Therefore, the antidotes to help heal the earth might just be the gratitude, compassion, love and joy.

It is interesting to then look at how our planet is a part of a much larger living system – our solar system, and the entire Universe. In this respect, our planet is only one small frequency within a much larger living system. However, some people say that it is a key acupuncture point in the Universe at this time.

Chapter 13 – Volume or Amplitude

Different volumes of sound affect us physically, mentally, emotionally, and Spiritually in dramatically different ways. For the most part, loud sounds are activating, soft sounds are calming – but not always.

Volume is a component of sound that is completely separate from frequency or pitch. They are independent of each other and normally do not affect each other.

Loud Sounds
Loud sounds can be negative or positive. On one hand they can shake us and annoy us tremendously – particularly if we have decided that we don't like the sounds. Some say that loud sounds can even drive the Spirit out of our bodies. On the other hand, strong vibrations can bring us out of depression or help to harmonize a stuck emotion. And for many, loud music can be extremely energizing and fun. In fact, it is just like getting a massage.

Whenever a sound matches the frequency of any part of the body it feeds it energy. If the part of the body is small and fragile – like a cell or kidney stone – loud sounds can cause it to break up. This is much like when a singer breaks a wine glass by matching its frequency and singing very loudly. In fact, if you can find the frequency of a cancer cell, it can easily be exploded with sound – without affecting any of the cells nearby.

Volume is measured in decibels on a scale of 0 – 140. 0 dB is a threshold of hearing. 130 dB is the threshold of pain. 90 dB is the threshold of where we begin to lose our hearing! The sound of a normal rock band is around 100 dB. Dance or Techno music is around 120 dB – although speaker huggers are getting well over 130 dB. A soft whisper is around 10 dB.

Strong bass frequencies can actually transform your whole nervous system into a state of peace. On a sound table, the speakers for the ears can be low, while the table itself vibrates your whole body intensely. This has been proven to help reduce any tension in the body, and has been used with fibromyalgia and Parkinson's. However, such strong vibrations are not helpful for anyone who is having a panic attack.

The only problem is that loud music can also destroy your hearing. Even gongs can get dangerously loud. It is important to be careful and not lay too close to a gong that is being played with full force. Crystal bowls can also be extremely loud when lying next to one. When sitting in front of a crystal bowl, the volume is 1/10th of the volume when lying with your head at the same level. Be careful, the little hairs inside the inner ear don't come back once destroyed.

The Ear
The ear actually has several mechanisms to help dampen down loud volumes. Here is a diagram of the inner ear.

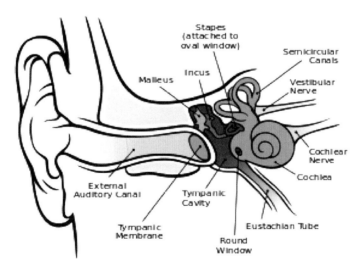

It has 3 bones that we laymen call the hammer (malleus), anvil (incus) and stirrup (stapes). The main function of these 3 bones is to turn the volume down when things get too loud. Whenever we hear a loud sound, the muscles attached to these bones tighten, turning down the volume. This is mainly to protect the fragile hairs within the cochlea or inner ear. If we were to unravel the cochlea it would be about 2 inches long. It has about 23,000 hairs on the inside. When the hairs move they create electricity that is then transmitted to the brain. The interesting thing is that all frequencies are spread across the

23,000 hairs, and each hair essentially picks up only one frequency.

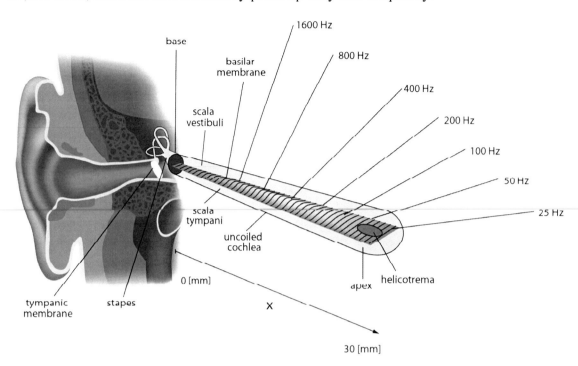

Cochlea with Frequency Spread

If you are at a concert and there is that feedback squeal (when a mic gets too close to the speakers), that one piercing frequency can practically demolish its corresponding hair in the cochlea. If the feedback is loud enough and long enough the hair will eventually die and you are then deaf for the rest of your life at that one frequency.

The hairs that pickup the high frequencies are smaller and more sensitive, so they give out earlier in life. Most people over 40 can't hear above 15,000 hertz – particularly if you played guitar or drums in a live band, or have gone to many raves or techno dance parties.

You must be careful because currently there is no cure or surgery to help fix these little hairs. However, what better modality than sound to help! I predict that within ten years we will have a way to use sound to regenerate these cochlea hairs with sound in order to bring our hearing back.

There is also another mechanism within the ear that actually turns down the volume of irritating sounds. For example, if a parent is constantly whining at a child throughout his or her childhood, the muscles in the child's ear that are connected to the hammer, anvil and stirrup will actually turn down the volume of the whining frequency.

The problem is that we now know that all frequencies are nutrients to our entire system. Therefore, when we move out of the home with the whiners, we are then deficient in those particular frequencies.

This can cause learning disabilities, or even problems with particular organs in the body that thrive on these particular frequencies.

There is a whole field of therapies based on the work of Alfred Tomatis who discovered this ability of the ear to turn down particular frequencies.

Soft Sounds

Just as loud sounds can be positive or negative, so can soft sounds be positive or negative.

A whisper with the right energy can be the most effective healing sound possible. Soft sounds enter our system without the resistance and tension that is created from loud sounds.

However, for someone with bad hearing (most people over 60), soft sounds can create a huge amount of anxiety. When you can't hear a sound clearly or can't hear what is being said, it is very stressful! You might be leading a most beautiful guided meditation while playing a crystal bowl with people lying on the floor, and completely stress people out because they can't hear a word you are saying above the crystal bowl. I must admit that I have come away from many wonderful guided meditations way more stressed out than before. Be careful about speaking too softly in volume; speak so people can hear you.

Envelope or Change in Volume over Time
The envelope of a sound is a map of its change in volume over time.

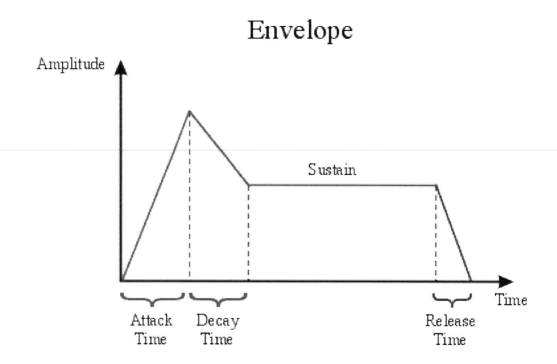

Envelope of a Sound

Sounds that rise in volume really quickly, like most percussion sounds, have been associated with anger. Sounds that rise in volume slowly are associated with love. In fact, the study of "Sentics" by Manfred Klynes has mapped out the full range of emotions based on change in volume of the sound over time. Manfred has even created software that changes the envelope of each sound in a recording in order to create different emotional effects.

Even more important is the envelope of the sound of the breath. A panting breath has an envelope with a very quick and sharp attack, whereas a relaxed breath has a much slower attack and release time. Breathwork specialists say that the different types of breath can activate every single state of consciousness. When you see breath in this way – from a sound perspective – you are given another tool for changing your consciousness.

Slow Fade of a Crystal Bowl

**One of the most powerful and profound components of
sound and music is the slow fade,
where the volume fades out over a long period of time.**

When a sound takes a long time to fade out, as it goes to complete silence, an unusual phenomenon happens. It seems like the sound continues "silently," as if you can still hear the tone in the air. And when you just listen for this sound and keep it going in your head, it leaves you in a place of profound peace.

As mentioned:

**A consistent sound that ends on the home note
is the definition of Peace.**

**And when you add a slow fade…
it seems to keep on humming consistently.**

Technically, there is no such thing as silence. There is always some vibration going on. When the home note continues in the silence in the room one can continue to meditate on it. Normally, for me, meditation has been very difficult; I have had to continually come back to focus as my mind wandered. However, when focused on this home note at the end of a slow fade, meditation became easier. It is so easy to simply hold that frequency in your head – seemingly forever.

If a sound stops abruptly, you are left with a bump – instead of the sound still hanging in the air.

In "silent retreats" I have easily been able to hold that one note peacefully in my mind for over an hour.

The other interesting aspect of this peaceful stillness at the end of the fade is the fact that it is actually very powerful.

For many years I had a booth at Earthdance, a major festival. And, every year, my booth was right in the middle of 4 stages with different bands playing on each of the 4 stages simultaneously. It was the most intense cacophony of noise you could ever imagine. However, we always would have several crystal bowls at our booth and people would be playing them constantly. As they played, the consistency of the sounds created a wonderful peaceful vibration in the middle of this chaos. We would often have a large group of people mesmerized in front of the booth.

Occasionally, I would signal everyone playing the bowls to stop all at once and their sounds would fade out slowly – into the cacophony. However, the amazing thing was that everyone listening would go to that same state of peace and stillness. Even though there was a cacophony around us, we could all hear the sound of the bowls still floating in the air – and the peace and stillness was profound – right there in the middle of the most intense cacophony of 4 overlapping songs playing at once.

This was a major revelation as to the power of a slow fade.

I have found for myself (and for many others I have talked to) that about 15 to 60 seconds after the sound goes to complete silence, I get chills and waves of energy moving through my body – as though I'm getting a download of healing energy.

Since then, I'm always careful to honor the silence at the end of the fade of a crystal bowl or piece of music that ends on the home note.

**In fact,
the best part of sound
is when it ends.**

**Honor the Silence.
It is where the magic is.**

There are many other instruments besides crystal bowls that also do slow fades (but none as slow as crystal bowls): Tibetan bowls, string instruments, and some drums all have the same power. It is actually difficult for the voice to do a slow fade, but it can get pretty close. Even shruti boxes and harmoniums don't fade out slowly, so I prefer to not end a song or chant with them.

You can simulate a slow fade with drums by getting slower and slower in tempo, sparser and sparser in notes, and softer and softer in volume.

In that this induces such a profound state of peace, it is surprising that so many people don't know this simple secret. So often, I hear music that might even be profoundly beautiful and heart opening, only to be left with an abrupt bump at the end – which completely obliterates the peaceful resolution of the slow fade.

Also, the more bass the song or instrument has, and the longer the fade, the more profound the state of peace. When a slow fade happens on a sound table that vibrates your whole body intensely, it seems that every cell in your body continues to resonate with the peace of that last home note, sometimes for hours.

This is vitally important because <u>so many people</u> are unable to go to a state of peace in this chaotic world. Yet, it is so simple.

Finally, when this state of peace is shared in groups (large or small), it connects everyone in the group. Sharing peaceful vibrations together opens our hearts.

SECTION III – FREQUENCIES IN AND AROUND US

Chapter 14 – Music Perception versus Direct Physical Effects

We perceive and receive sound and music in 3 main ways (and in so many other ways that we certainly don't understand yet):

1. The vagus nerve is connected to the eardrum and goes directly to every organ in the body except the spleen. The vagus nerve also goes directly to the heart. In this pathway, sound and music bypass the judgmental brain and directly affect all of the organs.

2. Sound and music also enter our body via the sound waves physically hitting the cells in our body – again, bypassing the wiley brain. Dr. Emoto's work with freezing water has shown this, but the clearest evidence is Cymatic visuals of water being vibrated with sound. Here are different water molecules being vibrated with different frequencies.

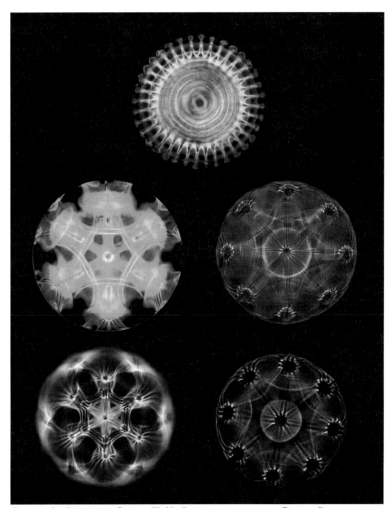

Cymatic images from Erik Larson – www.CymaScope.com

These patterns are actually animated, and are formed in every water droplet in our body whenever any sound hits the body.

3. Sound goes into our ears and is transmitted as electrical impulses into the brain. At this point the brain interprets it as either a positive or negative experience. It then sends information to the rest of the body based on its subjective judgment of whether we like the music or not. A recent research project showed that if we like the music, we get multiple positive physiological responses throughout the body. Our veins open up, our heart functions better, and our nervous system reacts positively. If we don't like the music, we get negative responses. As we know, one person's blissful music is another person's hell.

At the Sound Healing Institute we have feedback equipment to monitor the heart and galvanic skin response (measurement of tension). For our Sound Healing students, relaxing music, crystal bowls or consistent rhythms would totally relax them. Hard rock would certainly not relax them. However, we then hooked up one of our Rock and Roll students who was taking our Audio Recording program. When we played some heavy metal music his heart rate slowed down, and the tension in his system totally relaxed.

What we like is good for us. What we don't like isn't. To a certain extent!

Many people really like sugar. But research clearly shows that it is not good for us (particularly for the liver). However, it is interesting to note that based on the previously mentioned research there is still a positive reaction in our body when we first eat the sugar – simply because we like it. However, if we believe the sugar is bad for us, it is bad for us in two ways – realistically and based on our perception.

Our beliefs are more powerful than reality.

Even if we like music, it could still have a partial negative effect on us if it is innately bad for our organs and cells. However, even if a sound is exactly what we need, if the brain doesn't think so, it will send out its own negative frequency. This negative energy normally overwhelms the innate positive aspect and we ultimately don't get the healing from the sound.

When we hear music as a style that we recognize, our previous experiences and preconceptions of the musical style make a major difference as to how we experience the music based on any biases we might have developed. Sometimes our biases are even based on opinions of others. More often, these judgments are based on previous experiences of listening to the type of music. Most often, the judgments are based on a concept of the music being "too much" one-way or the other. These judgments can easily – and commonly do – result in a negative physiological response.

On the other hand, music can trigger a previous positive response. In a way, sound and music can be timeless. If you have music that reminds you of a time when your heart was completely open and hearing the piece opens up your heart once again in the moment – more power to it and you. If you have music that connects you with Spirit, use this music joyously.

The cool thing about much of the music within the field of Sound Healing is that it often escapes easy categorization. Often, it is so unlike normal music that we have no box to put it into. Perhaps as Sound Healing music becomes more mainstream, the boxes will be built, however currently many people don't know what to think of most Sound Healing music. Therefore, a person's mind does not get in the way. When the judgmental part of the brain is absent, sound travels into the body through two main physical avenues unimpeded – the ear and the brain.

With most Sound Healing we have no idea what to expect. Therefore, the mind remains awake, always waiting for whatever might happen next. Without our normal structure, we are often left with just the sounds. And when we really tune into the messages from the sounds themselves, we go to a deeper level of listening and feeling the music.

Sometimes with Sound Healing, people can't slow their mind down enough to get into the sounds and music that are offered. In fact, they may even feel the music is boring, often because they have become addicted to excitement and always needing something new. When you allow yourself to slow down and sink into the sounds, a whole new world opens up. A world of subtlety that is not boring at all – a world where other realms unveil themselves – a world where the essence of Universal Love and pure light of Spirit is hiding in between the notes.

Your Sound Medicine Cabinet

It is important to categorize your music so you know the best time to pull out a particular album or song. I believe that one of the main reasons people stop listening to music (God forbid) is that they have played the wrong music at the wrong time and had a bad experience. I feel it is important to find the full range of music that you play for a full range of times (of course, silence is also OK for each of these): waking up, getting going, getting out of a rut, sad times, frustrating and angry times, worrisome times, playful times, celebratory times, loyous times, loving times, sacred times, times of loss, going to sleep, making love, meditation and peaceful times.

Start categorizing your music based on what you need at the time in a more detailed manner. Then you can use your sounds and music as your own subtle way of therapy. I say subtle, but the truth is your choice can be the most effective and powerful therapy in the world when the selection is appropriate and the timing is right.

When you add specific sounds to your music collection you have a deeper set of therapies that can be even more effective than the music. So effective that perhaps a disease may disappear. Or, a deep-rooted pattern in your psyche that has been holding you back all of your life, dissolves – never to come back again. Or, your heart opens so fully that it never closes again – and from then on you end up lighting up every person you meet with love. Sound is so powerful, because we are sound beings – we are made of sound and frequency – so almost anything is possible with the law of resonance.

Chapter 15 – So-Called Positive and Negative Sounds

From a higher perspective there are no good or bad frequencies – all frequencies are perfect. They are only frequencies. All is perfect in Heaven and Earth.

On the other hand, there are some sounds that can be detrimental to our health. Therefore, it can be important to be aware of when these sounds are getting to us, and take action to protect ourselves or help transform the so-called "bad" sound itself.

A bad sound is one that creates negative effects on us physically, mentally, emotionally or Spiritually. A good sound is one that does the opposite. As previously mentioned, some sounds may be determined to be good or bad based on our unique individual perception and what we might need or be sensitive to at the time. For example, bad sounds can explode cancer cells or kidney stones. Good sounds can possibly lock us into a rut so that we never expand our consciousness.

Appropriate Action with Sound

The first step in using sound is to see everything as vibration – as it really is! You can then choose to live in harmony with those vibrations or choose to change those vibrations. Sometimes it can be fruitless to try and change the vibrations around you – especially those of other people. However, when you resonate certain positive vibrations and energies, those around you can often change dramatically (based on the laws of resonance). If you can bring to bear the right vibrations while working with others in a therapeutic session, you can certainly help facilitate their healing or transformation.

When you focus these positive vibrations with the intent of changing yourself, the transformation can be dramatic – physically, mentally, emotionally and Spiritually.

The first step is to be aware of the vibrations around and inside you and how they are affecting you. You must also become aware of your own natural vibration so you know when something has affected your energy. This generally means getting to know how you feel when you are at peace, clear and present. In Chapter 41, "Using Sound to Achieve Presence and Mindfulness," I explain several ways to use sound to bring about these states of consciousness.

Once you become familiar with your own home vibration (many of you already are), you can easily detect when an outside vibration has gotten in, and is distracting you from your core, flowing inner peace. As you become aware of your own personal sound landscape, you then have a choice to harmonize or use your own sounds to protect yourself.

There are two types of vibrations – those that break down your system (at any level) and those that feed your system. Many sounds and vibrations are detrimental to our health. They are not in alignment with nature's natural musical flow and they tend to break down our system. Other sounds are completely in alignment with the healing patterns of nature and the Universe and thus they support our health and can even cause positive transformations in our being. The key is to be present enough to recognize the difference. We commonly cruise through our world oblivious to how a particular vibration has affected us. The sounds, music and energy that are detrimental to our health often are those created by technology, engines, and people who themselves are disconnected from nature and Spirit.

If we look a little deeper at so-called "negative" sounds they actually manifest at each of the five levels of vibration: pure frequencies, timbres, music, and energy.

Bad Frequencies
From my perspective I have come to believe there are no "bad" pure frequencies. Perhaps there are certain frequencies that might trigger specific issues in people when they are not ready to deal with them; but I have never seen or heard of this happening. If you have too much of one frequency perhaps you can get out of balance, however this can happen with any frequency.

Technically, if you match the frequency of a cell and then turn up the volume, you can explode that cell. However, normally the volume needed is far beyond the volume that the voice can usually create.

The military has a specific frequency that is called the "brown" frequency because it makes you have to poop. However, even this frequency is not necessarily "negative." Clearing out your digestive system is not necessarily negative at all.

Some say 12 hertz is a frequency from the moon that can make people crazy. But I don't believe that that one frequency by itself will hurt anybody. I really just can't imagine any pure frequency on its own as being negative in any way. However, I leave the door open to learning a deeper truth I may not know yet.

Bad Timbres
On the other hand I do believe there are certain musical intervals and chords that can have extremely detrimental effects.

I believe this is what the military and police are now using as sound cannons.

Certain musical intervals and chords can create binaural beats (Section IX) that can easily cause havoc on certain parts of the body or psyche.

Technically, dissonance is not bad. It is simply activating. However, certain odd harmonic dissonance and annoying timbres can easily trigger a panic attack in someone who happens to be prone to them at the time.

Just as a car horn or the emergency broadcast system tone can grate on someone's nerves, so a screaming electric guitar can do the same to a sensitive person's nervous system.

However, these same timbres or chords can be blissful rock 'n roll to another.

Bad Music

Boy…what a can of worms to dive into, huh? Of course, one person's heavenly music can easily be another's hell.

I do believe there is certain music that can bring you into a down and depressed state with no hope of getting out. This is rare though.

As mentioned, when it comes to Sound Healing music, the focus is on smooth flow and going to the home note often.

Bad Energy

This is one of the most powerful and detrimental of all aspects of vibration by far. Negative or evil intentions can carry with them unusual power.

When any musician brings in dark energy into a song (sometimes done in "death metal") it can be extremely harmful. A similar thing can happen with the sexist, racist and violent energy of some Rap music. I feel it is important to remember that it is not the Rap music itself; it is the energy that the musicians bring to it.

Of course, there are many people in our society that get entrained into negative energies and then pass these energies on. It is also a large part of our language itself.

Bad Noises

At the risk of confusing the term with our previous definition of noise, we are now using the term to refer to sounds that are deleterious to us physically, mentally, emotionally or Spiritually.

Most sounds that we may think of as noise come from the city and technology. Just the sound of a car driving by is unbelievably loud and distracting compared to the common sounds that you would encounter in nature. The sound of a loud motorcycle or siren is not so intense these days because we are so used to them.

Motors also have an oscillation that is not like a pure tone. To hum to the sound of a car is actually difficult because it is not a single tone – it is an oscillating tone – one that goes back and forth between two tones.

Fans are also a huge distraction in our homes. A fan is normally a combination of White Noise and an oscillating frequency. It is not a pure tone. Not only does it entrain us into a certain frequency, it is not perfectly consistent, so it is not consistent with a feeling of peace.

Disruptive noises generally exhibit one of the following characteristics:

1. Two sounds oscillating back and forth from one to another – particularly at an inconsistent rate. This is like a scraping sound.

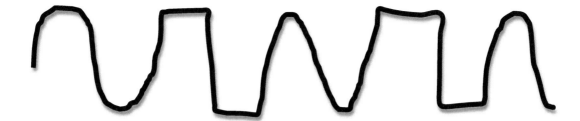

Waveform that is Going Back and Forth between two Sounds

2. Sounds that jump randomly from one sound to another. This resonates chaos. The best example of this is a person whose thoughts are scattered – jumping from one to another. This could be someone else you are around, or your own thoughts.

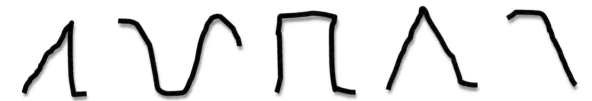

Random Scattered Frequencies

3. Abrupt sounds, such as a door slamming.

4. Multiple sounds at once. Even if the sounds are low in volume we sometimes have to actively tune out the sounds around us. The problem is also that our attention jumps from one sound to the other. If we stop and listen to all of the sounds at once we can often hear an interesting interplay between the sounds. However, when the sounds are louder they can create a cacophony that is difficult to deal with. It's like being on a busy street in the city (New York with all the honking cab drivers is an extreme example). Those who work in noisy factories simply get exhausted from all of the stimulation. Even if you wear headphones the sounds are creating little cymatic patterns in the water of every cell in your body.

5. Sounds that have excessive distortion or dissonance (odd harmonics), especially those that carry the intention to annoy.

6. Sounds that have frequencies in them that don't fit into the normal harmonic structure of sound mathematically.

7. Sounds with random noise injected into them.

8. Sounds that are too loud. Normally this is based on a person's sensitivity. But technically, a sound that is over 90 dB (a police siren driving by you is around 110 dB) for a sustained amount of time is causing ear damage. The best example of this is a jack hammer, motorcycle without a muffler, some loud rock concerts, or a Techno Rave.

Chapter 16 – Frequencies Around Us – Your Sound Environment

"Man's music is seen as a means of restoring the Soul,
as well as confused and discordant bodily afflictions,
to the harmonic proportions that it shares with the world soul of the cosmos."
- Plato (Timaeus) (429-347 BC)

I want to go into a bit more detail about the frequency and energy of sounds around us because they affect us in such dramatic ways. Even if you are completely centered in your own frequency many of these frequencies are so powerful that they can easily affect us in both positive and negative ways.

First, the negative ones:

Electricity
Electricity in our walls is one of the most prominent frequencies in our environment. Even though it is not very loud or strong in intensity, it still affects us dramatically. There was a study done in the United States where they asked people to choose the frequency that felt the most natural to them. Out of a whole range of frequencies over 70% of the people chose 60 hertz. Sixty cycles per second is the frequency of electricity in the walls. They did the same study in Europe and found that over 70% of the people felt that 50 hertz was the most natural frequency. Fifty cycles per second is the frequency of electricity in the walls in Europe. Because this frequency is so consistently present around us we have become entrained to it. Electricity in the walls is not a very strong vibration, but it is always there.

Actually, 50 and 60 cycles are not inherently bad frequencies at all. In fact, they can be quite healing. The problem is that they are not consistent frequencies. Graphically, they might look something like this:

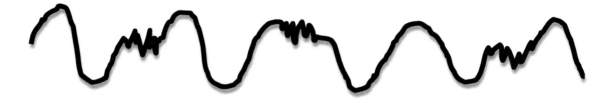

Inconsistent Electricity

Electricity is extremely erratic, jumping around all over the place. It is entraining us into a completely erratic and unstable state. The electricity in Europe is actually more stable. Many people are now using power conditioners to smooth out the frequencies that surround them in the home and office.

Electromagnetism

Electromagnetism is similar to electricity, however it is thousands and thousands of jumbled frequencies filling the air around us. These are much higher frequencies so some feel they don't affect us as much; however we are electromagnetic beings so they definitely still affect us. If we could hear these frequencies we would be driven mad by the overwhelming din of noise.

Dimmers

Besides cell phones, dimmers also affect us drastically – those light switches that turn the lights up and down smoothly. Though they can be quite romantic, dimmers are way worse than cell phones. They put out an incredibly powerful electromagnetic field that will peg out an electromagnetic meter. They can create havoc in our system. If the dimmer is turned all the way up (or down) it is not a problem.

Cell Phones

Cell phones are just another electromagnetic field. Again, there are thousands and thousands of frequencies swarming all around us and inside us. We are inundated with a complete cacophony of chaotic frequencies. However, with cell phones we often hold them up to our head. The unusual aspect is that cell phones use a carrier frequency that is the same as the Schumann resonance, so we are often entrained by this positive frequency. However, this makes us like moths attracted by a flame.

City Noises

City noise is all about inconsistency, which, on one hand, keeps us awake. On the other, it is devastating to our system. It is distracting, shocking, and exhausting at all levels of our system. Most city sounds are breaking down our system.

Other People's Energy

One of the noisiest sounds we encounter throughout the day is the energy of others around us. This mostly comes from the scattered and inconsistent frequencies created by people's thoughts. Often the problem comes with the sound of the resistance to the thoughts and expressions of other people. The sound of resistance is not a nice sound.

You've probably been around a "negative" person and after awhile have found yourself to become negative yourself. If you have ever lived or worked with a strong-willed person you know how easy it is to take on their traits or to be overwhelmed by them. This is so obvious. We all know how a strong-willed or intense person can affect not only one person, but can control an entire group. Hitler was the extreme case of negative resonances entraining a whole society into the same vibration.

Commonly, we also see people righteously upset at the negativity of others. Even though it may seem valid, they are now vibrating at a similar negative vibration.

One of the most difficult frequencies to contend with on the planet is the collective energy of people in fear and anxiety. There is so much on the planet that it has created a powerful resonant field that easily affects us. It happens locally when we come across someone resonating fear, but it also happens globally. It seems that this fear energy is really compacted in the city. Many are so sensitive to this field of energy that they can't even visit the city, much less live here.

Other People's Music
Sometimes we get to listen to music that we have not chosen, and this music might entrain us into a place that we would not prefer.

This can happen when a car drives by with blaring music or an exceedingly booming bass. Or, it can happen when you are with someone who plays something that is just not appropriate for you at the time.

There are also many positive sounds around us that affect us in many profound ways.

The Sun
When it comes to powerful consistent frequencies the sun is one of the most powerful. It is always bringing us life-giving frequencies. There are many sun worshippers that get higher levels of Spiritual energy from the sun. No wonder – if it weren't for the sun, there would be no life on earth at all.

The Earth
The earth is an incredibly powerful sustaining frequency – both in its overall frequency and in the immense complexity of life and beauty on the planet. When you really tune into this amazingly powerful and consistent frequency of the earth it is beyond words. Especially when you realize that our entire body is made up of the earth's materials. We are part of this powerful frequency.

Nature
As part of the earth nature is doing something with frequencies that is way beyond our comprehension. Just like it is difficult to grasp the incredible detail of being a living breathing human with all the harmonious systems working together, the details of how all the sounds in nature affect us is yet to be made clear.

There are nature sounds such as wind, water, fire and even earth movements. However, the world of animal and insect sounds is a complete healing and consciousness-expanding world in itself.

The Schumann Resonance
As previously discussed the Schumann Resonance, around 7.83 hertz, is a frequency resonating in the atmosphere that is entraining every brain on the planet into a brainwave state between theta and alpha. It is has been in the atmosphere since the beginning of time on earth, so much so that it is part of our being and existence. 7.83 hertz is also in our DNA. It has become a very powerful positive frequency for humans. Because it is so much a part of us, we now miss it when it is obscured by the electromagnetism

rampant in our cities.

Other People
When around someone who is really positive, we also get entrained into their energy. Just seeing a person smiling can make us smile. Many people go to see and sit with Spiritual leaders such as the Dahlia Lama, Eckhart Tolle, or Braco who are resonating a really powerful vibration of love and light just so we can get resonated into the same vibration. Many believe Jesus to be the best example of entraining large groups of people into love and light.

Just as people create fear and anxiety fields on the planet, so do they create resonant fields of love. Everyone that is living in their heart, even part time, is contributing to the field. And it is affecting us all, bigtime.

Circadian Rhythms
The spinning of the earth, rotation of the earth around the sun, the movement of the moon, and even the stars all affect us in profound ways that we are not yet completely aware of.

Astrological Frequencies
Of course, these can be positive or negative. They manifest mostly in the relationships (musical intervals and phase relationships) between planets.

Spirit and Source
Spirit and Source are all frequencies in the Universe.

There is no more powerful frequency than Spirit and Source. It is a frequency that has consciousness. When we tap into it, this frequency has the ability to unravel problems and issues in our system at all levels, and bring them into complete harmony.

Chapter 17 – Frequencies Inside Us - The Gene OM of the Human System

"Pythagoras based musical education in the first place on certain melodies and rhythms that exercised a healing, purifying influence on the human actions and passions, restoring 'Pristine Harmony' of the Soul's faculties. He applied the same means to the curing of diseases of both body and mind…"
- Porphyry (233-309AD) 2nd generation disciple of Pythagoras

The body is an unbelievably complex symphony of frequencies. There are over 70 trillion cells in the body but only 210 types of cells. Each cell completes 250,000 reactions per second. There are 206 bones and 640 muscles. The heart beats about 101,000 beats per day and we take around 23,000 breaths. The liver has 500 functions. We create 500 billion new cells per day and have over 100 billion neurons. There are 60 hormones in the endocrine system and your circulation travels 60,000 miles. We have 1,000 thoughts per hour and 80% of them are the same.

The complexity of the symphony in the body is overwhelming. Not only the number of frequencies, but also the relationships of all the frequencies…not to mention the most important aspect of all – the musical and energetic flow through the body.

The good news is that we have charts and charts of frequencies that people have come up with and we have included many of them in the index and provided links to even more detailed lists. However, the bad news is that no one agrees on any one frequency for any part of the body. No one!!!

Additionally, hardly anyone that has posted these frequencies explains in detail how they were derived. Was it clinical research or a psychic? Was it based on research on one person or 1,000's of people? Worst of all, the frequencies might just be part of someone's marketing plan or agenda. Without this information it can be difficult for many people to trust the frequencies.

We need more research. Not that every frequency has to be researched to be valid! For example, there are many miracle stories of healings and transformations from many sources and we don't have a clue how they happened. I certainly don't want to miss out on some powerful techniques just because they haven't been researched and these lists are a good place to start – many miracles have occurred and been documented. However, if we are to bring Sound Healing more into the mainstream, we are going to need proof.

In order to help we are conducting ongoing research at the Sound Institute in San Francisco. Called the "Gene OM Project," this is a major research endeavor to map all the frequencies in the body from cell to soul. It is an open resource project so we will be accepting any research from the field regardless of its source, and all information will be shared freely, as long as the details are provided to the Sound Institute.

We will be placing the research into 3 categories, based on the quality of the research.

1. Clinical Research – This is data that has been collected through quantitative research and is repeatable. We will also share information on the credibility of the research including number of people researched, and quality controls.

2. Not So Clinical Research – This is data collected by means that are not so well accepted by the mainstream. These will include techniques such as Kinesiology (muscle testing), rife boxes, and quantum devices that send signals through the body and "ping" different parts of the body. These techniques often still come up with really useful information.

3. Psychics – Data collected from intuitives and higher beings. We will especially be looking for data that corresponds with other psychics or with any of the other types of

research above.

It is really quite amazing that we really don't know the frequencies within our own human system. We haven't even begun to meet the orchestra players yet.

Some of these frequencies are the same from person to person. We know that certain materials in the body will have consistent resonant frequencies from person to person. For example, the resonant materials of bones should be quite similar. Bones will also have another frequency that resonates higher or lower based on the size of the bone. However, the bone material itself will be consistent based on physics (perhaps there could be slight variations based on ethnic groups or body types). Other materials in the body should also be consistent from person to person, such as muscles, tendons, ligaments, blood, etc. It is actually a simple process to find the resonant frequency of these parts of our system.

However, most of the frequencies will be different from person to person based on the size of the organ or body part and other detailed variables. Nevertheless, we will still be able to define a particular frequency range within which any part of the body will fall.

If you would like to contribute to the "Gene OM" project, please contact David Gibson at 415 777-2486.

Healthy Musical Intervals
Although many of the frequencies will actually be different from person to person, we assume that the relationships between body parts will be the same person-to-person in healthy people. The relationship of one frequency to another is a musical interval. As mentioned, our assumption is that the body is a symphony where every single part is working in perfect harmony with every other part.

For example, we assume that the liver in relation to the heart will have the same relative musical intervals from one healthy person to another healthy person – even though the actual frequencies may vary.
Ultimately, we will have a template of perfect health for the musical relationships between every part of the body. Ideally, once in hand, we can use these musical intervals to resonate the parts of the body back into harmony.

We can then find specific frequency markers in a person and tune the musical intervals to the divine template of perfection that he or she was born with.

These frequencies could be applied in an iPhone or a sophisticated virtual reality system we are working on. Check it out at www.soundhealingcenter.com/inside.html

The whole Gene OM mapping is too complex to include here (and many would be bored by it). The link to the site is www.GeneOM.com

As mentioned our system is unbelievably complex (who designed this anyway?). To give an example, consider the frequencies within the heart.

The heart has 4 resonant chambers, each of which has a resonant frequency based on the distance between the walls of each chamber. The materials of the muscles in the heart also have a resonant frequency. There are even neurons within the heart that have their own frequency. The blood in the heart has its own frequency, and there are cells which have their own particular resonant frequencies. Then, there is the energy of Love that is associated with the heart. There are probably many more frequencies that only a heart specialist might know about. Together, all of them create a particular timbre, or combination of frequencies that make up your particular heart.

However, all in all, the heart has one overall resonant frequency, which is actually **the home note or key of all the frequencies within the heart.** Then, this frequency will have a specific relationship to all the other organs in the body. It will also have a musical interval relationship to the whole cardiovascular system. The overall cardio-vascular system frequency also has a specific musical relationship to all of the other systems in the body: the nervous system, muscular system, endocrine system, lymphatic system, digestive system, etc.

And, it's all in harmony (when it is healthy).

**The basic concept of the GeneOM project is
to focus on what is right, instead of what is wrong.
Then, using the basic laws of resonance,
we resonate each part of the body back into harmony.**

We currently have major funding to get the research project underway. If you know of anyone that has research to share, or would like to help fund the project please let us know. This is major!

Let's now take a little deeper look at each of these parts of the human system.

Of course, if you have a particular issue, or are working on someone with a particular issue you can use this section as reference.

Once we have the frequencies mapped, you could also download a tone generator and use it to find the exact frequency for toning vocally or electronically.

Just imagine if our entire medical system were based on getting all the frequencies in the body back in harmony. The remedies would be more precise and therefore less invasive, with fewer side effects.

Below is a list of 25 aspects for the basic outline of the Gene OM Project information that will be mapped and presented; however, this layout might change as we gather more information from reliable sources. More details can be found in Appendix C online.

In the next chapter, we look at the hierarchy of how music flows through the whole body.

"It struck me recently, that one should really consider the sequence of a protein molecule about to fold into a precise geometric form as a line of melody written in a canon form & so designed by Nature to fold back into itself, creating harmonic chords of interaction consistent with biological function"
- Anfinsen (1916-1995) (Renowned Biochemist/Nobel Prize Winner)

1. Cells – 210 different types
Each of the different types of cells has a very specific resonant frequency. Scientific studies have now discovered and measured the actual frequency of sounds emitted by a cell. In fact, research projects have been done that show that when you apply the resonant frequency of a cell to itself, it triggers the cells natural metabolic process.

Recent studies have shown that cells use sound to communicate with each other instead of electro-chemical reactions.

2. 206 Bones
Bone material has its own specific resonant frequency that we assume is mostly the same between humans (although perhaps even this frequency differs slightly). Perhaps different nationalities might have slightly different bone material frequencies. The bone marrow also has its own frequency. The blood in the bone has its own frequency. And, there is a specific resonant frequency based on the size of the bone. Then there is the overall frequency of a particular bone in a person.

In her book, "The Song of the Spine," June Wieder has found the different frequencies of each vertebra in the spine.

3. 640 Muscles
There is the muscle material (of which, there are many parts to one muscle), the size of the muscle, the blood flowing into the muscle, and the overall muscle frequency.

4. Tendons, Ligaments, Cartilage
There is the home note, overall frequency and relative frequencies of each.

5. Organ Frequencies

- Heart
- Liver
- Kidneys
- Pancreas
- Stomach
- Gall Bladder
- Spleen

6. Endocrine Glands
There is the frequency of the hormone and the frequency of the secretion pulses.
There are 3 chemical types of hormones.
Overall and frequency makeup of each gland
Musical Intervals between glands

- Pineal
- Hypothalamus
- Pituitary
- Thyroid
- Thymus
- Adrenals
- Pancreas
- Testes
- Ovaries

7. Neurons
- Sensory neurons
- Motor neurons
- Interneurons

8. Brain
- Cerebral Cortex
a. Frontal Lobes - Most anterior, right under the forehead.
b. Parietal Lobes - Near the back and top of the head.
c. Occipital Lobes - Most posterior, at the back of the head.
d. Temporal Lobes - Side of head above ears.
- Brain Stem - Deep in Brain, leads to spinal cord.
- Cerebellum - Located at the base of the skull.

9. DNA and Gene Frequencies
It is interesting that our DNA has genes in it that are defined with different combinations of letters – A, C, G, and T – representing the four nucleotide bases of a DNA strand: adenine, cytosine, guanine, and thymine. Of course, each of these nucleotides carries a specific frequency. Also, occasionally more than one of these nucleotides will occupy one spot on a particular section of DNA – creating a timbre or harmonic structure. And, the 2nd strand of DNA has the opposite sequence of frequencies so there are musical intervals at play at every step of the DNA. Since the order of the letters on the DNA is so critical to each individual person, it follows that our DNA strand is simply a song moving up and down the DNA.   Perhaps this particular song is our true Soul song.

It is interesting to note that there are four core frequencies that make up all of the music in the DNA.

10. Acupuncture
Every acupuncture point has a frequency. Also various charts show the note or pitch

associated with each meridian. Because this system is based on good flow through the meridians, once we know the frequencies and notes of each acupuncture point, we can then map out a detailed song as energy flows from one acupuncture point to another. Each meridian is also known to have its own associated frequency.

11. Metabolic Rhythms

It is assumed that all of the rhythms within the body are in synch with each other in a healthy person. It would make no sense for any rhythm in the body to be off from the rest of the rhythms.

Since every rhythm is technically a pitch, then even the pitch of the rhythm must also be in harmony with the other higher frequencies in the body.

- Basic Metabolic Rate - This is the rate or speed at which our cells work. It is controlled by our Endocrine Glands in reaction to our environment, age, and genetic make-up.

- Heart

It is interesting to note that a healthy heart is not necessarily about stability. In fact, a healthy heart goes up and down in tempo quickly in reaction to any stimulus that comes into the body. However, when a person is in a state of heart coherence (gratitude, love, joy, etc.) then the heart will go up and down in tempo precisely to an "s" curve.

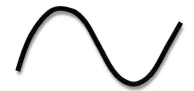

Heart Rate Variability in Coherence

It just so happens that this ideal "s" curve exhibits golden mean ratios.

Also, when in a state of coherence, the heart puts out harmonics that are in golden mean ratios.

The most common healing heart rate tempo seems to be between 40 and 60 beats per minute. However, some people have higher resting rates and can be quite healthy.

- Respiration

23,000 breaths per day.

An average adult breathes 12-20 times per minute. Here are average breath rates by age:

- Newborns: 30-40 breaths per minute
- Under 1 Year: 30-40 breaths per minute
- 1-3 Years: 23-35 breaths per minute
- 3-6 Years: 20-30 breaths per minute
- 6-12 Years: 18-26 breaths per minute
- 12-17 Years: 12-20 breaths per minute
- Adults Over 18: 12–20 breaths per minute.

- Brainwave Rhythms
All rates in cycles per second.

- Deep Delta < .5
- Delta   .5 – 4
- Theta   4 - 8
- Alpha   8 – 12
- Beta   12 – 30
- Gamma   30 - 100

- Cranial Sacral Frequencies
6 to 12 cycles or oscillations per minute

In the disharmonious individual who is out of balance, the craniosacral rhythm might behave like a stormy sea. Areas of tissue restriction will energetically pull and distort the waves, causing the craniosacral rhythm to be upset, uneven, and out of balance. This disharmony adversely affects the entire body.

- Natural Strolling Rhythm
From paying close attention to these rhythms for many years, I've noticed that there seem to be three main rhythms:

1. Walking at a slow pace totally connected to your surroundings – this tempo is our slowest natural walking rate.

2. Walking to get somewhere – this tempo seems to be practically double the natural gate and is the rate that most people walk when on a hike or when focusing on the destination.

3. Running gate – there are probably even different running tempos but there is one main natural rhythm.

- Circadian Rhythms
Technically, you might say Circadian rhythms are rhythms outside our bodies that we are more or less attuned to – particularly, the spinning rhythms of our planet, its rotation around the sun, and the rotation of the moon around the earth. However, in truth Circadian rhythms are not outside of us – we are part of them.

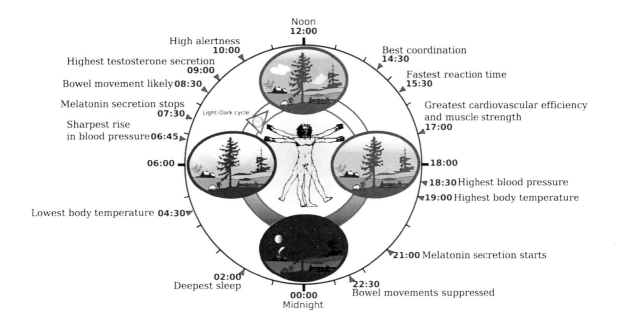

12. Fluid types

    - Water

    - Blood

The different blood types account for the primary differences in the human blood frequency. There are many components within the blood that also have frequencies of their own, including white and red blood cells.

        1) A

        2) O

        3) B

        4) AB

    - Lymphatic

    - Saliva

    - Mucus

    - Gastric Juice

    - Tears

    - Sweat

    - Aqueous and Vitreous Humors of the Eye

    - Cerebrospinal Fluid

    - Semen

    -Vaginal Secretions

13. Body Cavities

Whenever you have an enclosed space there will normally be resonances that are setup based on parallel walls. Sometimes resonances might bounce around 3 or more walls to create the sound. Technically, these resonances are much higher in pitch inside the body because the sound is traveling through water instead of air. The speed of sound is 4 times faster in water than in air.

Technically, there are 3 frequencies in each cavity.

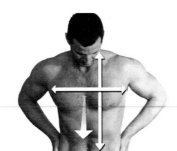

Three resonances in the chest

14. Body Systems
Generally the body systems are all about energetic flow. Each body system is made up of multiple frequencies and timbres that must all work in harmony.
- Circulatory system
- Digestive system
- Endocrine system
- Excretory system
- Integumentary system
- Lymphatic system
- Muscular system
- Nervous system
- Reproductive system
- Respiratory system
- Skeletal system

15. Brainwave Frequencies
The brain vibrates at various frequencies from less than 1 cycle per second to around 70 cycles per second. We look at these frequencies in detail in Section IX. All of the numbers are in cycles per second (cps), which is the same as hertz.

- Deep Delta < .5   Deep meditation
- Delta   .5 – 4   Deep sleep (about 1.5 hours of the night)
- Theta   4 – 8   Dream state (whether asleep or awake). Very creative state.
- Alpha   8 – 12   Relaxed attention
- Beta   12 – 30   Normal day to day thinking and processing.
- Gamma   30 – 100 High state of meditation

It is known that brainwave rhythms synchronize with the heart rhythms when in high emotional states such as love or any type of bliss. It seems obvious that these rhythms would have to also be in harmony with all the other rhythms of the body. We believe that this rhythm is in direct relationship to your Root/Soul frequency.

16. Morphogenetic Frequencies
Science has discovered that there is no way that our brain can control 70 trillion cells and the interactions between them in even the simplest dance move. Not only is the brain not complex enough, the speed that information travels through neurons and the like is too slow to get the messages back and forth from the brain.

Scientists have now discovered non-local brains around each part of the body that actually control that part of the body down to the cellular level. The information about how the body part is to function and move, and the way it communicates with other parts of the body, is all carried in the Morphogenetic field.

This field is described as an informational field. However, when you get right down to it, the information is simply frequencies arranged in very specific geometrical patterns.

Nutri-Energetics is one of the leading companies on the forefront of these studies. There is also a great movie called "The Living Matrix" that interviews all the scientists in this field. I highly recommend it. Go to www.TheLivingMatrixMovie.com

17. Quantum Frequencies
These are frequencies that do not exist in our normal physical world. However, they make up much of the vibrational world we live in. Quantum physics is just now beginning to provide explanations so that the scientific world can embrace this information. Regardless, these frequencies can dramatically affect us physically. Many believe it is in this world that all healing (and raising consciousness) should start.

The biophysicist, Stuart Grace Greene, explains the quantum world as the world of harmonics, whereas our world of 3D reality is the melodic world that requires time to exist.

The physicist Macho Kaki puts it this way:

> "Subatomic Neutrons, Protons, Quarks are musical notes on strands similar to tiny little rubber bands or little violin strings. When the rubber band is twanged, each of the subatomic particles changes from one frequency to another – electron to neutrino. When the rubber band is twanged enough times, it can change into all the subatomic particles you see in the world.

> Therefore, all the subatomic particles in our body are nothing but different notes on many little vibrating strings.

> Physics is the law of harmony among the notes of these vibrating strings. Chemistry is the melody that you can play on these strings. The Universe is thus a symphony of

strings. And the mind of God is cosmic music resonating through 11 dimensional hyperspace."

18. Voice Frequencies

- Key of Your Voice
Every song is in a particular key – every song has one home note. Everyone also speaks in a particular key and their voice has a home note toward which it naturally gravitates.

We can often recognize someone by the key they speak in. If someone were to speak in another key – we wonder what is going on with them.

As we'll discuss later in Chapter 45, "The Sound of Love," most people go to the root frequency of the key of their voice, when in love or when speaking of love.

- Your Natural Toning Frequency
Everyone has a particular note that is the easiest to sing – the one that takes the least amount of energy to produce. Just open your mouth and make a sound with the least amount of energy possible. Don't stretch your vocal cords or mouth – just let it out – as if you are simply breathing the note (sometimes professional singers have more of a problem doing this than anyone). Play with different notes and you will find that there is one that is the easiest to make.

This note is different for different people. This particular note is really important for you, because it is the note that you can tone ("OM" / "AH") the longest without getting tired. It is also a really relaxing and peaceful note for you to sing.

It is also the easiest note to use to practice bringing power through your voice.

- The Notes We Speak and Songs We Sing When We Speak
When we speak we are singing a song. Everyone does it. Every syllable is normally a different note. Some people are extremely expressive with the way they sing each word. Some sing more subdued songs. The songs we sing when we speak say a lot about who we are. It is the number one way we resonate vibrations into the world.

We are all professional singers! Often people come to the Institute and say that they have no musical background and are tone deaf. So I then sing back to them the notes that they just sang while speaking to me. We are all professional singers!

Sometimes this song does get constricted when people sing. Sometimes it does go out of pitch but normally only when we are extremely emotionally distraught or not feeling well.

Some people are very flamboyant singers and go up and down the scale dramatically. Probably the most dramatic word singer of our time was Martin Luther King. His words used musical intervals and melodies that were as inspiring as it gets. On the other hand,

VoiceBio research by Kae Thompson Liu has shown that someone who is on his or her deathbed commonly only sings one note over and over – like a monotone. Certain cultures are more expressive than others and sing melodies that cover the full range of notes available.

It's also interesting to notice the types of music we sing when we are enveloped in certain emotions. There is a whole science to this that is taught in theater classes. We sing completely different melodies when charming someone, when angry, when teaching, when critical, when in love, and when at peace. The key to greater authenticity is learning how to sing songs with your words that correspond to the emotion being expressed. This awareness is especially important when expressing love. However, when mastered, this technique can be abused (politicians are a good example).

The songs that people sing together are even more extraordinary. What duets we sing. In loving relationships, even more important than completing someone's sentence is completing their melody (with the perfect rhythm and timing). You can hear how close two people are, in any type of relationship, by how well they sing together when they are simply speaking.

For the next week pay attention to the songs that you and the people around you are singing when speaking. This is important because once you become aware of the songs you sing with your words, you might find that you would like to sing a different song. Perhaps something sweeter, perhaps something with more power, perhaps with more integrity.

Once you learn how to use your songs effectively, there comes a great responsibility to use your songs with integrity. There are many people (particularly politicians) who use their songs to be manipulative or controlling – or deceitful.
Most important, is to pay attention to the songs you sing when expressing love, affection, or kindness. Listen to yourself, and see if the songs you are singing are in alignment with the emotions you are expressing. Many people have grown up with songs in their voice that barely change when expressing certain emotions. When you really get it down your melodies come from the heart and are totally in alignment with what you are expressing.

Listen to others and learn the songs you would like to be singing. We already do this in huge ways. When in a relationship, especially a friend with whom we spend a lot of time, we commonly pick up their inflections – sometimes our whole speech patterns change; sometimes we pick up a line here or there.

The music we sing with our words is a huge part of the frequency that we send into the world. Adjust this frequency by putting out music that you like.

- The Timbre of the Voice
Of course, the tonality of a person's voice is a huge part of who they are. Again, the tonality is made up of the harmonics in a person's voice. Some say the timbre of your voice is related to the makeup up of the frequencies of your organs – particularly the

strength or weakness of each organ.

- Voice Analysis

There are around a dozen companies that look at the frequencies in your voice and provide an assessment of your system at many different levels. Some programs show weaknesses in organs; some show the balance of your physical, mental, emotional and Spiritual bodies, and some show missing nutrients.

Then these systems suggest you either tone or playback the frequencies that are the weakest (or overly strong) in your voice to create a healthy balance of all the frequencies in your system.

Some voice analysis systems look at the notes you speak; most systems look at the harmonic structure of your voice. The Aspire system by Don Estes also looks at the envelope (change in volume over time) of the sound of your voice, and the sound of your breath!

We discuss the various systems online in Appendix D "Sound Technologies."

19. The Frequency of Words

Words are a heavy thing...they weigh you down.
If birds talked, they couldn't fly.
- Sy Rosen and Christian Williams, Northern Exposure, On Your Own, 1992

Besides the sound of the voice, there are frequencies that are carried in the words we choose to use. These frequencies not only affect others in very deep ways, but also affect the speaker internally. Negative, condescending and judgmental words not only affect others, but they also resonate through our own system. Uplifting, positive words do the same thing.

Not only are your words affecting people and the world around you
(some would say the whole planet),
they are affecting every organ and system within your body.
The words you sing are a huge component of the frequencies
that you are putting into your body –
and therefore affect your health.

Also, of course, our words often come back to haunt us vibrationally as people then treat us differently.

There are many classes I have seen advertised that are now focusing on cleaning up the vibrations of the words we use. For example, "This is killing me," carries a very serious vibration even when one is kidding. Pay attention to the meaning of the words you use because every one of them is putting out a particular vibration into the world.

The Buddhist tradition calls this "Right Speech."

20. Frequencies of Thoughts

Most people's thoughts are simply their own voice speaking silently. Therefore, thoughts normally have the same word music as normal speech. Think about it, or just pay attention to the music of the words in your thoughts. Just like your speech, your thoughts are transmitting frequencies of music into the world, and your whole system.

As with speaking, the intention and information within each thought carries specific harmonic information that affects others and the individual. The frequency of our thoughts is also affected by the quality of words that pass through our mind.

Even more important than the actual thoughts themselves is the rhythm and tempo of the thoughts – ultimately the quality of the flow of the music of your thoughts. If our thoughts are imbued with tension, they can create enormous amounts of stress. If the thoughts do not complete by going to the home note, we are once again left in a state of tension and stress.

It seems there are 3 types of thoughts.

1. Normal thought which occurs in our speaking voice (sometimes in the voice of others).

2. Pure music. We are not thinking, we are simply singing a song in our head. We can also use sound and music to simply replace our thoughts and go into this flowing place of pure music.

3. No thought at all. There are two types: Stressful unsettled silence, and a complete state of inner peace and stillness. Some people also talk of a void, which can be positive or negative. We can also use sound and music to get to this place of "no thought". Listening to or repeating tones, chants and mantras is very helpful, as are sounds that fade out slowly on a home note – which leaves us in a place of profound peace.

We also can go to this place of "no thought" by simple being totally present with all of the vibrations in and around us simultaneously. In this state of perfect presence our thoughts actually become the music of our surroundings.

Some people think that as long as you don't take wrong action, it's okay to have negative thoughts. However, looking at this from a frequency perspective and considering the Law of Resonance, we see that this is completely false. Any vibration is going to affect the vibration of anything close by. Therefore, our negative thoughts seriously affect every bodily function – from the heart to our nervous system, and every organ.

However, the big obvious problem is that most of us have difficulty controlling our thoughts. Often, there is no telling what's going to come streaming through next. It's

107

really important to not go to the negative thought vibration of frustration or guilt over this. Be easy on yourself. Ultimately, however, one aspect of higher consciousness is to hold positive thoughts in your mind as much of the time as possible. The key to this is presence! Simply be as aware as possible of thoughts passing through, and learn different ways to simply and easily change your thoughts whenever you find them resonating bad energy. Sound and music are some of the most powerful ways to change your thoughts. Energy and intention are even more powerful. Two other techniques that are handy are focusing on gratitude and compassion. Both of these carry transformative vibrations – not only to your whole body, but also to the world.

Buddhism calls this "Right Thought."

The rest of the list of frequencies inside us is addressed in later chapters.

21. Frequency of Emotions
There are two types of emotions:

1. Emotions that create distorted and inconsistent vibrations, which break down our physical body and create all types of maladies.

2. Emotions that create completely coherent and consistent vibrations that not only can be healing, but also can take us into higher realms of consciousness.

We explore these in detail in Chapter 44, "Resonating Higher Emotions with Sound."

22. Frequency of Chakras
Each chakra has a frequency, timbre, music, and energy that people have associated with it since the beginning of time. We explore these in detail in Chapter 42, "Harmonizing Chakras with Sound."

23. Frequency of Auras
Even Auras have been associated with specific frequencies. We explore these also in Chapter 43, "Harmonizing Auras with Sound".

24. Frequency of Your Soul or Signature Frequency
Your Soul frequency is explored in detail in Chapter 46, "Connecting to the Soul with Sound".

25. Frequency of Vitamins and Minerals
It is now known that you can use frequency to create all of the vitamins and minerals out of thin air. We explore these frequencies in Chapter 30, "Using Sound to Create Nutrients".

Chapter 18 – The Hierarchy of Frequencies in the Human System

The key question when looking at frequencies in the body is "What is the hierarchy of sounds?" The assumption here is that not only are all the frequencies relating to each other, but also certain frequencies affect other frequencies more. It often means that energy will flow in a certain direction based on the order of the frequencies. It is our guess that there are specific musical progressions that Source likes to take – and these are commonly found in nature as well as the body. In other words, energy flows from one note to the other using very specific intervals.

Within the Gene OM project we are asking for papers on this hierarchy to get various systems that can be tested. Here is my theory:

I believe it all begins with the Soul. The frequency of the Soul is the home note that every other frequency in the body is based on. It is the "key" of the whole human system at all levels.

Next are the auras, which are all in harmonic relation to the Soul note. In fact, Barbara Brennan talks about the 7th aura (Ketheric Template) as being the Soul or higher self, and this the divine template for the whole system. The frequency of the 7 chakras are then in relation the frequency of each of the 7 Auras. The frequency that activates each of the endocrine glands is directly triggered by the frequencies of each of the chakras. The frequency of each endocrine gland directly affects the organs in two ways: with hormones and with energy. From there the organs go to all of the cells in very complex ways.

Here is a beginning diagram of the hierarchy:

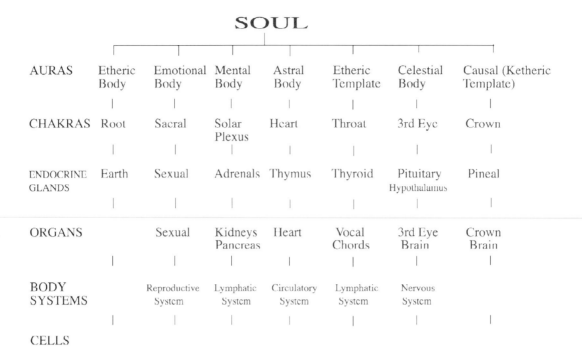

				SOUL			
AURAS	Etheric Body	Emotional Body	Mental Body	Astral Body	Etheric Template	Celestial Body	Causal (Ketheric Template)
CHAKRAS	Root	Sacral	Solar Plexus	Heart	Throat	3rd Eye	Crown
ENDOCRINE GLANDS	Earth	Sexual	Adrenals	Thymus	Thyroid	Pituitary Hypothalamus	Pineal
ORGANS		Sexual	Kidneys Pancreas	Heart	Vocal Chords	3rd Eye Brain	Crown Brain
BODY SYSTEMS		Reproductive System	Lymphatic System	Circulatory System	Lymphatic System	Nervous System	
CELLS							

Once we have the flow of energy through the system mapped out,
we will be able to track down the root cause of any illness
and know precisely where to apply the sound to heal or harmonize the issue.

SECTION IV – How It All works

"Reality is an illusion,
but it is a really persistent one."
- Albert Einstein

Chapter 19 – The Laws of Resonance and Entrainment – The Keys to Creating Change

Only by observing and absorbing the true nature of things –
by apprehending the rhythms and cycles that guide all creation –
can we discover the laws that apply to our own individual lives.
- I Ching

When we understand the basic laws of resonance, we can work with the laws of nature instead of against them, in order to manifest what we want and what the world needs. If our intention is strong enough and pure enough, it can overcome the laws of physical reality and amazing changes and healing can take place. When we are in complete alignment with how it all works, we get extra help, and our Sound Healing tools work better.

Many people, if they don't understand how something works, often won't believe that it works. If you don't believe something will work, chances are it won't. If you do believe it will work, chances are it will. This can be the case for both you and the patient or client.

Also, understanding how things work helps us to get the masses on the bandwagon of changing our whole medical system so that we can get sound and energy healing into hospitals and homes, and take back our power to heal ourselves and others.

All of the laws of resonance in this chapter come from physics.
They are based on proven science.

Resonance
Resonance is the ability of one thing to cause another thing to vibrate. It is not only the basis for making changes in your life, it is how we feel and merge with higher energies of nature and Spirit.

Entrainment is when one rhythm causes another to synchronize. However, many people use the term entrainment to mean resonance.

Based on physics there are many laws of resonance that affect us physically, mentally, emotionally and Spiritually.

First, here is the outline:

1. Resonant Frequency - Everything vibrates at its own natural frequency

2. Resonant Fields - Two objects that have the same resonant frequency create a Resonant Field

3. Resonant Dominance - A stronger vibration will overcome and entrain a weaker vibration into the same vibration as the stronger.

4. Transformative Resonance - A stronger vibration can actually transform the resonant frequency of an object so that its resonant frequency becomes that of the stronger vibration.

5. A Consistent Vibration is More Powerful - The more consistent a vibration without distortion or distraction, the more powerful it is.

Now let's look at each of these laws of resonance in more detail:

1. Resonant Frequencies - Everything vibrates at its own natural frequency

Resonance was discovered by Galileo Galilei
with his investigations of pendulums beginning in 1602.

First, everything in the Universe is vibrating, and I mean everything – from physical matter to thoughts, emotions, and consciousness. Science has proven this and we seem to know this intuitively. But more importantly, everything in the Universe has a frequency that it naturally wants to vibrate at. This is true for a rock, a cell, an organ, an entire body, a state of consciousness, and even our Soul, Spirit and Source. Basically, everything in the Universe has its own note to sing, and it is naturally vibrating at its own particular frequency. In fact, this is what makes the particular object what it is!

The interesting thing is that the resonance frequency of something actually stores energy in that object, and when you match its resonant frequency it releases this energy.

This is the most basic component of how Sound Healing works.

When you hit the resonant frequency of something it releases this energy. Your body naturally uses this energy for the healing process. This is what people refer to as the body's natural healing response. In the case of a cell, it simply feeds the cell energy. In fact, scientific experiments have shown that when you play the resonant frequency of a cell, it triggers the cell's metabolism.

Every single organ in the body also has a resonant frequency. When you resonate that frequency, you are not only releasing stored healing energy, you are giving that part of the body a massage. This is especially effective in muscles. When you find their resonant frequency they naturally begin to relax.

This is a perfect example of resonating what is "right" in something. In the body, it is normally a matter of finding the resonant frequency of a healthy part of the body, then helping it to return to this natural healthy vibration. Often sickness and disease are a result of some part of the body becoming out of tune, or distorted, or distracted from its own natural frequency. Resonating its natural frequency helps retune the body part to its natural state of health.

In the quantum realm of thought forms, feelings, emotions and energy, resonance works exactly the same. Resonating the energy of an emotion like love amplifies it. But even more powerful is when you make the sound of love. It makes the emotion much stronger.

Each thought form resonates a frequency. The Buddhists speak of "Right Thought" knowing that there is a frequency that is emitted from every thought. Not only are your thoughts resonating out into the world (even when not expressed), but also they are resonating through your whole body.

There are also resonant frequencies for each of the emotions – good or bad. When we find their actual frequencies, it amplifies their energy dramatically. There are resonances for fear, anger, worry, and even depression. On the other hand, there are resonant frequencies for gratitude, joy, love, compassion and Spirit. Some believe there are archetypal frequencies for these higher emotions. Some believe that we each have our own personal resonant frequency for each. The key is that if you can associate a sound or frequency with each of these emotions, you can then use that sound or frequency to invoke that emotion at will. We already commonly do this with music. If we want to be happy, we play a happy song.

At the quantum level of energy each chakra has its own resonant frequency. Because everything has a resonating frequency, each Aura must also have its own natural frequency.

When you resonate your own home note or the frequency of your soul, you return to your own innate frequency – a place of perfect peace and harmony throughout your whole system. When you are in touch with your core frequency you are also perfectly present.

Resonance at the quantum level is still being explored, researched and understood. One of the basic concepts is that whenever there is a resonant frequency within us that matches a resonant frequency in another we are "entangled." In the beginning before the big bang, everything was one resonant frequency. So in a way, we are still all one. Science has proven without a doubt that once something is entangled, when you change one component it affects all the other resonant components across the Universe (in real time with no delay). Therefore, you could say that resonance accounts for the fact that we are all one!!!

To find the frequency of something and to resonate at the same vibration is the basis of connecting to anything. At its most profound level, this is love.

On the other hand, oddly enough – resonance can be used as a weapon. If you find the resonant frequency of a cell and turn the volume up loud enough, you can explode the cell. Such power can be used for negative purposes as the military does, but it can also be used to break up stuck energy and blockages in the body. As mentioned, this is how ultrasound works to destroy kidney stones, and how cancer cells can be destroyed with sound.

How to Find the Resonant Frequency of Something
In order to learn how to find the resonant frequency of something it is important to understand how resonance works.

There are 3 main types of resonance:
1. Resonance in Spaces
2. Resonance in Materials
3. Resonance in the Quantum world (thoughts, emotions, intention, Spirit, etc.)

Resonance in Spaces (Acoustic Resonance)
Every space has its own natural resonant frequency. This includes spaces within rooms (including temples and pyramids), spaces in hollow instruments, and spaces within body cavities and organs.

Resonance in spaces happen when the wavelength of a sound equals the distance between two parallel walls. So let's look at what a wavelength of sound is.

Wavelength is simply the physical length of a wave traveling through the air. The wave-length of waves in the ocean is the distance from one peak to the next peak. In the air, sound waves are made of compressed air and spaced out air.

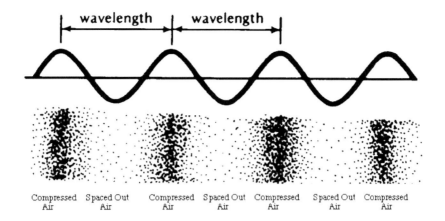

Compressed Air and Spaced Out (Rarefied) Air

Therefore, the wavelength is the distance from one area of compressed air to another.

The compressed air is created when a speaker pushes out. The spaced out air is created when the speaker pulls in.

If you have 100 cycles per second (also called hertz) that means that the speaker is going in and out 100 times per second. Every time the speaker pushes out it compresses the air so it is denser than normal air (higher air pressure). Every time the speaker pulls in it generates spaced out air. This fact is not completely intuitive. Imagine pushing the water in the tub. It then creates a wave peak. When you pull your hand back, the water doesn't come back – instead, it creates a trough. The same thing happens in the air. The speaker pulls back and creates spaced out air.

Therefore, if the speaker is going in and out 100 times per second you will get 100 sets of compressed air and spaced out air per second – traveling through the air at the speed of sound.

Now, the higher the frequency – that is, the more times the speaker goes in and out per second – the smaller the wavelength of the sound. The lower the frequency, the longer the wavelength of the sound.

At the risk of triggering trauma from math class…here is the formula.

Wavelength = $\dfrac{\text{The Speed of Sound}}{\text{Distance Between Two Parallel Walls}}$

The Speed of Sound is 1130 feet per second.

At 100 cycles per second (speaker going in and out 100 times per second) we get:

$$11.3 \text{ ft.} = \frac{1130}{100}$$

That means that we have 5.65 feet of compressed air when the speaker pushes out, and 5.65 feet of spaced out air when the speaker pulls back in. The complete waveform is 11.3 feet.

Now play (or sing) a frequency of 100 hertz in a room with two parallel walls that are 11.3 feet across…Voila, we have resonance – and we hear that one frequency gets louder.

This is the essence of what resonance does – it makes that one particular frequency louder in volume.

At 1 cycle per second the wavelength is 1130 feet. This is big enough to knock down a building, break a wine glass, or easily break up a cancer cell.

The lowest frequency we can hear is 20 cycles per second, which is 56 feet in length (28 feet of compressed air, 28 feet of spaced out air traveling through the room at 770 mph).

At 1000 hertz (about the highest note we can sing), our vocal cords are going in and out 1000 times per second creating a wavelength of 1.13 feet. That's 6 inches of compressed air, and 6 inches of spaced out air.

The highest frequency we can hear is 20,000 cycles per second, which is .565 feet (about ½ inch). At 20,000 hertz the speaker is going in and out 20,000 times per second, and our eardrum is going in and out 20,000 times per second. Not only that, every water droplet in our body is creating a dancing cymatic pattern based on this frequency.

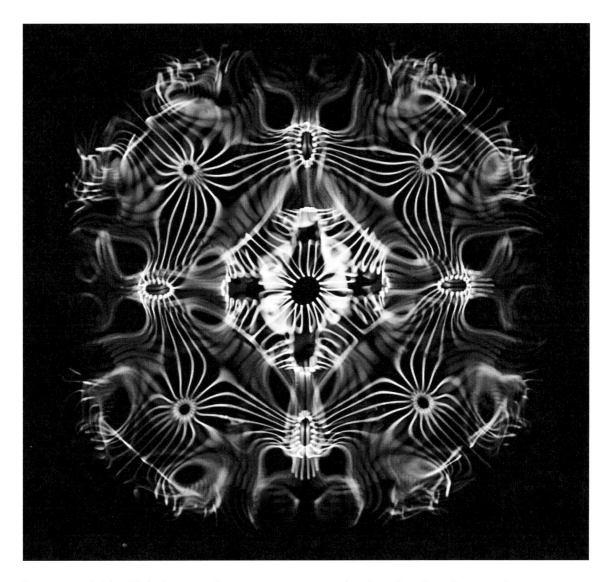

Because of this, high frequencies are way more activating than low frequencies.

Below is a photograph of a 2000 hertz wavelength traveling through the air (done with smoke and lasers). Notice the wavelength is about 6 inches long from one white section (compressed air) to the next.

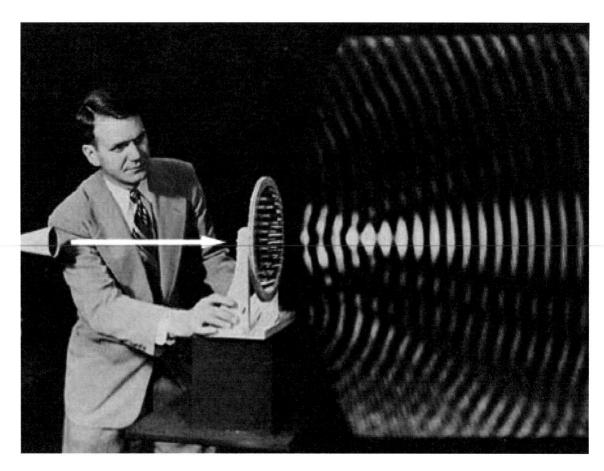

2000 hertz

The full range of wavelengths ranges from 56 feet long to about ½ inch. This means that low frequencies are <u>huge</u> physical waves traveling through the air. High frequencies are little tiny waves.

Thanks for hanging in there.

Now...here's the importance of all this.

Any instrument that has a hollow space uses that space to help create each note of the instrument. This is particularly true in the wind instruments (voice, flute, clarinet, saxophone, tuba, etc.). When you resonate the frequency of certain rooms in temples and pyramids you can be transported into higher states of consciousness. You can also resonate chambers in the body such chest, head, or heart for health purposes. You can actually resonate the spaces within any organ to help massage it into a healthy state. You can even resonate the aorta as though it were a flute. When you resonate these cavities you are feeding energy to that part of the body or organ. You are also giving it an internal massage, which helps it to relax.

Technically, you can find these resonant frequencies by measuring the distance between the two parallel walls. Here's the formula for that:

$$\text{Frequency} = \frac{1130}{\text{Distance between the walls in feet}}$$

This might be helpful if you are creating a specific healing technology, or if you are designing a room to resonate at a specific frequency or note.

However you can also find this frequency of a space by doing a frequency sweep.

You may have experienced this in the shower. When you sing certain notes they are way louder than others – because you just so happened to have hit the resonant frequency of your shower – based on the distance between the walls of the shower.

To find the resonant frequency of your shower do a frequency sweep like the sound of a siren. Using your voice, sweep smoothly from the lowest frequency you can make up to the highest frequency, then back down again. While sweeping with your voice, listen closely for the sound getting louder. In the shower, it will get <u>really</u> loud when you hit it. If you don't notice it, move to a corner of your shower (if you have a shower curtain it won't work…you must have two shiny parallel walls). When you hear it, zone in on it! Go up and down in pitch ever so slightly until you get right on it. The sound will then be unbelievably loud. So loud, it can take you out of your body (and into higher states of consciousness).

Stop reading now and go get in your shower and try it.

This is resonance in a space. It makes the one frequency that is equal to the distance between two parallel walls louder. Your voice is triggering the resonant frequency of your shower.

You can also easily find the resonant frequency of your chest cavity. Put your hand on your chest and do the frequency sweep up and down until you find the frequency that vibrates your chest the most – you will be able to feel it in your hand. Again, zone in on the frequency by going up and down in pitch ever so slightly until you have your chest cavity resonating intensely.

You have now found the resonant frequency of your shower and chest. These are the frequencies that each naturally wants to vibrate at.

Now let's play a little more.

Put your hands on your neck.

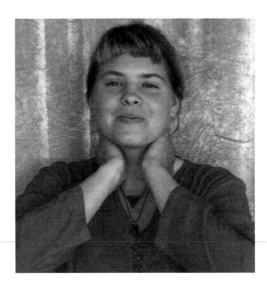

Now do a frequency sweep to find the resonant frequency of your neck. Again, zone in on it so you feel your whole neck vibrating intensely (you may notice multiple frequencies).

Now, put your fingers in your ears (this one is the most intense of all). Again, do a frequency sweep until you find the resonant frequency of your skull cavity. As you will see, it is unbelievably loud.

Now, one more test. Put your hand on your heart. The heart has four chambers that are all about the same size. Do a frequency sweep until you find the frequency of these four chambers in your heart! This one is much more difficult because it is quite hard to feel these small chambers resonating in your hand. You almost have to do it intuitively. Again, zone in on the frequency until you seem to feel your heart vibrating. Don't feel bad if you can't find it. But know that with practice you can find it quite easily. Just about everyone in our classes gets to this point by the end of the semester.

You can now use this technique for any organ in your body. And remember, when you vibrate an organ you are giving it more energy physically, and you are also giving it a massage – both of which are really healthy for the organ.

You can also use this technique on the Endocrine Glands. Endocrine Glands are especially responsive to resonances. When you hit the frequency of an endocrine gland it can trigger the release of its particular hormone. However, even more importantly, it triggers the energy that is associated with that gland – for example, the thymus is associated with Universal Love, the pineal gland with a direct connection to Spirit. We'll be exploring the endocrine glands and their associated chakras in detail in Chapter 42, "Harmonizing Chakras with Sound."

There are actually 3 resonances in a room: left to right, front to back, and ceiling to floor. These 3 resonant frequencies create a musical chord.

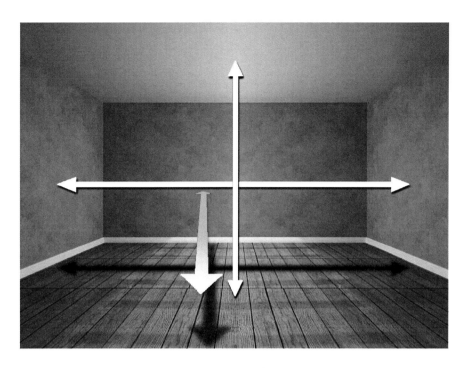

Three Resonances in a Room

Some chords created by rooms are harmonious. Others are dissonant and annoying. The quality of the chord created by the resonances in a room drastically affects the energy of the room. You've probably noticed that certain rooms have a really nice "feel" to them, while others seem a little strange. Sound Healing architects are now creating rooms in buildings that create very harmonious chords.

Even more interesting is that certain ancient temples and rooms in pyramids have been designed so that the three sets of walls create a resonant chord which then takes you into higher states of consciousness – particularly when you tone the notes of the chord while in the room. I know many people (including myself) who have had amazing experiences where after toning the notes of the room the ceiling opens up and love and light pour into the heart. Normally it takes around 15 to 45 minutes of toning for such experiences to happen. Oh my God!

It is well known that the King's Chamber in the Great Pyramid in Egypt has a resonant chord that can open portals to higher states of consciousness and other dimensions. Various people say that the low frequencies of the male voice are the best for opening the portals; however, I have seen female voices open the portals also. When I was there I was able to easily find these resonant frequencies with a simple frequency sweep.

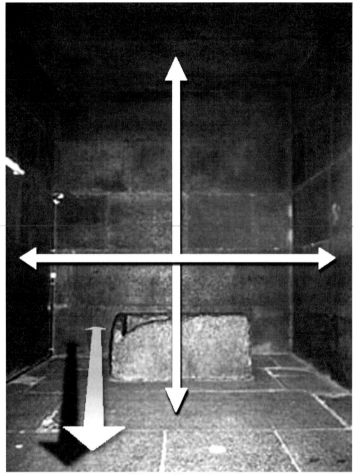

Kings Chamber

But what is even more amazing is the resonant frequency of the cement sarcophagus in the chamber.

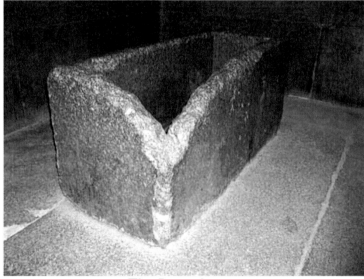

The Sarcophagus

When I hit the resonant frequency of the sarcophagus it rang as if a humongous bell was lighting up the whole room. I then lay inside the sarcophagus and toned its resonant frequency – and immediately went out of my body into the akashic records beneath the pyramid. Energy (and information) came up from below the pyramid and poured through my whole spine. I have never been the same since!

Of course, it also follows that each of the chambers and organs within the body also normally has 3 resonant frequencies that are creating a specific musical chord. As we'll discuss later, this chord or timbre is even more important than the overall frequency of the organ or part of the body.

While in Egypt I also made another resonance discovery. Most of the temples in Egypt have images carved into the walls – often thousands of them. While toning in the temples it occurred to me that these reliefs make the distance between the walls vary. Therefore, when you tone in one of these rooms the information from the reliefs on the walls break up the sound waves bouncing off the walls and the information goes directly into your body (and the water within each cell of your body). Toning in these temples literally resonates the carvings on the walls into your body!

John Reid got some interesting results when his team stretched a thin cloth over the sarcophagus in the Kings Chamber and used a tone generator to vibrate powder on the cloth. In his book, "Egyptian Sonics" he explains how the hieroglyphs formed in the powder that lay on top of the cloth when they hit the resonant frequency of the sarcophagus!

If interested, you can actually figure out the resonant chord of your own room. Measure the distance between the walls and divide the number of feet into 1130. Then look up the notes that correspond to the frequencies in the online chart Appendix B, "Frequency to Pitch Charts."

Resonance in Materials (Mechanical Resonances)
Besides spaces, materials also have resonant frequencies. The materials in bones, tendons, ligaments, blood, nerves, and skin all have specific resonant frequencies. Therefore, an organ not only resonates based on the size of its chamber, but also on the material in the organ. In the heart, not only is there a resonant frequency for each of its 4 chambers, but the muscles also have their own resonant frequencies. Even the blood in the heart has its own resonant frequency. Still, the heart has one overall frequency, which is its home note – and all the other frequencies in the heart are in direct harmonious relation to this home note.

In instruments, strings (as on a guitar, violin or piano) and drumheads are examples of resonant materials. In a violin, there is a resonance in the hollow body and a resonance in the wood that makes up the instrument. However, the most important resonating material is the strings.

In the voice, the primary resonant frequency comes from the material of the vocal cords. However, all of the chambers of the throat, mouth, nose, head cavity and chest cavity also affect this core resonance.

Different materials have drastically different resonant frequencies. Wood, metal, air, fire, and water all vibrate at different frequencies. This accounts for the difference in sound between metal and wooden flutes. The resonant frequencies of different materials have also been correlated to different parts of the body and different chakras (as we'll discuss later).

Technically, the resonant frequency of a material is a function of the size of the object, the tension, the thickness, and the density. Muscles make the vocal chords more or less taut to create different frequencies.

The pitch or frequency of an instrument varies:

- Inversely with the length (double the length, half the frequency)
- Directly with the square root of the tension (9 times the tension, 3 times the frequency)
- Inversely with the thickness
- Inversely with the square root of the density

It is interesting that the resonant frequency of a crystal bowl is based more on the material than the space. The resonant frequencies of both crystal bowls and Tibetan bowls are based on the thickness of the glass (or metal) instead of the size of the space in the bowl.

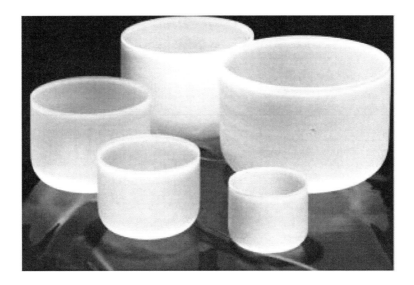

Set of Crystal Bowls

This explains why you can actually buy a particular size of bowl tuned to any specific note you like! For example, you can buy a 14" bowl in any of the 12 keys (C-B), because its note is totally based on the thickness of the glass.

If you pour water into the bowl, the pitch goes down. You would expect the pitch to go up as the space in the bowl gets smaller. However, because the pitch is based on the thickness of the bowl's material, the water contributes to a greater thickness, making the pitch go down. The same thing happens with a wine glass. The more water you pour into the glass, the lower the pitch. It is not the size of the space that determines the frequency; it is more the amount of mass (thickness).

There is also the resonance of cells and atoms. Research has found that each cell actually has its own resonant frequency that can be picked up with an extremely sensitive microphone. As mentioned, if you resonate the frequency of a cell it opens up that cell to receive energy. If you can find the resonant frequency of a particular cell for a specific disease, you can then turn the volume up and explode the cell (much like breaking a wine glass).

Both John Reid and Fabien Maman have demonstrated how to find the resonant frequency of a diseased cell, and by turning up a sound that matches the frequency you are able to explode the disruptive cell. None of the other cells in the body are affected because they don't match the resonant frequency of the sound being transmitted.

Research cited in Lynne McTaggart's book, "The Field has now shown that cells communicate with each other by sound, instead of through electromagnetic and chemical reactions.

Understanding the different types of resonances in the body (acoustic and mechanical) becomes really important later when we discuss how to vibrate them with instruments and with the voice in order to break up stuck energies or resonate higher vibrations.

Quantum Resonances
Then we have resonance in the ether (for lack of a better term). Technically this should be referred to as resonances in the quantum field. We're talking about resonances of thoughts, emotions, intention, and higher energies of Soul, Spirit and Source.

It is not exactly clear what the physics are of these types of resonances. Alice Bailey says that when we find the matter that makes up Chakras there will be a major shift in the science of Spirit. Scientists do talk about the resonances in chemical reactions and electromagnetic processes when thoughts and emotions occur, but there is little talk of the thought or emotion having its own frequency.

Science tells us that everything in the Universe is vibration, so it makes sense that thoughts, emotions and even Spirit have resonant frequencies.

The most important resonance in the quantum field is that of intention. It has been proven over and over scientifically that intention does affect matter – and one's health. (See Lynne McTaggart's book, "The Intention Experiment" for details of the scientific experiments.)

Again, it is all frequency – high or low.

2. Resonant Fields

You can often trigger something's resonance by feeding it energy. For example, if you hit a bowl (crystal or Tibetan) with a wand or stick, it will sing out at its own resonant frequency.

Of course, this is not the case with everything. If you hit a person, they don't vibrate at their own natural frequency.

If you sing or play a note at the resonant frequency of something you can get it to sing its note, so to speak.

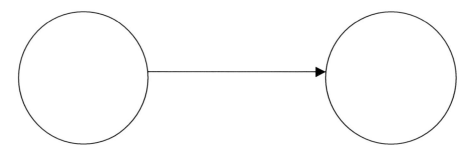

You can generally sing into an acoustic guitar and some of the strings will start vibrating – that is, if you happen to sing the same note that the string is already tuned to. You can do the same with a wine glass.

Another example of this type of resonance is that whenever we hear a word, our brain searches its database for a word that resonates the exact same structure or frequency. This is how we understand things. The same process happens when we see anything. When we see a car, our brain searches its database and looks for resonances that match a car. We then recognize it as a car. Of course, this happens at a speed faster than light.

However, the most amazing thing of all is when two things naturally have the same resonant frequency. Then, they both trigger each other.

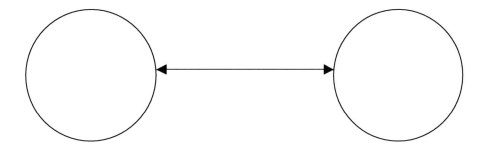

Then the most amazing thing happens – they actually create a field of energy around the two of them that is greater than the two of them resonating separately.   It's called a "resonant field."

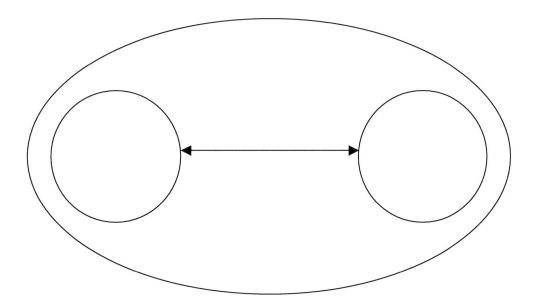

The best example is that of love. One loves another and the love is returned in a beautiful circle of love. This resonant field then creates an entire energy field around the two. You can feel it when people are in love…it lights up the whole room. You also feel it when you are in love; it seems that there is a bubble of love surrounding the two of you wherever you go. It affects everything around you – not to mention every cell in your body.

Another good example is when two people have the same resonant frequency or Soul frequency. There is an instant chemistry (for better or worse).

Furthermore, the more objects or people you have at the same frequency, the stronger the resonant field.

When more than two objects vibrate together in a resonant field the effect can be incredibly powerful. The best example is when a small group of people resonate a higher emotion like love. However, when an entire audience comes into complete harmony with each other at a concert the effect can be huge. Ultimately, when a large number of people on the planet are all resonating love and light at the same time, the field is overwhelming.

3. Resonant Dominance - A strong vibration will overcome and entrain a weaker vibration into the same vibration as the stronger.

This is the ability of one vibration to change another vibration and is the key engine for change and transformation in the Universe – whether physically, mentally, emotionally or Spiritually. And, the stronger the resonant field, the more powerful the effect.

This manifests in both positive and negative ways.

Negative resonances are one of the biggest problems we have to contend with day to day. There are many so-called "negative" vibrations around us that entrain us into their frequency. Electricity, cell phones, noise of the city, and even other people's frequencies (vibes, voices, thoughts, movements) are constantly interrupting our consistency.

We are commonly entrained into so-called "negative" vibrations from people – particularly those that are scattered and inconsistent.

If you have ever lived or worked with a strong-willed person who has a less-than-high vibration, you often find yourself being entrained into his or her energy. You might find yourself becoming negative (if only negative over their negativity). Sometimes you even start taking on some of their speech patterns or behavioral ticks. We all know how a strong-willed or intense person can affect not only one person, but can control an entire group. Hitler was the extreme case of negative resonances entraining a whole society into the same vibration.

Electricity is another perfect example. They did a study in the United States and asked people, "What is the most natural frequency for you?" They played the full range of frequencies and over 70% of the people said that 60 hertz was their favorite. Sixty hertz is the frequency of electricity in our walls! They did the same study in Europe and again played the full range of frequencies. Over 70% said the 50 hertz was their favorite. Fifty hertz is the frequency of electricity in the walls in Europe.

Electricity is not loud, but it is consistently present around us all the time.

**Consistency is as powerful
as a loud volume,
probably even more powerful.**

Actually, the frequencies of 50 and 60 hertz are not bad frequencies – they can be very healing. However, the problem is that electricity is not stable or consistent. It is extremely erratic, jumping around all over the place. It is entraining us into a completely erratic state. The electricity in Europe is actually more stable. Many people are now using power conditioners to smooth out the frequencies that surround them at home and in the office.

Sounds from technology including automobiles and fans can easily entrain us into an inconsistent vibration. One of the biggest culprits in the home is the refrigerator. Cell phones and the cacophony of electromagnetism around us have the same basic effect on us through Resonant Dominance. We are around so many vibrations in this world that are vying to distract us from our own natural vibration.

Even the powerful resonant fields of fear and anxiety in the astral field entrain us into these states without our even knowing it.

First, negative vibrations often entrain us into negativity, and it can happen at all four levels of existence – physically, mentally, emotionally and Spiritually.

On the other hand, Resonant Dominance manifests in positive ways and is the most powerful tool there is for healing and transformation.

When around someone who is really positive, we also get entrained into their energy. Just seeing a person smiling can make us smile. Many people sit with Spiritual leaders who are resonating a really powerful vibration of love and light in order to get resonated into the same vibration. They go to see people like the Dalai Lama, Eckhart Tolle, or Braco in order to be entrained into their vibration. Jesus was the extreme example of entraining large groups of people into love and light.

First, there is a huge resonant field that we call the Earth. The earth and all of nature are powerfully entraining us back into its harmony all the time. We see its effect when we spend more time in nature or live in more rural areas. If only we weren't so distracted by other chaotic frequencies.

The Schumann resonance is a consistent frequency in our atmosphere that is triggered by lightning – and lightning strikes every second somewhere on the earth. This frequency of 7.83 hertz is a powerful positive frequency providing perfect consistency. We'll discuss it in more detail in Chapter 39, "The Schumann Resonance and Nature's Entrainers."

Another powerful resonant field that is dominating us is the Sun. The sun...the life giver!!! The sun resonates life into us and everything on the planet. The moon, the profound level of order in the planets, and certainly the Milky Way and the entire Universe, also affect us.

Even more powerful is our Soul. Our Soul is resonating a powerfully peaceful frequency. We only need to build the bridge of resonant connection (or reconnection) for it to change our lives dramatically.

But probably the most powerful resonant frequency of all is that of Source and Spirit. It is more powerful than we know.

Even more importantly we are entrained by the overwhelming amount of love on the planet. There are so many consistent vibrations in and around us vying to help bring us back into alignment with nature and Spirit.

As mentioned, the more powerful the resonant field the more powerful the Resonant Dominant effect. As you can imagine, this is the key way to make changes not only in yourself and others, but in the world as a whole.

Getting large groups of people entrained into the same vibration can do it. It is especially powerful when it is done at the same time all across the planet – such as World OM Day. Based on these laws of resonance, the more people we have in states of love and light, the stronger the resonant field and the more other people are entrained to the same vibration. You see this effect locally every day. When we come across someone who is in a high state of energy or someone who is caring, loving or giving – it affects our energy – often dramatically.

However, it also happens globally. A strong resonant field of love and light affects everyone on the planet through the mechanism of entanglement in the quantum field. This is how we are all connected. Resonant Fields combined with Resonant Dominance is the key to planetary transformation. And this is not "woo-woo". These laws of resonance are well known and have all been proven scientifically with the laws of physics.

4. Resonant Transformation - A stronger vibration can actually transform the resonant frequency of an object so that its resonant frequency is the same as the stronger vibration – forever.

The most interesting aspect of resonance is that if a vibration is powerful or consistent enough it can actually restructure the second object so that its resonant frequency becomes the same as the first.

In one experiment a laser beam was focused on a frog's egg. The beam went through the frog's egg into a salamander's egg. The salamander egg was then transformed into a frog's egg and birthed a frog!

It often takes a really loud or strong vibration to transform the weaker vibration. However, even a perfectly consistent vibration can transform something over a long period of time.

The most striking example is that of Spirit or Source transforming a disease into a totally harmless benign cell.

Anita Moorjani (who has been touring with Wayne Dyer) is one of the most profound examples of this. She had 4th stage lymphoma, which means the cancer had metastasized throughout the entire body. On the final day, all of her organs were shutting down and they called the family to say goodbye. She then went into the light and she got the message that she still had work to do. Within one month all of her cancer was completely gone.

As the most powerful Resonant Field in the Universe,
Source has no trouble using Transformative Resonance
to transform the cancer cells into different types of cells.

There are many stories of people having similar experiences. I believe Transformative Resonance accounts for the myriad of healing miracles where tumors and diseases simply disappear overnight.

We are all quite familiar with the way that music resonates through our whole system. We've all been entrained by songs we like. Both sound and music work on all levels of resonance. Both sound and music can create sympathetic vibrations within our body, emotions, mind and even Spiritually. But most interesting is they can actually transform stuck energies, including diseases. Sound and music can also resonate higher emotions such as love and Spirit, which then can also transform our systems down to the cellular level.

The benefits of all these laws of resonance are far reaching – into many levels of reality. On the most basic level, this concept can be utilized to resonate the good in something. We can find the natural resonant frequency of a cell and vibrate it into its healthy state. We can find the frequency of an organ and resonate its healthy natural frequency. We can use instruments to resonate a state of coherence and consistency in every system of our body.

This whole concept becomes incredibly powerful when we use vibrations to resonate our system into higher emotions, such as gratitude, compassion, love and joy. We are simply using vibrations and our intention to trigger these emotions that then resonate through our whole body.

5. A Consistent Vibration is More Powerful
This law of resonance is also based on physics. It basically states that the more consistent the vibration, the more effective it is in affecting other vibrations around it.

Consistent vibrations like the earth, sun, Schumann resonance and even the noise of cell phone electromagnetism are extremely powerful. Also, it is easier to understand someone when they are consistent and focused. The consistency of a Spiritual leader has an incredible subtle power.

Again, this reinforces the concept that consistency is the definition of peace. In fact, the more consistent a vibration, the more peaceful it is.

This concept is the most applicable when we are doing healing work on someone. The more consistent our own vibration is, the more we resonate that energy into our client. Also, most importantly, the more consistent an intention is held, the more effective the intention.

Coupled with the concept of resonate fields –

**the larger the group holding a consistent intention,
the more powerful it is.**

You get a large group that is holding 100% focus, and you can practically heal anyone or anything!

Chapter 20 – Using the Laws of Resonance to Deal with "Good" and "Bad" Frequencies (So to speak)

Overcoming Negativity

When you encounter a negative (so to speak) sound or vibration you have two choices. You can let it be and resonate with your own positive sound. Or, you can create a sound to break up, transform, or harmonize the negative vibration. The two choices allow you to tune into positive vibrations that are within yourself, or create your own positive vibrations by using voice, instruments or music.

The power you hold to do either of these is based on the laws of resonance, basic laws of physics that essentially give you the power to control your world – if you so choose.

However, as the Hobbit has taught us, with any power comes responsibility. Trying to change something comes with huge responsibility. How do you know that what you are doing is really the best for the thing or person you are changing?

If you have permission from a person (as in a healing or therapeutic environment) you can use sound to breakup stuck energy or blockages. You can also use sound to slowly transform negative energies into positive vibrations. You can harmonize a dissonant vibration into frequency that is no longer detrimental, like resonating a cell into health. We'll go into each of these techniques in detail later in the book.

Resonating your own positive sound when encountering a so-called negative vibration is very effective. Simply create a powerful positive sound so that you are not affected by the negative energy. This sound can be found by tuning into your own body or by connecting with the frequency of your own Soul. Ultimately, as you create your own positive vibrations with sound and are able to easily find your way home to precious presence, your system becomes stronger and able to manage negative energies more effectively. The more you can establish and resonate a grounded, centered, and loving vibration in yourself, the less outside influences will adversely affect you.

The key is to be present enough to know when you are entrained to a frequency that you don't like, or that is harmful to your system. In that moment, with intention, you have the power to change your own vibration with your own sound.

On the other hand, when you encounter positive (so to speak) sounds or vibrations that are in alignment with the healing patterns of nature or Spirit you can choose to resonate with them. Ultimately, you can use sound to consciously tune into these higher and more consistent energies at will.

Ideally, the key is to become a transmitter of consistent frequencies. When you learn to do this all the time, you are no longer at the mercy of inconsistent frequencies around you.

As you resonate more with patterns that are in tune with nature or Spirit, or simply resonate more with your body and soul, you are adding a more consistent and peaceful frequency to the vibrational soup of the world. Based on the main law of resonance (a strong vibration naturally entrains a weaker vibration), you are actually helping to transform the world. On a local level, when you come in contact with another person, they will be affected by your higher vibration. Of course, whomever they contact will also be affected. However, as mentioned, quantum physics has shown how we are all connected through the process of entanglement. Even if we don't come in contact with someone, the quality of our own vibration affects everyone on the planet.

> The highest goal of all is to resonate peaceful vibrations of
> gratitude, love, joy, and direct connections to Spirit and Source,
> in order to create stronger resonant fields on the planet –
> eventually creating fields so powerful that everyone
> is naturally entrained into these higher vibrations
> without having to work at it.

This is the essence of Sound Healing. Our tools include our voice, most instruments, music, higher emotions, nature, Soul and Source. Healing might be as simple as chanting "OM." If you are a musician you can create resonances with your instrument. The nice thing about Sound Healing instruments is that you don't need to be a musician to play them. You only need focus of attention and intention.

In the next Section we will cover most of the traditional Sound Healing tools.

It's all Sacred

Ultimately, from a higher perspective, there are no good or bad vibrations. All vibrations are a part of Spirit and oneness – including those of technology and engines. This is why I have been using the term "so-called" negative or positive vibrations.

When you see everything as frequency, timbre, musical intervals, music and energy – there is no judgment. You see things as they really are. There are no critical filters to color your perception. The frequency is either high or low or in between. It is either an activating or calming musical interval, chord or timbre. The music is just what it is – moving vibrations. The energy is just what it is – an interesting combination of frequencies.

I have been using the term "so to speak" because in a different context a negative vibration may actually be positive for someone else. Also, there are times negative vibrations may be good for us without our realizing it. Perhaps a negative vibration is actually helping to break down a negative pattern within us that is unhealthy. Often vibrations that we think of as negative are triggering a stuck emotion or issue for good reason – bringing up the issue gives us an opportunity to finally resolve it. Ultimately, there are no positive and negative sounds or vibrations.

When we see everything as vibration
the world takes on a clearer focus –
there is no good or bad.

From this perspective it is easy to allow things
to be what they are,
without our resistance or reaction.

SECTION V – Your Sound Healing Toolbox

Introduction - The Sound Tools

Now, let's take a look at how we can use our sound, music and energy vibrational tools to make changes in ourselves and the world around us. In this chapter we give a brief overview of how the instruments work, how they affect us at different levels, and some tips on how to use them. Some considerations are also offered for buying an instrument. There are many books available on how to use instruments, so we only give highlights. If you are drawn to any one instrument, you may search for more detailed information and dive in completely.

One important component of the effectiveness of an instrument has to do with the number of parameters that you can creatively control. A keyboard gives you only a few: the particular note, the volume, and a couple of wheels that control pitch and modulation. A violin gives you quite a few more: the particular note, in-between notes, the many ways you can draw the bow across the strings or pluck the strings, and the way you hold your fingers on the frets (or move them to create vibrato). A guitar has a similar number of parameters including the ability to bend the strings. Wind instruments also have a large number of parameters, the most important being the detailed way that you can change sounds and volumes with your breath. Instruments played with the breath seem easier for the musician's essence and Spirit to come through the instrument. Wind instruments seem to be the closest to the most powerful instrument of all – the voice.

The voice has the most parameters of creative control by far. There are literally thousands of ways you can manipulate your mouth, tongue, throat, and your whole body to create an infinite number of sounds. Spirit has provided the voice with way more creative flexibility than any other instrument – by far. The voice is itself the instrument, so there is a direct connection between Source in both the being and the instrument.

One of the other most important parameters has to do with the construction and basic technique of playing an instrument. You can categorize all instruments relative to Air, Water, Fire, Earth and Ether based on the materials they are made of and how they are played. Also interesting to note is whether the timbre or energy of the music created approximates the energy of these elements:

Air – The voice, woodwinds, flutes, and anything that is triggered with air.

Earth – Particularly instruments made of clay, wood and metal.

Fire – Not too many instruments made of fire, but some instruments can produce very fiery sounds.

Water – There are actually a few instruments that have water inside them and there are rain sticks that make a sound similar to rain. There are also instruments that are more watery sounding than others – like the alto sax – and of course, many synthesizers include the sound of water.

Ether – These instruments include string instruments or any other sounds (often high frequency sounds) that access the angelic realm.

Don't forget, of course, how you play any instrument and the energy and intention you bring to the playing is as important as the sound of the instrument itself.

The truth is there are no rules. You might find that you are called to make sounds or do techniques that follow no particular protocol and that very likely might be the best Sound Healing treatment ever done in the Universe.

However, for many of us, it is nice to have guidelines. And, for those of you who are already performing miracles there is always room to expand on what you do.

The key to doing any type of Sound Healing session is to get out of the way and let Spirit and inspiration take over. You can use your mind to figure out what sounds to start with, but then just allow the sounds that are best for the person to come out. Just trust that Spirit will come up with the right sounds for the person. As we commonly say,

"Spirit is much smarter than we are.
Much smarter!"

Who is the Healer?
Some people say that you are in danger of creating karma for yourself if you heal someone because you might be removing the person's opportunity to learn the lesson that is being given to them with the illness. Even if they are healed the underlying issue is still there and will again manifest symptoms in another way.

Therefore, it is critical that the healing session involves the person being healed. It is a co-creative process. They have to want to be healed. Some people are not ready to be healed and going forward with the process can actually be detrimental to their overall path.

In certain cases, perhaps it is the time for the person to die, and performing the healing might only cause more suffering.

Therefore, the key is to ask the person if they want to be healed. And, listen to your own intuition.

You can ask for permission to heal. You can also ask that the work is to only be for the highest good of both you and the person you are working with.

Ultimately, the best thing you can do is to resonate the template of perfection in yourself.

Based on the laws of resonance, this may trigger the divine template of perfection in them.

Healing vs. Raising Consciousness

These days, many people believe that we should never be doing any healing. We should only focus on raising one's consciousness – bringing ourselves and others into a higher vibration. In fact, often when you bring people into Love and Light, issues do just fall away on their own.

Anita Moorjani is the perfect example of this. Just by releasing fear and remaining in the energy of love and light, she new that her body would heal – and, it did!

Chapter 21 – The Voice

Because the voice is by far the most powerful instrument in the Universe (and the cheapest too), we devote a whole chapter to it.

All the Sounds the Voice Can Make and Their Effects

The voice is the most powerful healing tool in the world. Let's look at the full range of sounds that you can create with the voice and the general effects each can elicit.

All of these effects are general and not definitive. You might find that Spirit calls you to do a completely different sound than indicated here – and it could be exactly what the client needs. Again...Trust!

To practice, make each of these sounds with your lips on the back of your hand (preferably the left hand). If you have a partner practice on each other to really know how they feel.

Frequencies and Pitches

High Pitches - High frequencies activate. They can be good for opening up higher chakras, especially above the head. One instructor says they are good for breaking up congestion.

Low Pitches - Low frequencies calm the body. They are especially good for tight and tense muscles, and can be very effective on bones. Lows are often used to help ground people. I use low frequencies whenever someone has a problem from the hips down, particularly if they have a problem with the knees or feet.

Odd vs. Even Tones

Odd Harmonics - Odd harmonics are activating. As previously discussed, they can be really good for breaking up stuck energy and blockages. They can also help with depression, lethargy or feeling overwhelmed. Reed instruments including bagpipes, shruti boxes, and harmoniums, produce odd harmonics. Instruments or strings made of metal also contain odd harmonics.

Even Harmonics - Even Harmonics are calming, soothing, and loving. Therefore, they can be good for someone who suffers from panic attacks, or struggles with issues around love and loving relationships, or for someone who is dying. Instruments with even harmonics include those made of wood and those made with nylon strings, particularly the harp.

Vowels - uu, oh, ah, eh, ee. Vowels tend to be soothing because they are the essence of a consistent sound. Their use is especially good for harmonizing trauma, fear and anxiety. UU is the most calming. EE is the most activating. It is also sometimes fun and effective to slowly transition from one vowel sound to another.

Consonants - Da, ga, ha, ja, ka, la, pa, ra, sa, ta, va, wa, za. Consonants can be good for breaking up stuck energy, especially when explosive (if appropriate). They can also be used to create effective rhythms.

Overtone or Throat singing (including Tibetan or Mongolian sounds) - These are especially good for clearing chakras. I often like to use them while moving up and down the chakras in order to facilitate the smooth flow of kundalini energy.

Pure vs. Rich Tones

Pure Sounds - Whistles and pure vowels in the high frequency range are often good for activating a specific organ or cell.

Rich Sounds – Use of the full voice (like and opera singer) is very good for instilling a sense of power and confidence. I often use such sounds when someone seems to have blockages around the throat chakra.

Long vs. Short Duration

Staccato Sounds - Good for breaking up stuck energy.

Long Sustained Notes - Good for instilling power and a sense of security.

Noises

White Noise - Shhhh, water or wind sounds, whispers, or soft breathy sounds are extremely helpful in blowing away blockages and releasing stuck emotions.

Other Languages - These are known and not known including gibberish and light language. Such silly sounds can be really good to scramble emotional issues. It can also help someone break through creative blocks.

Sounds Based on Previous Experience

Human Sounds - Baby sounds, sighing, wailing, and crying are appropriate for bringing up and releasing deep emotional issues.

Animal Sounds - The effect can be dramatic.

Musical Intervals

Octaves, fifths, fourths, thirds, etc. - Using the intervals of the harmonic structure of sound is even more effective. The list of benefits can be found in Chapter 9, "Musical Intervals and Chords."

Music

Humming - Humming often allows you to synchronize with subtle emotions in order to transform them.

Half-tones or Flat/Sharp Singing - This includes Vedic or Hindu chanting and is very good for breaking up a dissonant cell or getting a stuck energy to move.

Songs - Made-up or known. Sometimes a known song comes to you during a Sound Healing and you find that it is an important song for the recipient, perhaps from their childhood, or maybe it is associated with a trauma. You never know. Stay open and share. Sometimes you might find that you are singing the person's Soul song.

Rhythms

Vibrato - Sounds that go up and down in pitch create movement, flow, and balance. A full frequency sweep from low to high and back again provides the person with all frequency nutrients, from which their body can choose. Also, it creates the energy of flow through their whole system.

Tremolo - Sounds that go up and down in volume also create flow. Because the oscillation of volume up and down creates a rhythm, it is also affecting heart rate and brainwaves.

Combinations

Multiples/Combinations of Sounds - Using combinations of all the sounds above, morphing from one to the other, can help to break up stuck patterns and move energy. It can also remove emotional and creative blocks.

Toning

Toning is simply the elongation of vowel sounds. Toning any vowel sound can help with all of the following:
   - Creating consistency and peace
   - Deeper breathing and more oxygen for your system
   - Better sleep
   - More creativity
   - Resolving emotional issues and trauma
   - Accessing higher states of consciousness to get answers to important questions
   - Toning has been proven to slow down heart rate and respiration, and is good for our nervous system.

I'm sure there are many other benefits that haven't been discovered yet.

The most powerful benefits of toning are gained when you do it for long periods of time. Although even one minute can help center and ground you, it is said that a minimum of eight minutes can open a portal to a new state of bliss and sweetness. However, do toning for 20 minutes or even 8 hours … and … oh … my … God! You are in the zone big time.

There are no strict rules when it comes to toning, except one.

There are no "bad" sounds.
There is no such thing as out of pitch or off key.

However, most important is to set an intention while toning. It is especially effective if you make a sound that represents – and thus becomes – the intention.

The Institute offers a CD called "Holding Frequency" in which we have toned intentions of gratitude, compassion, love, joy, oneness, etc. It is a great CD to tone along with.

Chant
Chant is simply singing something over and over. When you repeat something with similar melodies and rhythms your thinking mind goes to sleep because there is not enough variation. This allows you to access deeper or higher states of consciousness associated with the right brain.

The rhythm of a chant also entrains your brain into a particular brainwave state – normally delta or theta. Also, the melody of the chant can activate certain states of awareness.

The key of the chant can also have a dramatic effect on the energy you receive. It is interesting to pay attention to how easy it is to sing in the chosen key. You might try singing a chant in a different key to see how it feels.

Chants can be in any language. However, chants in Sanskrit and Hebrew tend to be the most effective. That is because the words in the languages, when spoken correctly, actually are designed to access different parts of our body, chakras and energy states. However, sung with the right intention, any chant can be unbelievably effective.

Mantra
Mantra is the repetition of a sound or set of sounds over and over. Again, the sounds themselves have their own powerful effect – particularly when in Sanskrit.

The frequency in which you chant the mantra is also really important. Try different frequency ranges – high and low – to see how they feel.

Mantras can be spoken or sung. Regardless, the tempo at which they are repeated will powerfully entrain the brain into the same corresponding rhythm (brainwave states are covered in detail in Section IX). In fact, mantra means "mind tool."

Here are some of the most well-known mantras.

OM NAMAH SHIVAYA
Fire of Transformation

OM SHANTI SHANTI SHANTI OM
Peace / Recovery

OM SHRING MAHA LAKSMIYE NAMAHA
Abundance

OM GAM GANAPATAIYE NAMAHA
Removal of Obstacles

OM KLEEM KRISHNAYA NAMAHA
Enhance Relationships (including the Divine)

OM AIM SARASWATAYEI NAMAHA
Inspiration / Creativity

OM DUM DURGAYEI NAMAHA
Boundaries / Fierce Compassion

TAT TVAM ASI
I Am That I Am

OM MANI PADME HUM
God is the Jewel in the Lotus

There are many books that go into detail on toning, chant and mantra. If you are interested, I highly recommend the following:

• "The Yoga of Sound – Tapping the Hidden Power of Music and Chant" by Russill Paul

• "Sound Medicine: The Complete Guide to Healing with the Human Voice" by Wayne Perry

• "The Healing Sounds" by Jonathan Goldman

• "Being and Vibration" by Joseph Rael

Chapter 22 – Other Sounds, Instruments and Vibrational Tools

First, here is an outline of the other sounds we'll be focusing on. There are so many sounds and instruments in the world and most of them can be used for healing and raising consciousness when used with the right intention. Therefore, this is only a small list of those most commonly used. Notice that we have included other vibrational energies besides sound. Often using combinations of different vibrational modes can be especially effective in a treatment.

Crystal Bowls
Tibetan Bowls
Tingshas
Chimes
Tuning Forks
Didgeridoo
Gongs
Shakers and Rattles
Drums
Woodwind Instruments
String Instruments
Tone Generators
Synthesized Sounds
Other Instruments
Sounds of Nature
CD's
Frequency of Silence and Peace
Thoughts
Intention
Higher Vibrations such as Gratitude, Compassion, Love, and Joy
Pure Spirit and Source
Food and Water
Light and Color
The Frequencies of Shape - The Relationships between Geometry and Sound
Crystals and Gems
Flower Essences
Electromagnetism and Magnetism
Lasers

You can find and listen to many of these instruments in our online store:
www.ResonantHarmonySF.com

Crystal Bowls

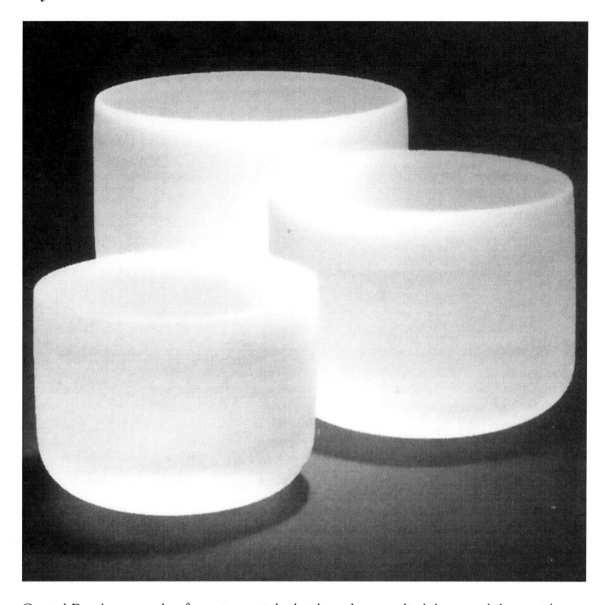

Crystal Bowls are made of quartz crystals that have been melted down and then put in a form to cool. The quartz is heated to around 3,000 degrees and then becomes soft and flexible; (if the temperature goes much higher the quartz crystals actually evaporate). Quartz crystal has a unique capability to resonate sound and often keeps going for as long as 5 minutes after you stop playing them.

They actually come from "ancient" San Jose...California, that is. There are a few drawings of what people say are crystal bowls from ancient Egypt, but the crystal bowl was actually created in the heart of the computer industry. Quartz crystal tubes are used to create computer chips. The chips would move along a railroad track inside the quartz crystal tube filled with a poisonous gas, which actually caused them to grow. Then, someone noticed that when they tapped the quartz tube it created a nice tone. Someone then put a bottom on it and Voila! the crystal bowl was invented – in "ancient" San Jose (around 1960).

<u>What They Do</u>
Sometimes called Singing bowls, crystal bowls do many things. Their harmonic structure is quite pure so they tend to be quite activating. They are often quite loud which also tends to make them more activating. You don't usually use crystal bowls to help someone go to sleep. When using Galvanic Skin Response tests (which measure tension in the body), many people do not completely relax when using bowls. However, people do go into profound states of coherence – peace and bliss. People's hearts often synchronize in a state of coherence where the heart rate smoothly goes up and down in speed. This "s-curve" in heart rate variability often occurs when a person is resonating a state of love or many other high states of consciousness.

There are several other characteristics of crystal bowls:

1. Delta Inducing – Most bowls have a very slow oscillation that is normally less than 4 cycles per second (often less than 1 cycle per second). This slow oscillation entrains you into a delta brainwave state. Less than 1 cycle per second takes you into deep delta, which is the state that has been seen with EEG on people who are in deep states of meditative bliss and stillness.

2. Phasing – The sound of bowls commonly seems to float around the room. This is based on the fact that the bowl normally has a curve in it, which produces multiple frequencies. The interaction of these frequencies creates an effect called phasing, a subtle and slow oscillation that makes the sound of the bowl seem like it is floating around the room. When you perceive a sound to be moving around the room in 3D it is actually quite activating in a positive way. It helps you to be present in 3D reality.

3. Consistency – Probably the #1 benefit of crystal bowls is the fact that they are resonating a consistency that is akin to the consistency of Universal Love, Spirit and Source. These higher energies are as profoundly consistent. This effect is enhanced tremendously when you also tone along with the bowl – doing so brings a deep sense of stillness.

4. Slow Fades to Peace – As previously mentioned, my favorite thing about crystal bowls is the way they slowly fade out. Because the sound fades into silence so slowly and smoothly, it is as though you can still hear the bowl's frequency even after it has completely stopped vibrating. The **space** in which you are still hearing the consistent sound is a profound **state** of peace. **It is the whole deal in Sound Healing.**

This is so important because so many people are not **capable** of stopping and going into a state of complete peace.

5. Singing with the Bowls – Because the bowl is so loud, it is easy to sing along with. It is quite interesting and spiritually activating to hear how your voice interacts with the sound of the bowl. Singing with the bowl also allows timid people the freedom to sing

144

without being heard very much, because the bowl is so loud.

People who sing with the bowls are commonly transported into other worlds where all kinds of sounds being heard are healing in ways that are more powerful than you can ever imagine. I have seen people go into complete trance over and over. It's nice to aspire to such states when playing the bowls.

Tips on Using Them

Crystal bowls can be played in two ways. Using a felt wand or rubber mallet, you can simply tap the bowl, or you can stroke the top outside edge in a circular motion. It is normally best to tap the bowl lightly in order to get it going a bit, before you begin going around the edge. Remember the bowls are very fragile so don't ever hit them hard.

As you get to know the crystal bowls you will find that each has its own specific tempo or speed at which you stroke it. You can recognize the right speed, as it seems to feel a bit easier to play. Technically, when this happens you are moving at a tempo that matches the actual note of the bowl. Each bowl also has its own pressure that it likes.

Different pitches and sizes of the bowl will activate different parts of the body: organs, glands, and chakras. We believe that the best pitch is a bowl that matches your Soul note. We explain how to find your own Soul note in Chapter 46, "Connecting to the Soul with Sound."

As previously mentioned, do be careful when playing a bowl next to the head while someone is lying on the floor. The volume of a crystal bowl is quadrupled when you are at the same height of the bowl. When sitting next to a bowl this is not a problem.

If small enough (less than 15 inches) you can place bowls right on the body – usually on the abdomen, chest or back (normally the lower back). Of course, you have to be really careful so that the bowl does not fall off. The effect on the body can be quite physically transforming. Be sure to have the person let you know if it is uncomfortable or painful.

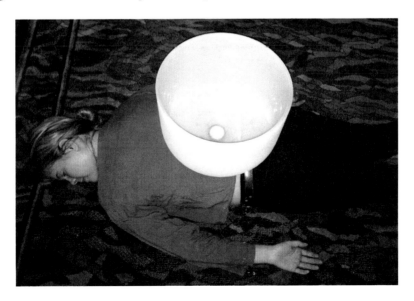

145

Crystal Bowls (Singing Bowls) are commonly tuned to specific pitches that correspond to Chakra frequencies or to the frequencies of the rotation of the planets around the sun.

When you order a crystal bowl you get to choose the note, but the actual frequency is up to Source ... so to speak. You don't get to choose the actual frequency or tuning system unless you pay more money. Therefore, they can often sound out of tune with normal music. However, you can tune them by pouring water into them. The more water, the lower the pitch becomes.

There are three general types of crystal bowls.
1. Classic Frosted - These bowls are by far the most common and least expensive. They also often have "deeper" sounds than the other types of bowls. Classic bowls can also be created in very large sizes where the other types cannot. Larger sizes give you lower octaves.

2. Practitioner Bowls - These are bowls that have handles on them so they are easy to hold over the body.

3. Alchemical Bowls

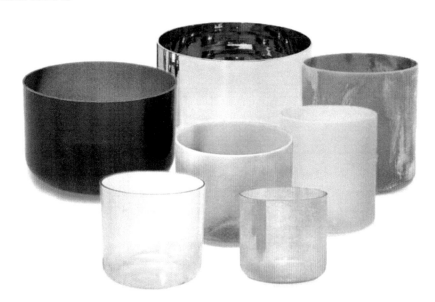

Although these bowls are quite a bit more expensive, their sound is heavenly because they have different minerals and gemstones embedded in them. For example, you can get one with gold, diamond, rose quartz, platinum, or other rare minerals embedded in the bowl. This alters the specific harmonic structure of the bowls to create a very specific tonality that can often take you into blissful states hard to imagine. Many see the bowls and their sounds as actual states of living consciousness that are affecting us at all levels of reality – similar to crystals and gemstones. In fact, the actual mineral or gemstone is being transmitted into your body as a sound frequency. You can listen to some great examples of these bowls at www.soundhealingcenter.com/alchemicalbowls.html

When buying a bowl the primary consideration is the size and pitch. You can get bowls from 6 inches in diameter to around 28 inches. The larger the size, the more low pitches it contains. Bowls under 10 inches are a little harder to play because they fall over more easily. Therefore, I often recommend at least a 10" or 12" bowl. I actually prefer the 14" bowls but at that size they get a little harder to carry around. 18" is wonderful, but you sure can't take them hiking with you.

As far as the pitch, as you know by now, I recommend that you get a bowl tuned to your own home note – your Soul note. We can help you find your note at the Institute: www.soundhealingcenter.com/throotsoul.html

People also commonly buy bowls that are tuned to the key of their voice. You can find this note by simply relaxing and, with the least amount of energy possible, make the sound "Ah." Don't sing the note or stretch your mouth in anyway to make the note. Simply let out whatever note wants to come out when you breathe out. This is the note that is the easiest for you to sing, and it allows you to sing with the bowl for the longest time without getting tired.

If you can hear the actual bowl before buying it, the most important considerations are: Does it speak to you? Does it give you chills and goosebumps? Does it help bring you to a place of peace and stillness? And, does it open your heart?

Tibetan Bowls

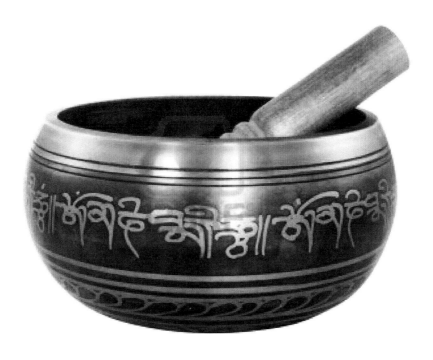

<u>What They Do</u>
Tibetan bowls have many of the same characteristics as crystal bowls with a few major differences. For instance, they still have a nice slow fade that can lead you into a peaceful state of stillness, but they don't ring out nearly as long as crystal bowls. Because the Tibetan bowls are made of metal, the biggest difference is that their sound has more activating odd harmonics than crystal bowls. And, the sound is actually much richer and more complex in Tibetan bowls because the timbre has many more harmonics in it (crystal bowls are more pure with fewer harmonics). This richness and almost edgy tonality is what makes them even more activating than crystal bowls.

Additionally, some Tibetan bowls have a whole other level of energy that is present in them. Because they are made by hand, there are certain bowls that are quite magical – particularly when the consciousness of the person who makes the bowl is connected to higher realms. It's like the consciousness of the maker goes right into the bowl with every little hammer stroke, and Spirit gets infused into the metal and the sound itself. Of course, the energy of this consciousness comes through whenever you play the instrument. When purchasing a Tibetan bowl look for this higher energy if you are able to perceive such types of energy (just trust your intuition). Crystal bowls are not made by hand.

Tibetan bowls commonly have very pronounced oscillations in volume that will entrain your brain into a specific brainwave state. They also have the "slow fade" component going – so remember to honor the silence at the end of the ring.

<u>Tips on Using Them</u>
Some Tibetan bowls are very difficult to ring by going around the edges. Sometimes wood wands are used, instead of rough felt. Therefore, some bowls are simply played by hitting them on the side with a wooden or rubber mallet. Larger bowls are often played with the softer mallets.

It is quite common to place Tibetan bowls on the body since they are generally much smaller. They can also be played and moved around the body – particularly around the head. I like to do a slow sweeping motion around the top of the head, ears and throat while the bowl is ringing. Most bowls, being smaller, tend to resonate upper chakras; however, placing the bowl on the root chakra can also be quite effective.

Another nice technique is to strike the bowl and then put it next to your mouth. Then, open your mouth just the right amount until you hear the bowl resonate within your mouth cavity. You can then change the size of your mouth ever so slightly to get a small sweeping "wah-wah" type sound.

When buying a Tibetan bowl there are a few main considerations. First, there are two main types: handmade and manufactured. The handmade ones can be good or bad quality. The really good ones not only sound more amazing, but the person that makes them often puts a healing intention from Spirit into the bowls while making them.

Purists sometimes don't like the manufactured bowls; however I have found them to be quite amazing. They often have much purer sounds with fewer harmonics and are quite a bit less expensive.

Another consideration is the pitch. Do you like the frequency of the bowl? Just feel into it. Second and even more importantly is the tonality. How pure and how rich is it? Again, does the tonality feel good? If you can get the bowl to sing while stroking it around the outside edges that is a huge bonus. However, most important is how long the bowl continues ringing after you stop playing it. The longer, the better.

Tingshas

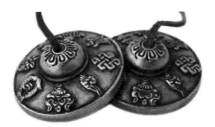

Tingshas are similar to Tibetan bowls in that they are handmade, and therefore can carry a whole other level of powerful energy within them whenever they are played. As with Tibetan bowls look for this higher level of energy transmission – I actually can tell when I get chills and goosebumps while playing the Tingshas.

<u>What They Do</u>
Tingshas are two small bells that are detuned a little bit from each other. This detuning of the bells relative to each other creates a "difference tone," which is a low frequency vibration (heard as a "flutter") that matches and entrains our brainwaves into the particular frequency (delta, theta, alpha, gamma, etc.)

They are also very high frequency instruments so they commonly activate the higher chakras – particularly the third eye and crown chakra. Therefore, they are often played around the head. They also have the "slow fade" component going – so remember to honor the silence at the end of the ring.

<u>Tips on Using Them</u>
Tingshas can be played on any part of the body and can be used to assess where energy is stuck in the body. As you move them across the body, they will stop ringing out when you pass a part of the body that is holding negative energy.

They are also really good for clearing any stuck or negative energy from a room. Simply play them throughout the room – and especially in corners.

When you hold the Tingshas so that one bell is over each ear, you can also synchronize the left and right brain, so this is the ideal way to hold them:

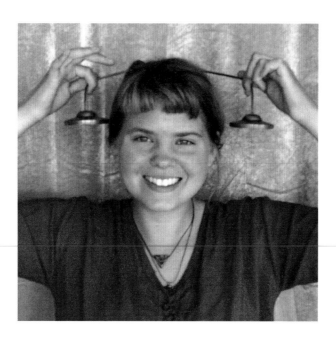

Tingshas around the Head

As with Tibetan bowls listen for the quality of the tonality and the oscillations created between the two notes. And, listen for how long they last.

Chimes

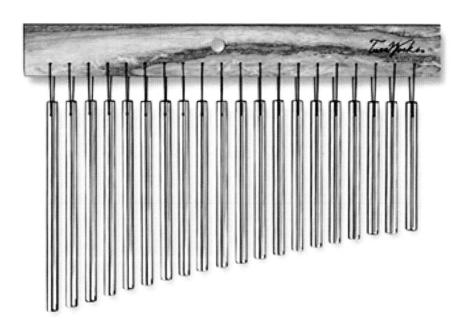

<u>What They Do</u>
Chimes are very similar to Tingshas in that they are very high activating frequencies. However, chimes have a major difference – the relationships between each of the tines on the chimes create individual musical intervals, which have associated states of consciousness. But more importantly, the overall tuning of the chimes in relation to each other creates a very complex chord that can be very powerful.

Chimes can be tuned to ancient tuning systems such as Pythagorean or Just Intonation, which are both based on the natural harmonics found in nature – therefore, re-aligning you with nature. One of our instructors, Randy Masters, makes chimes tuned to a full range of different systems found in nature including: the frequencies of the rainbow, the planets, the Fibonacci sequence, and the Golden Mean. You can find them at www.UniversalSong.com. All of these mathematical patterns resonate harmony into your own system at many levels when you play the chimes.

Chimes are quite activating – particularly for the third eye and crown chakras, which include the pituitary, hypothalamus, and pineal glands. They also have subtle oscillations in volume than will entrain your brain into a specific brainwave state, and they do have somewhat of a slow fade that leads you to a peaceful silence.

<u>Tips on Using Them</u>
Chimes are quite nice when played above the head (when someone is laying down). I like using them to begin and end a session. You can also play individual tones on the chimes or sections of the chimes. The energy you bring to the motion of your hand when playing the chimes is especially important.

Tuning Forks

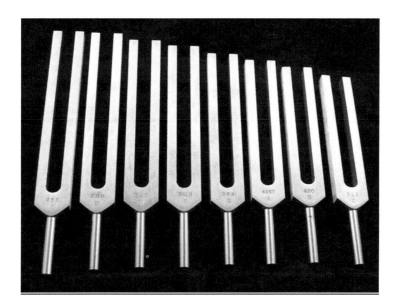

Tuning forks create very pure frequencies. In fact, they have one of the purest sounds of all natural instruments. If they do have other frequencies in them, they are normally so low in volume that they are hardly noticeable. People use tuning forks with very specific frequencies for many issues. People get tuning forks tuned to the full range of frequencies including: planets, solfeggio frequencies, vitamins and minerals, organs, chakras, and Soul frequencies.

What They Do
They can be played by placing the bottom stem of the tuning fork directly on the body, or by moving it around the body just a few inches away. Tuning forks are often placed on acupuncture points and many believe they are even more effective than acupuncture needles.

There are three key components in the sound of tuning forks. One is the particular frequency of the tuning fork. Particular frequencies can activate particular cells, organs, endocrine glands and acupuncture points. Second, when using two tuning forks (one in each hand), the musical interval between them is really important. The body really loves the Octave and the Musical Fifth, however other musical intervals are often called for. The third component of forks is the fact that they fade out slowly. Although they fade out much faster than bowls, when the fork is right on the body it is quite effective in instilling peace in that part of the body.

There are other components that come into play as well. The material that the fork is made of is quite important. Randy Masters has forks made of a specific combination of metals. Aluminum based forks tend to ring out longer. Steel forks don't last as long but have a more solid sound (less harmonics). Some forks also have resonators on them to help them last longer.

Because the fork is essentially an extension of your fingers, the energy that is conveyed in the movement of your hand in applying the fork to the body is extremely important. Just bring love and grace to the placement on the body and you'll be fine.

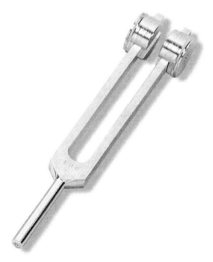

Tuning Fork with Resonator

<u>Tips on Using Them</u>
There are many complex systems of how to use tuning forks on the body and they vary wildly. These include Acutonics, Fabien Maman, John Beaulieu, and our own Randy Masters, to name a few.

Generally tuning forks are placed on the body like this:

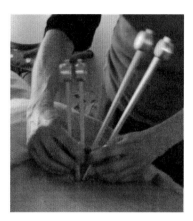

However, tuning forks are often simply held over the body, or near the ears like this:

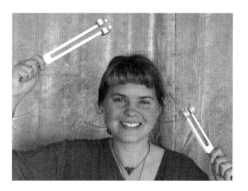

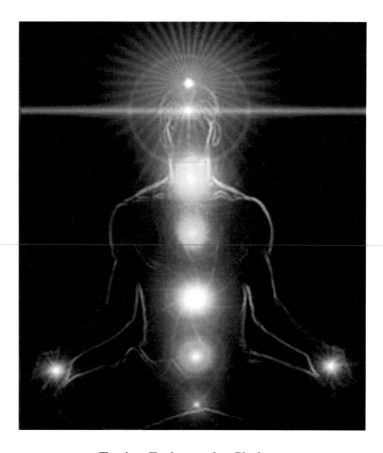

Tuning Forks on the Chakras

There are so many excellent books on how to use tuning forks that we won't go into much more detail here on how to use them.

Acutonics has identified specific frequencies based on the rotation time of various planets that are good for different acupuncture points in the body.

Randy Masters also offers tuning forks tuned to the following frequencies:
• Tree of Life
• The Rainbow
• Natural Tunings (Just Intonation and Pythagorean)
• Sacred Geometry
• Fibonacci
• Positive Emotions
• Archangels

Here is a simple technique that has proven to be quite effective.

First, find two forks that sound good together. You can use two forks that are at an octave or musical fifth. However, I often prefer to simply play various forks together and tune in to the combination that feels right at the time. If the client is a sound being (especially sensitive to sound and music, or just intuitive at all) you might even have them choose which two forks sound the best.

Hold the forks so that you don't interrupt the vibration in the tines.

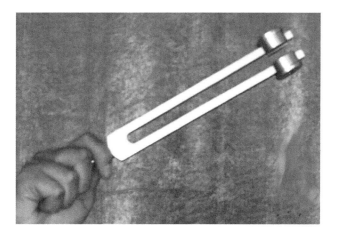

Holding a Tuning Fork Correctly

You can hit the forks on a rubber puck designed for ringing forks, or you can hit them on the floor or another solid surface. Hitting your knee or wrist to get them going may require you to get a treatment upon completion to get rid of the pain and injury – not recommended!

Start with two tuning forks around the whole body a few inches away. Move the forks up and down around the whole body as if smoothing out the aura of the person with the sound. I prefer smaller forks for this part of the process. The subtle fields or auras of the body respond better to high frequencies than low.

Then use two tuning forks on each vertebrae of the spine. Generally, larger tuning forks are better on the spine, simply because people often don't feel the smaller forks very well.

Place the two forks on both sides of the spine (not directly on the spine), and let them ring until they go to silence. Do this one by one next to each vertebra as you go down the spine. This simple technique is unbelievably effective – it is often as good as a full body massage.

You might also place forks on various acupuncture points (there are many detailed charts on the web). The general consensus is that if there is a pain in the body, it is best to place the forks around the pain to draw the energy away from the pain, instead of placing the forks directly on the painful spot. This is same when dealing with a headache.

Ultimately and ideally as you practice, you will find that you intuitively know right where to place the forks. It is always best when Spirit takes over. Until then, use the techniques above.

Always remember to transmit loving graceful energy with every placement of the forks.

Finally, you can also place the forks on a quartz crystal and put the crystal on the body. You can tape the crystal to the fork, or just lay it on a flat surface on the body. Quartz couples to the materials in the body much better than aluminum or steel, and it also amplifies the frequencies coming from the tuning forks.

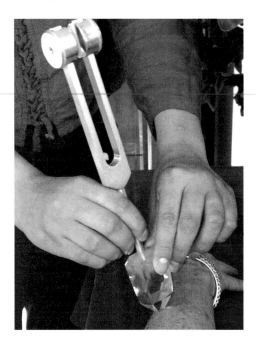

Tuning Fork through Quartz on the Body

Didgeridoo

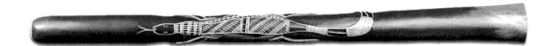

<u>What They Do</u>
Didgeridoos have a large amount of bass, which is really good for getting energy to move – particularly in muscles and bones. They also fluctuate in pitch, which is really good for breaking up stuck energy (technically, creating a binaural beat oscillation that breaks up the stuck energy).

Tips on Using It
A Didgeridoo is especially effective when played right on the body – particularly for muscles. They are also extremely effective for helping digestion problems and harmonizing all of the organs, chakras and auras. When the Didgeridoo is tuned to a person's own resonant frequency it is more effective at grounding them.

Gongs

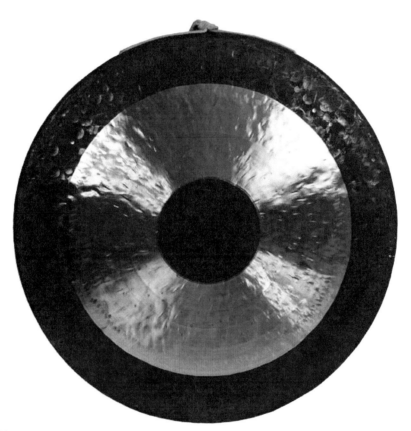

What They Do
Gongs are one of the few instruments that have some harmonics that are not mathematical multiples. Therefore, there is no better instrument for getting someone unstuck from any pattern or rhythm to which they have become entrained. There is nothing better than a gong for breaking up and releasing deep emotional issues.

Tips on Using It
As with all instruments, the intention that is held is especially important. Play with hitting the gong on different areas and notice the difference in how activating the sound is. The key to playing the gong is the smoothness of changes in tone as you play it. Think of it as playing a song – and the smoother the flow of the song the better.

Shakers and Rattles

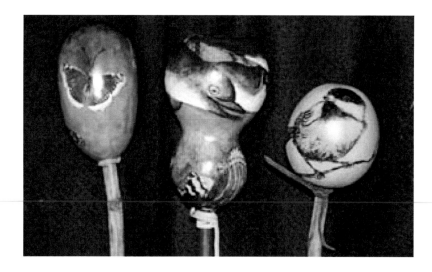

<u>What They Do</u>
Shakers and rattles are mostly white noise so they are really good for breaking stuck frequencies physically, mentally and emotionally. Native American shamans commonly use shakers and rattles to drive away evil Spirits and breakup blockages.

Depending on the speed at which you shake them you are also creating a rhythm that entrains the brain into a specific brainwave state.

<u>Tips on Using Them</u>
The quality of the energetic flow you bring to the playing of rattles and shakers is really important because the rhythm you play is such an extension of your own energy. Therefore, it is important to really be present with your own energy and the intention you have set for the person you are working on.

There are many rhythmic variations you can try. You can start with a slow tempo and smoothly build up to a faster tempo, then slow back down. Ideally, you will intuitively find a tempo that seems to resonate with what the person needs. Listen for this tempo. Similar to doing a frequency sweep, you can play at different tempos until you find the one that feels right for the person.

If you sense that there is a blockage in any part of the body, simply play the shaker or rattle over that part of the body with the intention of breaking up the stuck energy.

Drums

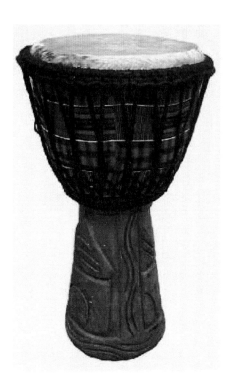

What They Do
Even more so than shakers, the rhythms you play on the drum will have very specific effects on the heart rhythm, brainwave rhythms and nervous system. However, by far, the #1 most important aspect of playing a drum is the consistency of the rhythm. If the rhythm is too inconsistent (or gets interrupted) it can stress out a person dramatically. This has been proven by playing drums on people while watching feedback from heart monitors and galvanic skin response (measuring tension in the body). A consistent drum rhythm does not stress the body. In fact, over many years of testing, we have found that a fast tempo is hardly more activating than a slow tempo based on this type of feedback. Again, only when the tempo varies wildly do people get stressed.

Faster tempos do speed up the heart a bit more, but volume intensity seems to be even more activating than fast tempos.

There are many other parameters that get very complex as to the material that the drum and drumhead are made of, the tuning of the drum, and the place on the head where the drum is played. Generally, metal drums are more activating. A handmade wooden drum also carries the energy of the person who made it. The material of the head even carries the energy of the particular animal it was made from (even those vinyl or plastic animals). When tuned correctly the drumhead will resonate the drum chamber quite loudly. Listen for this when picking a drum – again, just choose what feels right for you. Whenever any instrument works for you, it gives you more energy to bring to the client. Finally, the middle of the drumhead generally gives a lower, more resonant tone that generally works for lower chakras. When you play the edge of the drumhead, it is more activating.

The sound of drums also has some harmonics that are enharmonic – that is, some of the harmonics are not mathematical multiples (as explained in Chapter 7, "Timbres (Tones or Harmonic Structures"). These enharmonic frequencies act like white noise in that they help to activate and break up structures in our system that are not healthy and are not serving us. You can think of them as dissonance that breaks up patterns in us that are not in alignment with nature or Spirit.

<u>Tips on Using Them</u>
One of the most basic drum techniques is to simply play the sound of the heartbeat. This is often a perfect rhythm to start with. Listen and think about synchronizing the rhythm to the person's own heartbeat. You can then slowly change the tempo of your rhythm to slowly calm the person down, or give them more energy by speeding up the tempo.

The heartbeat rhythm is one of the most calming of all. The more complex the drum rhythm, the more activating it is. Remember that activation is often what is needed to move stuck energy and transform one's consciousness.

Woodwind Instruments

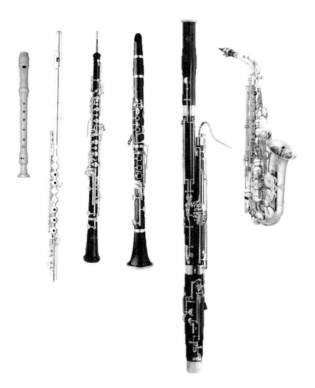

<u>What They Do</u>
As previously mentioned, instruments such as the saxophone, clarinet, flute, bassoon, oboe and trumpet have the major advantage of being able to manipulate sound with the breath instead of the hands. Our breath is closer to our own being and is way more expressive than the hands. I believe that it is more of a direct connection to Spirit (but, of

course, just about any instrument can be used as a pure conduit).

Woodwind instruments with reeds create very specific odd harmonic sounds that are quite a bit more activating than most other sounds. As mentioned, bagpipes are the extreme case. The shruti box and harmonium also use reeds and so tend to be more activating than calming (although, of course, the music played through them can be extremely calming).

Tips on Using Them
Woodwinds give the player a nice array of parameters for Spirit to come through. Of course, a little more work is often required to get to the point where one can really let go and have higher energies come through. When using woodwinds, it is really important to tune into the subtle energy that can be created by manipulating the volume on one note.

String Instruments

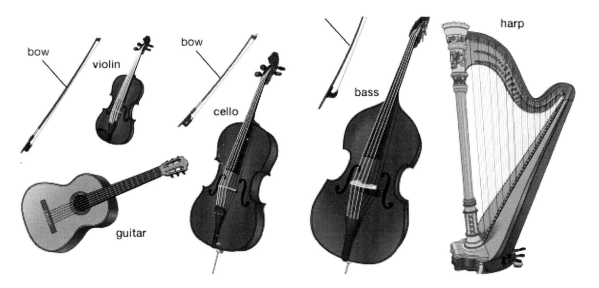

These include guitar, violin, cello, harp, piano, etc.

What They Do
Perhaps I'm expressing my own bias here, but I find that a string section sounds more angelic and opens my heart to Universal Love and Source more than any other sound. I also find that the cello has a tone similar to crying that easily opens my heart.

The harp is the instrument that is used the most to express love. The harp and the voice are the two main instruments used in Hospice for the sick and dying.

Technically, the violin and cello have a perfect balance of odd and even harmonics, and the volume of the harmonics fade to a perfect mathematical multiple series (1/2, 1/3, 1/4, 1/5, 1/6) so there is something auspicious in this perfection that comes through the sound. Also, both violin and cello are able to make sounds similar to crying. And, of course, the cello brings in the grounding low frequencies.

Although the piano has been used so much, it seems to have one of the least obstructive components to our consciousness. What I mean by this is that most people like it. Technically, its sound is a little more activating because it is actually a hammer striking the strings (versus a pluck on a guitar).

There is a large difference between acoustic guitars with nylon strings (classical or flamenco guitar) versus those with steel strings. The nylon strings tend more towards warm even harmonics, whereas the metal in the steel strings brings out more activating odd harmonics.

Tips on Using Them

Again, for many of the string instruments there is often a pretty steep learning curve, so it can take a while to get to the point where the instrument can be played in tune with Spirit. However, there are many string instruments that have no bad notes – examples are the Lyre (which looks like a miniature harp), the Sarod (like a sitar tuned to open tuning), and the zither. Instruments like these allow the beginner to immediately bring higher energies through without being worried about hitting wrong notes.

Tone Generators

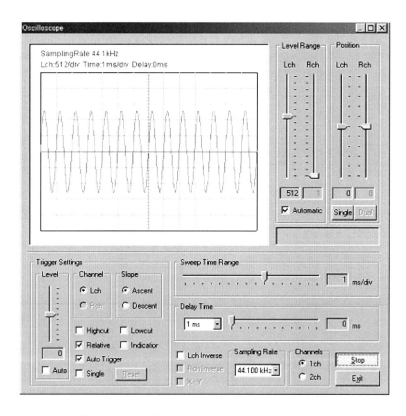

Tone generators (or signal generators) are electronic devices that create pure tones with no harmonics. You can check one out at:

Free online version (site that is selling Sound Healing Tinnitus treatment):

http://www.audionotch.com/app/tune/

Free software for Mac or PC (two week demo, then about $35)
http://www.nch.com.au/tonegen/index.html

<u>What They Do</u>
Tone generators are helpful for a few things. First they allow you take a specific frequency from a chart of healing frequencies and immediately use the frequency for its specific purpose.

They can also be used to create binaural beats to entrain a person's brain into a specific brainwave state (delta, theta, alpha, gamma, etc.), which we'll discuss in more detail in Section IX – "Mental Expansion with Sound."

Since tone generators have no Soul in the least, it is critical when working with them to add us much heart and intention as possible, which then gets carried on the waveform and frequency of the tone itself.

<u>How to Use Them</u>
Tone generators can be played directly on specific parts of the body (or just through speakers). However they are commonly used to simply find a frequency so that you can then use your voice or tune an instrument to the specific frequency.

You can also embed tone generators in the background of music and entrain the brain into any of the brainwave states: delta, theta, alpha, beta or gamma.

Synthesized Sounds

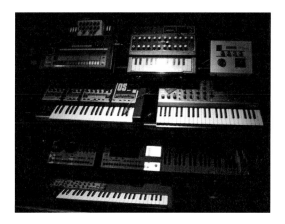

<u>What They Do</u>
Many people have an aversion to synthesized sounds, however, these days they are technically no different than listening to a CD (and actually often have better quality). Of course, there is nothing better than a live acoustic instrument, but again, let's not throw any babies out.

There are many nice things about synthesized sounds these days. First, of course, it gives us access to a wide range of natural instruments and unique sounds that we may not otherwise have access to.

Also, on the latest synthesizers there are many very complex sounds that can create a flow in us as they transform from one tone to another *within one sound.* This amount of complexity can be very pleasantly activating. Also, many synthesizers are able to play back beautiful nature sounds. Probably most importantly, it gives the musician a full array of frequencies at his or her fingertips. Most other instruments only give you one general type of sound. Synthesis allows you to completely transition from one sound or a whole group of sounds to another whole group of timbres – this creates a very powerful effect.

Tips on Using Them
Combining synthesis with acoustic instruments can be quite effective. Probably the most effective part of synthesizers that you can rarely get from other instruments is the low bass. Low bass can be really powerful in a session (or on a sound table) when it is consistent and particularly slow in tempo.

It is important to note that there are many bad synthesizer sounds that are cheesy-sounding and may not have much healing capacity. Therefore, it is critical to use some of the newer synths – the sounds from Software Synths in a computer tend to be the most versatile these days.

Go to www.SoundHealingCenter.com/music.html to listen to some cool and healing synth sounds.

Other instruments
There is a vast array of musical instruments – particularly from other cultures that often having amazingly powerful capacities.

Based on what you now know about the healing capacity of different timbres and the instruments we have outlined here, you should now be able to gauge how any unknown instrument might be used. First, focus on whether it has more even (calming) harmonics, or more odd (activating) harmonics. Then notice whether it is more of a pure sound, or a rich sound. Then simply feel into it – tune into how it feels in your body. Trust your own body and feelings.

Sounds of Nature

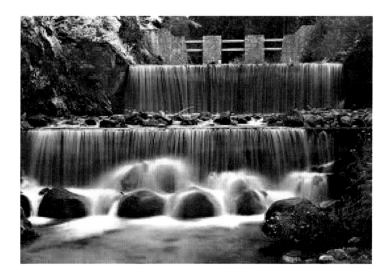

See deep enough, and you see musically;
the heart of nature being everywhere music..."
Thomas Carlyle (1795-1881)

What They Do
There is no better sound healer than nature. Nature has it down. Sounds in nature bring us back to harmony.

Nature sounds include those made by the elements of wind, water, and occasionally earth and fire, and the sounds made by animals, birds and insects. In all cases they run the full gamut from extremely calming to extremely activating. For example, you can have calm waves lapping on the shore, or huge waves crashing with a roar. You can have the soft murmur of a cat's purr or the intense roar of a lion.

It seems obvious that every sound in nature has many unique purposes that we have no awareness of. It has become clear that animal sounds are doing way more than attracting a mate! Scientific studies have shown that bird sounds actually activate the metabolism in plants. There are companies now utilizing the frequencies of bird songs to double and triple crop growth and create way more healthy vitamins and minerals in fruits and vegetables (check out www.OriginalSonicBloom.com).

Also, there have been studies done in the jungle showing that the sounds of all the animals in the jungle actually cover the entire sound frequency spectrum from 20 – 20,000 hertz. Every animal has its own frequency within the full spectrum. And, when an animal or species dies out, another animal will take over the missing frequency so that the full range is still covered.

There is something going on with nature sounds, something beyond our understanding. Every sound contributes to the entire frequency spectrum of our planet.

Nature is the most powerful sound healer there is... by far.
Nature has it down.

It becomes even more obvious when you listen to nature sounds slowed down.

Go to www.SoundHealingCenter.com/nature.html
to listen to the amazing angelic sound of crickets slowed down.

There is a whole world of nature sounds that are too fast for us to hear consciously, however we do hear them subconsciously, and the frequencies definitely go right into the water in our bodies and affect our cells directly.

Certain animal sounds such as whales and dolphins have been reported by huge numbers of people to precipitate complete personal transformations. There are dolphin therapy centers where you can receive healing treatments from dolphins. One kid with autism was walking and talking for the first time in his life after two days in the water with these dolphins.

There is a place in Hawaii where a mother can birth her baby in the water with the dolphins, and the dolphins transmit healing and transformative frequencies into the babies. (Some of the kids are said to have become Indigo and Crystal children.)

The sound of water is mostly white noise. Therefore, the sound of oceans, rivers, waterfalls and the wind has a powerful effect of clearing out stuck frequencies in us.

Then there are the unheard sounds of the rhythms of earth spinning, and revolving around the sun, and the movement of the moon, not to mention those of the planets. The frequency of 136.102 hertz is the most common frequency associated with the earth. It is often called the "Om" frequency and is a mathematical calculation based on the rotation of the earth around the sun. The frequency of 194.18074 is a frequency based on the spinning of the earth.

The Schumann Resonance is an electromagnetic resonance in our atmosphere triggered by lightning that is vibrating at an average of 7.83 cycles per second entraining every brain on the planet into a brainwave state around alpha and theta. It is so important for our health that astronauts are fed this vibration when in outer space. This frequency connects us to nature; however, it is obscured by electromagnetism in a city. Resonating with the Schumann Resonance or tuning music to it can return one to harmony with nature.

One of the key aspects of the healing power of nature is that it opens us up. When we are in nature we listen ever closer and closer, to hear sounds as quiet as the movement of a cricket walking on a dead leaf.

Tips on Using Them
Of course, the best way by far to benefit from the healing sounds of nature is to simply go

for a walk, hike, or camp out. However, because nature sounds somehow access a very deep part of us inside, simply listening to recordings of nature sounds can be quite transformative. It's like they have the key to various parts of our system. As previously mentioned, using your voice to make various nature and animal sounds can often be miraculously healing –

> particularly when you bring through the energy of a particular element or animal so that it "speaks" through the sound of your voice.

Here's a list of calming versus activating nature sounds. Note that some might be calming to one person and activating to another. The sound of normal crickets is very soothing to some, and stops others from sleeping.

Calming	Activating
Trickling brook	Roaring river
Small waterfall	Roaring waterfall (extreme case being Niagara)
Small ocean waves	Large crashing waves
Light rain	Intense hurricane
Lightning & Thunder in distance	Lightning and Thunder over your head
Small tweety birds, including owls, lark, wren, and the flutter of a hummingbird	Ravens, crows, etc.
Sweet little animals	Animals that can kill and eat you
Most insects	Bees, flies, and mosquitoes
Soft wind through the trees	Howling wind
Leaf falling from a tree	A tree falling over
A cat's purr	An angry cat screech or one making love
A dog's whimper	An angry barking and growling dog

CD's

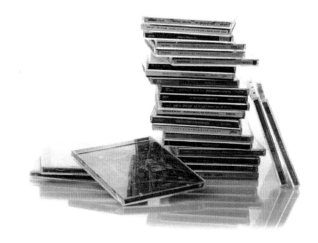

It is good to become aware of what each of your CD's is doing to you energetically. It is important to categorize your songs and music as to when you need them. You certainly already do this to a certain extent – you know what music to put on for dancing and which you put on to make love. However, you might create even more detailed music categories:

1. To wake up to
2. To get inspired
3. To calm down or go to sleep
4. To open the heart (without the nostalgia)
5. To connect to Source
6. For learning
7. To be productive mentally and/or physically
8. To meditate
9. Opening your creative channels
10. Helping you to focus on a project
11. Relieving specific pain
12. Working with a specific illness or disease

You can also categorize your CD's based on Chakras. Know which ones are good for:
1. Grounding
2. Clearing emotions or activating you sensually
3. Empowering you
4. Opening your heart
5. Creativity and expressing your heart or thoughts (also is it good to tone or sing with)
6. Opening the third eye and accessing your intuition about things
7. Connecting you to your Soul, Spirit or Source

As mentioned, not only should you be aware of exactly how the music of a particular CD affects you, but also notice that you very well might need different types of sounds and music at different times of the day. In India, there are specific Ragas for different times of the day. There might also be different music for different times of the year (or month).

Once you really tune into how any song is affecting you at each level –
physically, mentally, emotionally and spiritually –
you then also gain a wider perspective on
what sounds and music can work the best for
any healing or consciousness expanding session –
whether with live instruments or CD's

Frequency of Silence and Peace

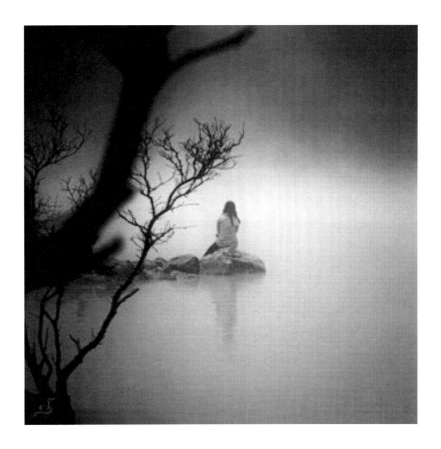

"The Medicine Man, taking his music with him, is passing quietly into the Great Silence, where the old songs were "Received in Dreams" by "inner-plane communication."
Francis Densmore (1867-1957) friend of Geronimo

Silence is Golden,
Peace is Pure White Light
- Anonymous

Silence is not always peaceful:

The eternal silence of these infinite spaces fills me with dread.
- Blaise Pascal (1623 - 1662)

Oppression can only survive through silence.
- Carmen de Monteflores

Silence is the most perfect expression of scorn.
- George Bernard Shaw (1856 - 1950), Back to Methuselah (1921) pt. 5

The cruelest lies are often told in silence.
- Robert Louis Stevenson (1850 - 1894)

However, silence that is peaceful is more powerful than all the bombs in the world.

Not merely an absence of noise, Real Silence begins when a reasonable being withdraws from the noise in order to find peace and order in his inner sanctuary.
- Peter Minard

In the attitude of silence the soul finds the path in a clearer light, and what is elusive and deceptive resolves itself into crystal clearness.
- Mahatma Gandhi (1869 - 1948)

Learn to get in touch with the silence within yourself and know that everything in this life has a purpose.
- Elisabeth Kubler-Ross

In fact, as we have previously mentioned, the best way to get to silence is by way of a song that ends on a home note and then fades really slowly. Also, the more bass the sound has, the more you end up in a profound state of peace.

This could be the most important piece of information in this whole book. So many people can never go to peace. They live their lives in a state of noise and anxiety – always looking to quell the boredom – always looking for something new to amuse them. However, there is nothing more wonderful in the world than true peace.

Silence is more musical than any song.
- Christina Rossetti (1830 - 1894)

A man's silence is wonderful to listen to.
- Thomas Hardy

True silence is the rest of the mind; it is to the spirit what sleep is to the body, nourishment and refreshment.
- William Penn (1644 - 1718)

Thoughts

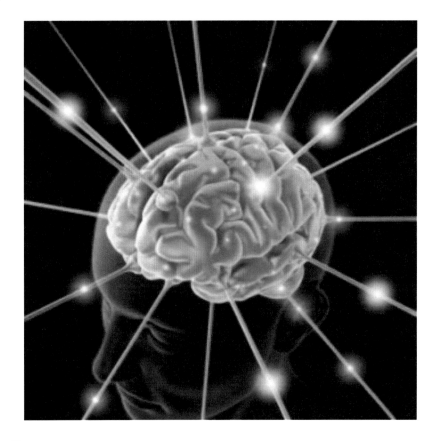

<u>What They Do</u>
As mentioned in the previous section, thoughts are made up of the frequencies of the music that our voice sings, or simply music or silence if we have no thoughts at all. Thoughts also carry positive or negative energy based on their content.

<u>Tips on Using Them</u>
There are several ways to change our thoughts with sound. The easiest is to simply replace our thoughts with sound or music. You can do this externally or internally. Monks actually replace their thoughts with non-stop prayer and chanting – often up to 12 hours a day.

You can also simply pay attention to the music of your thoughts and change the music whenever you notice that your thoughts are not flowing, or are flowing with an inordinate amount of tension and stress. When you notice such going on, add a little positive energy to your thoughts in the form of a focusing sound such as an "OM" or an "AH."

Intention

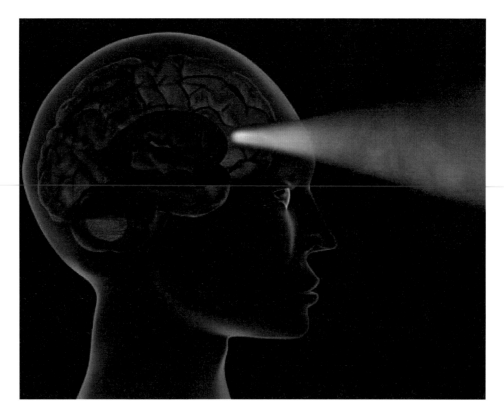

Intention is a very specific frequency. It can be as pure as one thought or as complex as an intention of flow and connection to Earth and Spirit through the Heart.

Dr. Emoto has demonstrated how our intention affects water. Also, "The Intention Experiment" by Lynn McTaggart brings together all the experiments that have scientifically proven that intention works.

Besides our words, the "intention behind our words" has a frequency that is being expressed in the world and throughout our body. If we carry a loving intention with our words, there is a second vibration that is being transmitted along with our words.

An interesting example is when someone honks a horn. The sound of the horn is actually a small part of the vibration being sent out. In fact, the sound of a horn without the negative intention of a driver could be considered to be a healing frequency that is activating. In Sound Healing dissonant sounds like this may be used to break up stuck energy. But when it is coupled with an angry intention behind it, it becomes a completely different frequency experience. It's interesting how a long horn blow is synonymous with a really angry intention. Next time you get blown at, separate out the sound from the intention. You might find that you have a whole different experience of the sound itself and it may not be annoying at all (thereby allowing you to have compassion more easily for the upset person).

<u>Tips on Using Them</u>

The key to a positive intention is to hold it purely and consistently without distraction – as if in a trance. And, remember, the more people that are holding an intention without distraction the more powerful it is. Not only can you likely heal a disease with such power, you can also change the world in very powerful ways.

And as mentioned, intention gets recorded and is carried along the sound waves every time the recording is played back.

Before, doing any type of session, set your intention for the outcome, then hold that intention consistently in your mind throughout the session.

Higher Vibrations such as Gratitude, Compassion, Love, and Joy

Similar to intention and thoughts, whenever you resonate gratitude, compassion, love or joy, you are naturally affecting others based on the laws of resonance. One of the most powerful healing frequencies you can bring to a session is Love itself. The energy of love can be more powerful than any sound.

Before doing a session, connect to these higher energies and bring them through the sounds that you are creating. (This may be the second most important thought in the book.)

Pure Spirit and Source

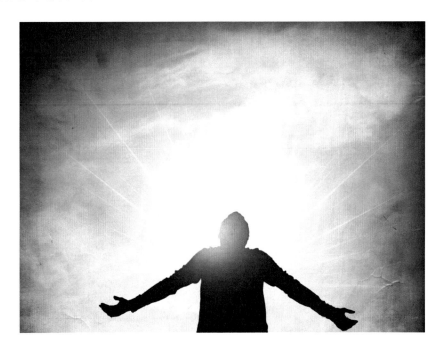

Even more powerful than Love is the energy of Spirit or Source. Source creates miracle healings everyday.

Food and Water

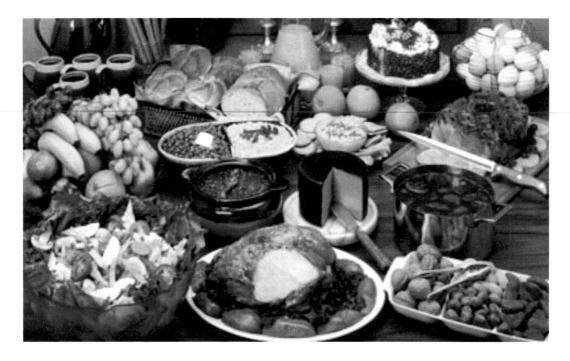

Everything we put into our body is a specific vibration or timbre. You can think of a meal as consuming a song one note or bite at a time.

Just as with sound and music there are two keys as to whether food and water are healthy for us or not. One key is whether or not we like the taste. Just as research has shown that music we like is actually healthy for us, so can we discern to a certain extent the health we gain from the food we like. Also, if we think that a food is not what we need at the time, or we feel that perhaps it has gone bad, just the thought can create the stomachache. On the other hand, regardless of what we think, certain foods are not healthy for us. Sugar may taste good, but it destroys the liver.

The key to healthy frequency food consumption is a balance of all of the nutrients or frequencies. If we get too much of anything, it can be bad for us. We can think of vitamins, minerals and all of the things we eat as providing the components of a balanced frequency diet.

When we are deciding what we would like to eat (or looking at a menu), we simply are doing a frequency sweep of all of the food frequencies and choosing, that which seems to "resonate" with our needs. Sometimes we choose things that we feel will be a healthy balance of frequencies for us. Sometimes we choose frequencies that are just fun and might actually hurt us a bit. Of course, the key is to be looking for resonances that we need in the long term for a healthy balance, versus resonances that make us happy in the moment, such as ice cream or chocolate (not to give them a bad rap).

Herbs are more specific frequencies that target very specific organs or systems in the body.

You can also look at the sustaining capacity of food based on its geometrical shape. Don Tolman talks about resonance of shape. For example, kidney beans are shaped like the kidneys and are actually good for the kidneys. Likewise, almonds are good for the ovaries, and tomatoes for the heart.

Water is more like our Soul frequency. I guess we can have too much water, but for the most part this is not a problem. The key here is to get the purest frequencies as possible. Fortunately, we can use filters to clear out all of the distracting frequencies and toxins.

There are now many devices that are also infusing frequencies into the water. The one we sell puts in the Schumann resonance of 7.83 hertz, which has been shown to not only resonate frequencies we need, but it also breaks up other negative frequencies. If interested go to www.SoundHealingCenter.com/GIA

Before you bring anything into your body, look at the food and water as a vibration. Notice its texture, its smell, and tune into the vibrational energy of where it came from. As you become more and more aware of all food and water as vibrational energy you become clearer about what items support your health as opposed to breaking it down.

Light and Color

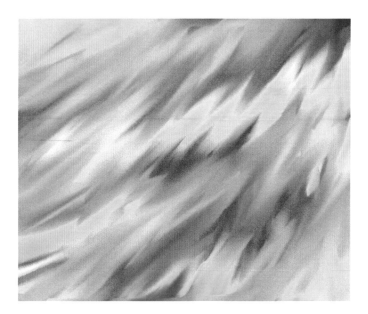

Color is a frequency, albeit one that is not heard. It is an electromagnetic frequency, which has different characteristics than sound. The key difference is that

175

electromagnetism is not carried through the air.

Color actually manifests in two ways: in pigment and in light. Pigment is the light we see reflected off of things. Light is, of course, colored light. The two actually mix together in different ways. Clear light is all colors. A black surface is a surface that reflects all colors.

In healing, colored light is the most effective; however some folks have gotten in trouble with the FDA for using colored light and making certain health claims.

The main researcher in this field was Dinshah Ghadiali. His son, Darius Dinshah, wrote the main book in the field of light therapy called, "Let There Be Light." It covers the full range of how different colors create different effects when used on the body. The book, "Color Medicine – The Secrets of Color/Vibrational Healing," by Charles Klotsche is a simplification of Darius' book and is much easier to read and comprehend. He even relates each of the colors to actual frequencies in the periodic table.

There is also a good book on pigment by John Ott, called "The Psychology of Pigment."

Below is an accepted formula for converting electromagnetic light into sound frequencies.

For those adventurous souls, here is the formula:

$$\frac{\text{Speed of Light (in nanometers per second)}}{\text{The Frequency of the Color (also in nanometers)}}$$

The ancients actually showed the speed of light to be 432 times 432, which equals 186,624 miles per second (another good reason to tune your music to 432 hertz instead of A 440). Amazingly, that comes out to exactly 300,000 kilometers per second. In nanometers per second that is 3×10^{17} (which is 3 with 17 zeros behind it).

Using red as an example, you divide its frequency of 656.1 nanometers in to the speed of light (get out your calculator). That gives you 4.57247×10^{14} or 4.57 trillion hertz. If you octavize that down (½, ½, ½, ½ etc.) 40 times you get a frequency of 415.864 hertz, which is a G sharp or A flat.

Here is the chart showing specific frequencies for the various colors, however even a slightly different shade of color corresponds to a slightly different frequency.

Note	Hertz	Equivalent Wavelength Angstroms/10 Nanometres	Approximate Colour
A	440	619.69	Orange-Yellow
A#	457.75	595.66	Yellow-Orange
Bb	472.27	577.34	Yellow
B	491.32	554.95	Yellow-Green
Cb	506.91	537.89	Green-Yellow
B#	511.13	533.44	Green
C	527.35	517.03	Green
C#	548.62	496.99	Green-Blue
Db	566.03	481.70	Blue-Green
D	588.86	463.03	Blue
D#	612.61	445.08	Blue-Violet
Eb	632.05	431.39	Violet-Blue
E	657.54	414.67	Violet
Fb	678.41	401.91	Ultra Violet
E#	684.06	398.59	Invisible Violet
F	705.77	772.66	Invisible Red
F#	734.23	742.71	Infra Red
Gb	757.53	719.86	Red
G	788.08	691.96	Red-Orange
G#	819.87	665.13	Orange-Red
Ab	845.89	644.67	Orange

There are many other people who have correlated frequency to color. The webpage here shows many of these correlations:

www.altered-states.net/barry/newsletter346/colorchart.html

What They Do
Just as with sound the different pure frequencies of color will affect us in very specific ways physically, mentally, emotionally and spiritually. Just as there are many charts as

to how different frequencies affect cells, and organs and various systems in our body, so there are multiple charts of how different colors affect us. Many people have psychically associated various colors with various frequencies, and just like with sound, no one seems to agree on a specific frequency or note for a color.

Certain colors are actually a combination of multiple colors – just like a timbre. These colors affect us in more complex ways.

Then, there is the movement of color in concerts, video, film and in certain healing tools. Now we are again looking at the quality of the flow from one color to another. This is really the color healing of the future.

Finally, we can add intention to the use of a color and we can use colors for specific intentions.

Tips on Using Them
Even though there is an accepted mathematical formula for color frequencies, there has been very little scientific research to prove that any colors have the same effects as sound frequencies. Therefore, just as with sound, I find it best to do a frequency sweep to find the best color for a specific issue. You can simply scan the full range of colors in your mind and listen for which one resonates the best for you at the time.

You can visualize colors around the whole body, inside a specific part of the body, organ or cell, or inside of a chakra.

The accepted colors for each chakra are:

1st Chakra (Root) – Red (although I like gold)
2nd Chakra – Orange
3rd Chakra – Yellow
4th Chakra – Green
5th Chakra – Light Blue
6th Chakra – Indigo
7th Chakra – Purple or White

You can use these colors, however I will often do a frequency sweep to find what color that chakra needs at any specific time.

Using colors and sound together creates a stronger Resonant Field. Again, the more ways you lead a horse to water, the more chances it will drink.

The Frequencies of Shape - The Relationships between Geometry and Sound

There is geometry in the humming of the strings,
there is music in the spacing of the spheres.
- Pythagoras (569-475 BC)

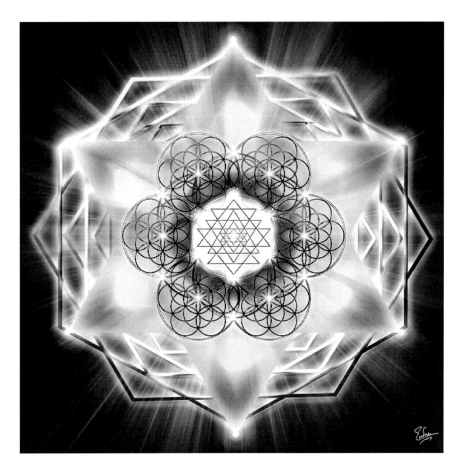

Sacred Geometries are archetypal geometric forms that are the basis of the physical world. This is a large field that has been written about in over 100 books. Again, we are just giving highlights here. If interested there are many ways to dive deeper.

There are many classic geometric forms that can be visualized inside or around the body. You can also buy these forms and use them to create energy in a room, or even place them on the body.

Here are some of the main geometric forms and their corresponding energy and colors, although you should always try and sense intuitively whether they work for you or the client.

Cube – Grounding, earth, green

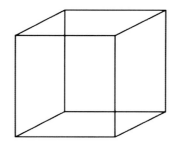

Tetrahedron – Four-sided pyramid (3 up sides) - Fire, red, mind, hydrogen

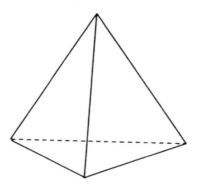

Pyramid – Five-sided pyramid (4 up sides) - Ascension

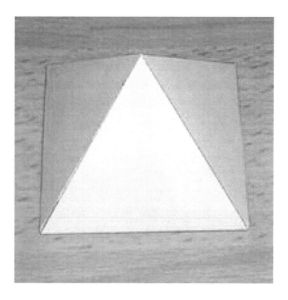

Octahedron – Two adjacent five-sided pyramids - Air, yellow, main form that straddles heaven and earth.

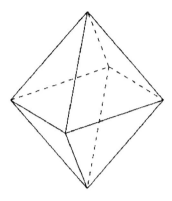

Icosahedron – 20 identical equilateral triangles - Blue

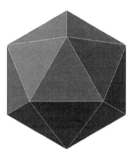

Dodecahedron – 12 pentagonal faces - Ether, gold, violet, white. Water also. Some say it is the shape of the Universe.

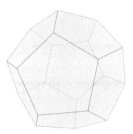

Torus – Primal form of all vortexes. Represents perfect flow within sacred geometry

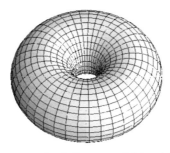

Flower of Life – Contains all geometrical forms within this one structure

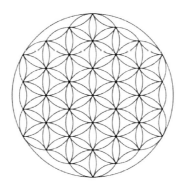

Technically every sound has a corresponding shape, and every shape has a corresponding sound.

Of course, some people intuitively get frequencies from shapes, but there are two very precise ways in which sound and shape correlate.

Cymatics
Sound creates little mandala-like patterns in the water in every cell in our body. The study of this is called Cymatics. If you place sand or water on a metal plate and vibrate the metal plate with sound you see very specific patterns in the sand. Hans Jenny did the most extensive research with Cymatics in the past and there are many YouTube videos that you can check out. John Reid and Erik Larson (one of our instructors at the Institute) have created the Cymascope and refined it to the point where you can see very clear images of water droplets being vibrated by sound.

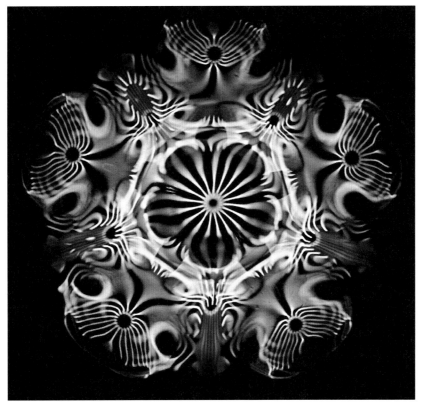

Sound of a Water Droplet (thanks to Erik Larson - www.cymascope.html)

The interesting thing is that with Cymatics you can create practically every shape in nature with specific frequencies and combinations of frequencies. Let me say that again...

> You can create practically every shape in nature
> with specific frequencies and combinations of frequencies.

I would venture to say that you could actually create every shape in the Universe with sound.

Of course, people who study and teach Sacred Geometry say that it is the other way around – that form creates sound. Once again, the chicken and egg vibrations ensue.

It could follow that

> The Universe was created with Sound.

The ramifications of this are enormous. What this means is that every single part of the body has a very specific frequency that maps to its physical shape and size – from cell to Soul. That shows how we can then use sound very specifically to break up negative cells, and resonate positive ones into their natural healthy state (and the same with every other part of the body).

We also see this same type of correlation happening in Dr. Emoto's images of snowflakes that have been created with sound.

Mathematical Mapping of Geometry to Sound
Every single geometric pattern can be broken down bit by bit into sound. Let me show you how with a simple example.

A line is like a frequency. The frequency of the line is based on the length of the line.

_____

Then, we can see musical intervals in the relationship between any two lines. For example, in this triangle the relationship between side A and side B is a musical interval. If the bottom is 3 in length and the side is 2 in length then it is a 3:2 ratio, which is exactly the same as a musical fifth.

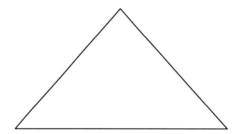

In the same way, every structure in the Universe can technically be mapped out in the form of music – no matter how complex – even the specific complex details of something like the heart.

So again, every part of the body is a timbre – in reality.
In fact, every single form in the Universe
can be mapped out as a combination of frequencies.

Our instructor, Randy Masters, has mapped out all of the musical intervals within the Sri Yantra

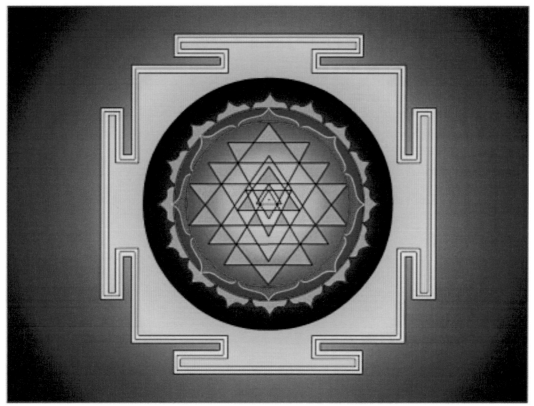

Sri Yantra

You can even see various rhythms in a flower. A flower with 4 petals is representing 4:4 time.

Tips on Using Them
You can use sacred geometry forms in many ways.

Protection – As previously mentioned you can visualize these images around yourself, an entire room or building or around the whole planet. As merkabas they create a frequency that protects you. My favorite is the Octahedron.

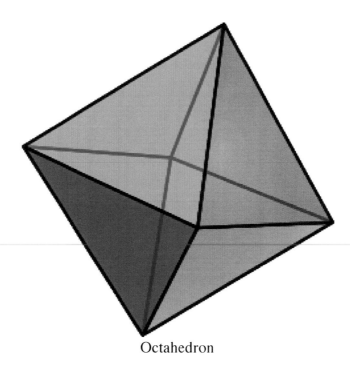

Octahedron

You can also place actual sculptures in a room or around the client. You can visualize these images inside the body – in specific parts or in specific organs. You can also place actual sculptures on various parts of the body.

When you incorporate the vibrational tools of sound, color and shape together you create an incredibly powerful resonant tool for healing and transformation. The possibilities have barely been tapped for concert production and plays.

Currently, we are working on using these technologies together in a Virtual Reality healing system where you can lie on the sound table and see a 3D graphic of the inside of your body. You will then be able to place a healing visual structure in specific body locations inside the 3D image. Sounds will then move up and down on the sound table, so that you feel them in your body right where you are seeing the visual.

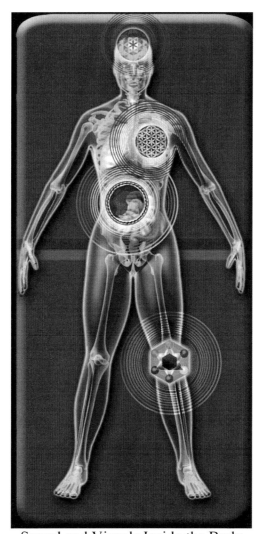
Sound and Visuals Inside the Body

You can check out more information at www.SoundHealingCenter.com/inside.html

Here are some of our favorite books on Sacred Geometry if you would like to explore further.

• "Beginners Guide to Sacred Geometry" by Michael Snider – Represents things in a really user friendly manner (good for those with math phobia).

• "Sacred Geometry – Philosophy and Practice" by Robert Lawlor.   Has some real substance with more math.

• "How the World is Made - The Story of Creation According to Sacred Geometry," by John Michell.   Amazing illustrations.

• "The Power of Limits," by Gyorgy Docci. Shows the golden mean everywhere in nature.

Crystals and Gems

Crystals and gems emit a very specific frequency based on the material and a second frequency based on its size. Then, the overall structure creates multiple musical intervals, which create an overall timbre. Technically, you could map the frequency to sound using specific mathematical calculations based on the size and lengths of sections; however you can also intuitively tune into the overall timbre and home note of the crystal or gem.

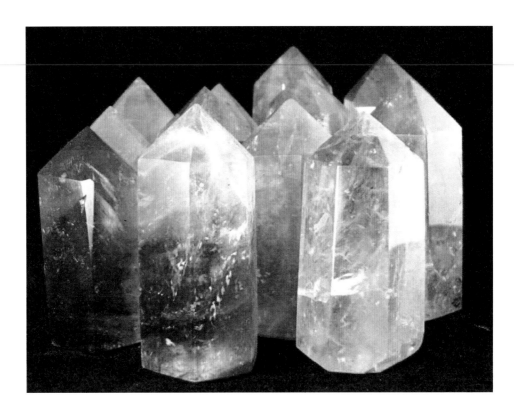

Flower Essences

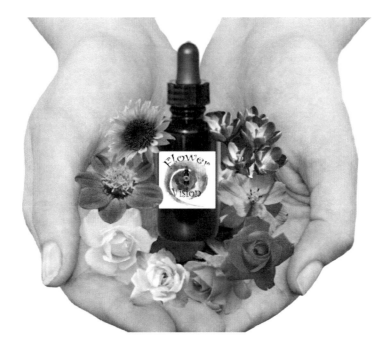

The same is true of flower essences. They commonly have multiple frequencies that create a timbre.

Electromagnetism and Magnetism

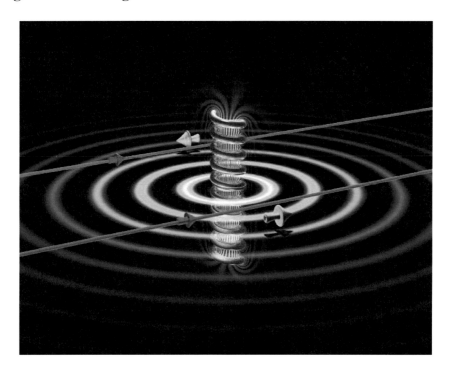

Electricity and all of the electromagnetic signals jamming the airwaves from phones, TV, and radio can create havoc in our system. However this same type of energy (including magnetism) can be extremely healing when used in coherent fashions where the frequencies are consistent and have a positive intention behind them.

What They Do
The key use is to pulse these energies to create a stable rhythm. The frequency can be used to transform cells and brainwaves, as well as to entrain the heart into healthy functioning. A healthy rhythm is one that breathes with the life of music. Therefore, the more you can instill a sense of human variation into the electromagnetic pulsing, the better.

Using the electromagnetism as carrier waves you can also transmit higher levels of information into the body and psyche. This information can come in the form of frequency, timbers, music, or pure energy.

Tips on Using Them
Generally we are talking about technologies that create these pulsing frequencies, although there are magnets that can simply be placed on the body. With these types of technologies, it is important that the rhythm of the pulsing be in synch with the sound frequencies also being used.

Lasers

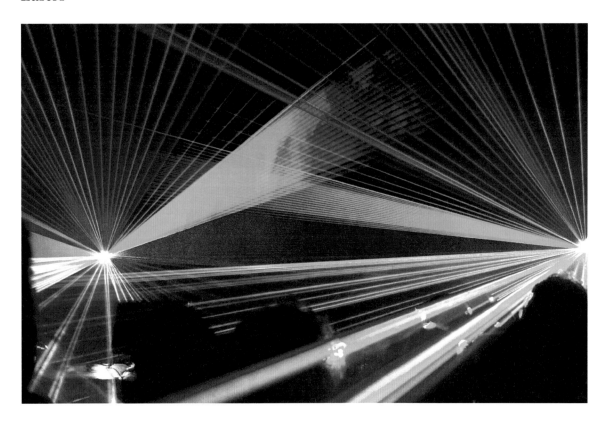

Lasers can be pulsed, but the frequency of the color coming out of them is also really important. As with electromagnetism and magnets, the pulsing frequency must be calibrated for whatever effect it is to create and must synchronize with any other vibrational methods being used.

The key aspect of lasers (and the reason they are mentioned here) is that they have a unique capability of entering the body and affecting it deeply at a cellular level. Many people believe there is no more effective way of getting sound and light frequency information into the body.

SECTION VI – Doing Sound Healing Sessions

Chapter 23 – Safety and Ethics

All sessions should be completely confidential. You want the client to feel safe in opening up and sharing.

Also, it is important to be very considerate when making suggestions. You don't want to sound as though you are telling them what to do.

> The ultimate goal when helping anyone
> is to empower them
> to be able to find their own answers
> to heal themselves.

Sound is an incredibly powerful tool. It has a power that must be wielded with full responsibility. It is really rare, but sound can bring up deep-rooted issues that can be very difficult for a person to deal with. It is important to be prepared in case anything happens.

People can have many types of reactions. Perhaps a memory of childhood abuses surfaces. Perhaps a deep fear comes to the surface. Perhaps someone has a panic attack. Perhaps someone has heart palpitations. It is important to know what to do.

1. The number one thing is to be calm. Do not react or go into fear or anxiety yourself. This is critical. Ground yourself, feel your own body; you might even tone silently to yourself in order to hold your own center. Be a pillar of peace for them!

2. Hold their hand, or if appropriate, give them a hug. If someone is having a panic attack there is nothing better than safe touch to help calm the body.

3. If appropriate, have them make the sound of how they are feeling. You might also help them make the sound. Do not use this technique if they are in fear, anxious, or having a panic attack, as sounding could make things worse.

4. Speak in really soft warm, loving tones.

5. Let them know that it's OK to feel what they are feeling, particularly if they want to cry. Often, I will say something like, "It's OK... let it out." If someone is crying, be quiet and hold space for him or her to complete the process on his or her own.

6. Don't be afraid to call 911 if things get really serious.

Generally, if you ask for guidance in the beginning of the session and set an intention for the highest good of the person, you should be fine, but it is always good to be prepared.

Chapter 24 – Performing a Sound Healing Session with Voice or Instruments

Voice Healing Session

Here are some suggestions for a procedure when doing any type of session. Use whichever ones feel comfortable to you and add your own techniques, as you like.

A voice session could be as short as five minutes or as long as an hour. Generally, I use my voice for about 20 to 30 minutes depending on the issue and situation. Ideally, you should trust your intuition as to the duration.

I actually prefer doing a voice healing session with both the client and myself standing up. It is easier to breathe and make sounds and you can get to all sides of a person's body.

However, it can just as effective to have them sitting or laying down. If lying down, it is better to have them on a massage table (if you have one) so you don't have to bend over.

Generally, you don't get closer than a few inches from the body. Some say you should never get closer than 6 inches because any less feels invasive for the client. However, if I am working on someone I know (or who trusts me) I will get closer – particularly if I am working on stressed muscles or bones. In fact, in such cases I might actually put my lips right on the body.

Tune in and make your own judgment calls as to how close you are going to get. Do what you feel is comfortable and right.

1. Set the Environment – This is often done before the client arrives. It is especially nice if you can dedicate a specific area or room for doing the treatments. That way you can really create a sacred space that feels healing to be in. Some simply create an open area. Some use crystals, soft materials, and other sacred objects to develop the space. This is not critical, so don't think you can't do powerful treatments within any space.

Some practitioners like to use sounds to prepare the space. Tingshas are known to help clear negative energies, as is playing a bowl. Playing music containing seven octaves is also a good way to clear a space. Some also burn sage or use essential oils, but be careful – some people cannot handle these strong aromas. It is a good idea to ask in advance if clients have any sensitivities.

2. Center Yourself – You can do this before the clients arrive or with them if they might be open to it. You might already have techniques you use to ground. You can simply breathe and feel your body. Then feel gravity in your body pulling you to the center of the earth. You might also play an instrument such as a crystal bowl or do any type of meditation that brings you into a place of peace and presence.

One of the simplest is to make the sound of "Om," or any vowel sound for at least a few minutes.

3. Invoke Sacred Space and Protection, and Ask for Help – I like to say something to the effect of, "I set sacred space <u>now</u>." I ask for the support and guidance of any higher beings, but only those that are of the highest good for both the client and myself. Some people like to invoke their guides, archangels, ascended masters, and/or unicorns. Others prefer to just ask for help from Spirit or Source. If it is your style, you might simply say a little prayer. This is also a good time to state an intention.

It is also really nice to visualize a sacred geometry structure around you and the client. Sometimes when doing a healing session you (or the client) might end up making some very intense and negative sounds. Just as beautiful sounds can get imprinted in the walls of a church or sacred space, so can negative sounds. Just as a Stradivarius violin actually reorganizes the cells within the wood over many years, so can sounds become embedded in the walls. Therefore, in case anyone needs to release any negative energy, it is critical that you protect the space.

There are many structures (sometimes called Merkabas) that you can visualize. Again, my favorite is the Octahedron:

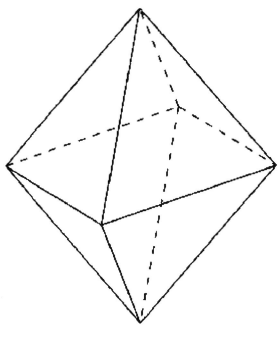

Octahedron

As with any sacred geometry structure, the visualized form actually creates a frequency. The relationships between the lengths of any two sides of a structure are actually creating a musical interval. In fact, the whole structure is just like a timbre or combination of frequencies. This structure you choose creates a stable and coherent frequency that imprints itself into the walls, protecting the room from any negative frequencies that might be emitted or released in the session.

Some people simply ask Spirit for help in protecting the space.

4. See the Person in Front of You as Beautiful, Perfect and Whole in Every Way.
Everyone is a pure, sacred Spirit in every way. There is a section in the book, "How Can I Help," by Baba Ram Dass where he meets a man who has been paralyzed on one side of his body for many years. The guy said that he had seen every type of doctor, healer and shaman he could imagine over the years. And his only wish was that **just one person would finally see him as whole instead of broken. Just one person!!!**

We are all pure perfect Spirits in every way. There is nothing wrong with any of us. Our "imperfect" symptoms are here to remind us of how to get back on the path of being connected to Source and Spirit.

Don't be attached to the outcome of the process. If healing is meant to happen, it will. If not, be humble. If it does, be humble.

5. Intake or Not – There are three different ways to do a session:

a) Ask no questions and proceed with the session. This technique can actually help get your mind out of the process.

b) Ask what their complaint or issue is. It is often helpful to know where to focus the sounds.

c) Use an assessment tool. You could do frequency sweeps on the person. You can also do a sweep up and down on the body with one consistent note, listening for where your voice breaks up. Some people actually use Tingshas or gongs on the body to see where the instrument seems to be muted or stops ringing out. These are all indications of blocked energy. There are a wide range of assessment technologies that you could also use that are discussed in Appendix A online, "How to Find Frequencies…"

d) Do a complete intake. This might include the following questions:

1. Any previous experience with Sound Healing?
2. What other types of treatments do you resonate with?
3. What brought you here? What would you like to work on?
4. Tell me about your day.

Daily Life
5. Any Health Issues?
6. Job and abundance?
7. Stressors?
8. How's your diet?

9. How's your sleep?
10. How much water are you drinking?
11. Any relationship issues?
12. What processes or practices do you do?

Favorites
13. What's your favorite style of music?
14. To what do you listen to feel at peace?
15. Favorite color?
16. What are your favorite instruments?
17. Do you prefer rhythm or no rhythm?
18. Prefer male or female voice?

19. How do you feel about your own voice?

When doing the complete intake, you may decide to focus on a specific issue or just do an overall healing session. Sometimes, you might even find that you are guided to focus on an issue other than what they are bringing up – perhaps a deeper issue behind the conscious issue.

6. Do a Minute of Silence – After doing any assessment, stop and let what they have said sink in.

7. Prepare to Begin – Tell them to let you know if any sounds are exceedingly uncomfortable and they would like for you to stop. This is really important so they don't ever feel out of control or overwhelmed. If you think you might touch them, ask for permission.

Some people like to actually think about the overall structure of the session, what instruments you might need, and get them ready. Always leave plenty of room for spontaneity.

8. Perform the Session – Get out of the way and let Spirit take over as much as possible. Trust that the sounds will come through you that are needed. **Trust!!!** You may also get the client to make sounds if appropriate and if they are open to it. Of course, don't force anything.

9. Do another Minute of Silence – Allow the sounds to sink in. I have found that most of the healing actually happens within the silence after the session has ended.

10. Give Thanks – Thank them and thank your spiritual helpers, including Spirit and Source Itself.

11. Get Feedback from the Client. Be quiet and listen.

12. Share What You Saw and Discuss the Next Step. If you got any information about what is going on with them, share it. This can help them focus on specific issues and integrate, and can also give them more confidence that something seriously healing just happened.

The ultimate goal is to empower them to heal themselves, so if you can, come up with some homework for them to do. This might be as simple as taking a bath, or as complex as doing a sound exercise such as toning or chanting daily. Chapter 50, "Living with Sound – Using Sound in Your Daily Life," has a complete list of sound practices that you might also suggest.

The more you do this process on others, the more comfortable you get, and the more effective the treatments become.

Sound Healing Sessions with Instruments

Of course, you can combine voice with this treatment. And, again, feel free to add in any techniques or modalities that you might already know.

A Sound Healing session could be as short as five minutes or as long as an hour and a half. Generally, I will do about 30 to 40 minutes depending on the issue and situation. I often start by putting someone on the sound table and vibrating them into bliss. Ideally, you should trust your intuition as to the duration.

The basic procedure is the same as for voice healing. However, sessions with multiple instruments can get to be quite complex, depending on your abilities and comfort zone.

Ideally, you want to follow your own intuition as to what to do in the session. The key is to figure out some basic things that you are comfortable doing. For example, toning on the body, using crystal bowls, using tuning forks, etc. Often, it is nice to have an array of sounds and instruments ready to go; however, if you have only one instrument, miracles can still happen.

Often, it is nice to plan out the whole session based on any assessment information you have received. It can be extremely helpful to plan out the overall flow of the session – even if Spirit ultimately takes over and takes you in a completely different direction.

There are several "flows" that are commonly followed in the field.

It is important to be aware of the flow of the session
in order to create continuity in the session.
This continuity provides the consistency
we are all looking for.

1. Meet people where they are, bringing them down into the depths, and then bringing them back up a bit at the end of the session so they can function and drive.

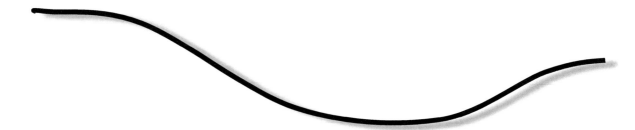

This flow is really good for someone who is having a hard time relaxing, and still has a lot to do after the session.

In this session format you begin by matching the person's energy level: high or low, centered or scattered, calm or anxious – wherever they are, try and find sounds that match their energy. Also, play the sounds at a volume that seems to match their energy.

Matching someone's energy and then slowly transforming it is called the "iso-principle." This technique has been proven to be extremely effective for transformation, particularly if someone is seriously stuck.

You might start with two or more crystal bowls at the same time, which can be quite activating. Then, play fewer and fewer bowls until you are down to just one bowl. You might then add your voice to the bowl's sound, singing more and more softly until you finally stop playing the bowl and are just singing, getting softer and sweeter the whole time. After a period of time, slowly bring the crystal bowl back in, or perhaps you might even play some Tibetan bowls to bring them out of the trance into an awakened state once again.

2. Deep Relaxation – Bring them down, down, down to a place of deep peace and presence.

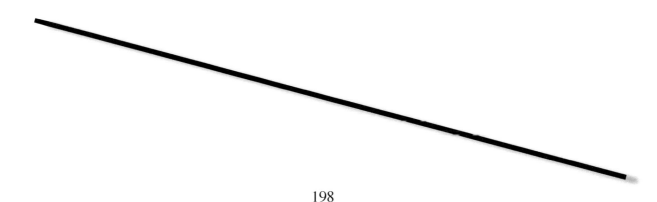

This flow is one my favorites. I often like to leave people at a deep state of peace. We are the most creative, productive and happy when we are at peace.

This type of session is ideal for someone that is dealing with stress. (Wouldn't happen to know anyone like that, would you? ☺) It is also perfect for someone who is anxious or having panic attacks. In fact, deep relaxation is good for just about any type of emotional issue. It is also good for most physical issues, because they are often exacerbated by a variety of emotions, especially fear.

3. The Stairway to Heaven

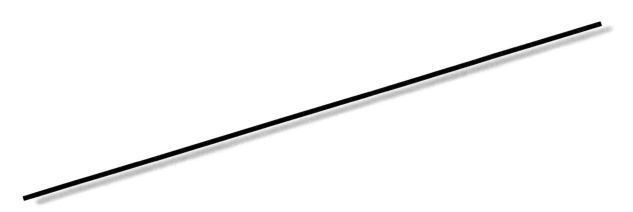

This flow is really good for anyone who is dealing with low energy, lethargy, depression or is having a hard time coping with a conflict or challenge.

4. The Mountain Journey

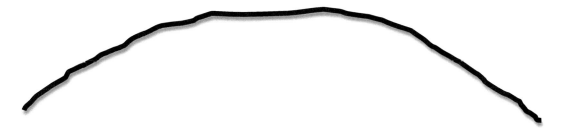

This type of flow is especially helpful for those that are overwhelmed or dealing with major challenges. It provides an opportunity to deal with intensity in a controlled way that then resolves.

5. Stability

This type of flow is good for those who simply need more stability and equanimity in their life. It is often quite useful for those who are hypersensitive to sound, or those who are over stimulated and can't handle much of anything.

There are many aspects of sound and music that create the ups and downs for each of these curves.

Sound and Music Dynamics

	Calming	Activating
1.	Even Harmonics	Odd Harmonics
2.	Complex (Rich) Harmonic Structure	Pure Sounds
3.	Harmonic Intervals or Chords	Dissonant Intervals or Chords
4.	Soft Volumes	Loud Volumes
5.	Fewer Instruments	More Instruments
6.	Low Frequencies	High Frequencies
7.	No Tempo; Slower Tempo	Faster Tempos
8.	More Sustain or Legato Notes	Staccato or Short Duration Notes
9.	Sub-Delta, Delta, Theta	Alpha, Beta, Gamma
10.	Simple Melodies	Complex Melodies
11.	No Harmony Parts; Unison Harmonies	2 or 3 Part Harmonies
12.	Simple Song Structure	Complex Song Structure
13.	Calming Nature Sounds	Activating Nature Sounds
14.	Sparse Mix; Reverb	Full Mix; Trippy Effects
15.	Vowel Sounds	Lyrics
16.	Male Vocals	Female Vocals
17.	Performing	Channeling
18.	Sound Healing Music (indefinable)	Normal Music or Known Song

Most of this chart is self-explanatory; however, some parts are not:

5. Fewer instruments are normally more calming, but if one instrument is extremely edgy and activating, then more instruments will actually mellow it out by making the one instrument less prominent

7. Tone generators don't create a tempo. You wouldn't think bowls do either, but they often have slow oscillations that actually do create a tempo.

8. Sustain notes are notes that last a long time. Generally, if you have a lot of sustain notes the tempo is slower.

9. These brainwave states are covered in more detail in Section IX.

11. Harmony parts simply mean singing or playing an instrument more than once at different notes simultaneously. A unison harmony means that more than one person sings the exact same note. This requires multiple people in a live session, but can be done with multitrack recording in the recording studio.

12. The song structure is the order of the sections of the song: Verse, chorus, bridge, lead break, etc. A crystal bowl playing by itself is the simplest song structure you can have – it has only one section for the whole song.

14. A sparse mix means an audio mix that has no effects added in the recording studio while mixing. There is a wide range of effects that can be created electronically in the studio.

15. When you have lyrics in a language that people can understand, another side of the brain kicks in. This side of the brain understands words and is also the judgmental side. Therefore, when you have songs that just use vowels or are in languages that we don't understand, like Sanskrit, our brains don't complain as much.

16. Male vocals are more calming because they are normally lower in pitch and have more harmonics. However, of course, there are many female vocals that are more calming based on the sound of the voice and the way the vocalist sings.

17. Channeled music is very activating at first, because you never know what is going to happen next. Therefore, it demands 100% presence. However, once you are present with the channeling they can take you deeper and calmer than ever.

18. Most styles of music we already have developed opinions about, and know the times and situations in which we would like to listen to it. Commonly, Sound Healing music defies categorization. Therefore, it often bypasses the judgmental brain and is allowed to go directly to all of our organs unmediated.

Treatments We Do at the Institute
To see all of the treatments done at the Institute go to
www.SoundTherapyCenter.com

SECTION VII – Physical Healing with Sound

Introduction – Physical Vibrations Changing Physical Matter

In this section we focus on how to use sound on physical parts of the body. Of course, the Newtonian way of breaking the body down into separate components can be quite limiting. As previously mentioned, emotional healing, mental enlightenment, and Spiritual transformation are as powerful if not more powerful in creating physical changes in the body. And often when we do treatments, we will bring in other aspects of healing than just the physical. They really can't be separated out. Ideally, all four aspects of physical, mental, emotional and Spiritual come together in a complete hologram so powerful that any pain, illness or disease doesn't have a chance.

However, in order to understand and apply the physical healing component of sound, we will be focusing only on it in this section. The information being presented can be especially helpful if you or a client has a very specific physical issue that you are dealing with.

The best part about sound versus other energy healing modalities is the physical component that comes to bear in the process. People often latch onto use of sound resources because science can explain the process very clearly. In fact, physics explains quite succinctly how sound works on matter. It has been studied for quite a long time now.

As previously mentioned, based on the laws of resonance, there are 6 main things we know:

1. Sound waves transmit energy into any matter they come in contact with. This is the most basic positive part of all Sound Healing, for receiving energy is practically always a good thing.

2. When you send a frequency that matches the resonant frequency of an object or piece of matter, it not only receives the energy transmitted, it also releases its own stored energy. This is key...for when you hit the resonant frequency of anything, you are feeding the object its own energy. In cells, this can trigger their metabolism.

3. Vibrating something is similar to a massage. We all need a massage – no matter whether we're a cell, an organ or a limb. Not only do frequencies feed us energy, but they also create more flexibility in us, which allows a more healing and enlivening flow of energy. Blockages are generally made up of things that are solidified or calcified, and vibrations can break up this rigid condition.

4. Sending a consistent frequency such as a vowel sound or a sustain note from an instrument, harmonizes the non-coherent state of a buzz in the body.

5. Loud vibrations transmitted at an object's resonant frequency can explode or break up the object or material. This doesn't normally happen with a person or individual organs, but it can easily happen with small and fragile matter such as cells.

6. Frequencies that are oscillating up and down in pitch ever so slightly create low frequency binaural beats that are powerful enough to explode or break up many things. This is more effective in small things like cells. We'll explain more about this later.

Chapter 25 – Buzz in the Body Syndrome (BIBS)

Given that our whole system is made up of pure frequencies, combinations of frequencies, flowing music, and flowing energy, it seems obvious that the key cause of any pain, illness or disease is simply disharmony at any one of these four levels. Ultimately, it can be disharmony at all of these levels.

Pure Frequency
Pure frequencies manifest as the home note in every cell, organ, limb, and in the chakras, auras and Soul. From a frequency perspective there are several "disharmonies" that can happen at this level:

1. Detuned – The cell or part of the body is simply resonating at a different note from the one it is meant to resonate at. It could be just slightly out of tune (the same note, just a little off pitch), or it could be detuned to a completely different note. It is my guess that this is not the most common problem, but until we do more serious research, no one really knows for sure.

2. No Frequency at All – I would guess that this is the most common problem of all. The cell or part of the body is just buzzing. It's kind of like the heart in defibrillation. It is not vibrating at any frequency at all, it is just sending out a noise similar to white noise.

In some areas of healing (particularly around the chakras) people talk about something being stagnated (not enough energy to vibrate smoothly) or over-activated (too much energy, also causing it to go out of smooth vibration). It seems that both of these states are like a buzzing sound – one subtle and the other more intense.

Timbre, Tone or Harmonic Structure
Every part of the body is actually made up of combinations of cells that create a whole "timbre" at which the organ naturally vibrates. Once again, there are only a couple of ways that the timbres can be in disharmony.

1. Detuned – The natural harmonic structure of any part of the body has its own harmonious integrity. If you could hear this, it would sound good and harmonious. If certain harmonics were to get out of tune, then there would be a dissonance. Dissonance in the system tends to block the flow of energy (or just slow it down). Any one harmonic could have gotten detuned, or a whole set might have gotten detuned. They might be too

high or too low in pitch.

The harmonics might actually not have gotten detuned at all, but if they are simply too low or too high in volume, that would also detract from the organ's natural ability to function.

2. Noise in the System – If noise or a buzz has gotten into the system, it can be seriously disruptive to the natural harmonic flow. One or more of the harmonics could be having problems vibrating because of an emotion or toxin, or there could simply be some outside noise that has entered the system.

Musical Flow
At this level, there are many things that can be out of whack. Of course, when the song moving through the organ is not flowing, this will also begin to interrupt the smoothness of the flow through the whole body.

1. Inconsistent Flow caused by outside forces interrupting the flow.

2. Buzzes in the song, just like static or distortion on an audio recording.

3. The song gets stuck or simply stops playing altogether. This can be a pretty serious situation depending on the organ.

Energetic Flow
Again, multiple problems all contribute to "rough flow" or "no flow."

1. Loss of connection to Soul and Source.

2. Distraction by negative energies.

At just about every level, one of the key problems is buzzing. I am using this term as a catch all for all of the distorted, jagged, scattered, icky sounds that occur physically in the body. Buzzes are pre-pain and therefore are not normally painful – although they can be extremely annoying and uncomfortable. Pain is actually the extreme case of a buzz – you might think of pain as a screaming buzz.

I'm sure you know what I mean about these buzzes. The best example is when you can't sleep because your whole system is buzzing. It is like there is a soft little bumblebee on coffee (or amphetamines) somewhere in your body. He's a little wired and he is not going to sleep.

I call this "Buzz in the Body Syndrome," or "BIBS."

I've come to believe very strongly that BIBS is the #1 beginning of any physical issue in the body. BIBS, over a long period of time creates all diseases.

I would guess that disharmony or detuning of a part of the body could be the cause of the buzz. And, I would guess that the cause of the disharmony is emotional stress and/or environmental toxins (including those in our food). We'll be discussing how to deal with the emotional stress in the next Section.

The good news is

Sound can easily
overcome and entrain
BIBS into
sweet harmonic vibrations again.

I have seen it happen hundreds of times. The bumblebee stops buzzing and starts humming again.

The first step is to track down the buzz. Where in the body is it? Often, when I thought my whole body was buzzing, I've discovered that it is actually one specific part of the body that is the prime culprit. It seems that this one buzzing part of the body is entraining the rest of the body into the wily buzz.

After many years of tracking down buzzes I have discovered that they normally occur in the endocrine glands – especially the thyroid, thymus and adrenals. I wouldn't doubt that the pituitary, hypothalamus and pineal glands in the head also get buzzes, but they are much more subtle to detect.

We will be exploring the endocrine glands in much more detail in Chapter 42, "Harmonizing the Chakras with Sound."

Buzzes also happen in the intestines. It is really hard to feel buzzes in organs and practically impossible to detect them in cells through feeling.

When you find a buzz in any particular part of the body, you can simply send a consistent tone to it. You could use your voice, an instrument or a tone generator; however, I believe the voice to be the most effective.

You simply tone a vowel sound and focus the sound on the part of the body that is buzzing. I find that my thyroid is the number one culprit, however commonly my adrenals are just crackling from being fried.

Chanting, mantras or any warm singing will also work. Simply focus your attention and the sound on the part of the body that is vibrating. Adding a positive healing intention makes it even more powerful.

I would say that this technique works more than 95% of the time for me. Perhaps I'm a little more experienced, but even if it works 60% of the time, it is worth a try.

**The buzzing simply stops
and I feel harmony in my body once again.
If I couldn't sleep, I go right to sleep.
Amazing!**

**Would that all of my aches and pains would go away
and not come another day
Lord, I promise, I would be
so grateful.**

Chapter 26 – Stress Relief, Anxiety, Panic Attacks, Fibromyalgia, and other Stress Related Issues

The most obvious benefit of sound and music is stress relief. It is one of the most effective, and because it is also so enjoyable and often pleasurable, it ranks at the top of all stress relief activities.

It is important to note that many sounds and music can easily create stress. At the risk of alienating a large number of people, I believe that very little Classical music is relaxing. It does not get really mellow, and it rarely has intention embedded in it (perhaps intention from the master who wrote it, but not from the conductor or musicians).

However, different people often react differently to various sounds and music. In fact, music that relaxes me one day sometimes bothers me the next day. As mentioned, certain sounds might work better in the morning; others are better in the afternoon or evening. The key is to develop your own sensitivities for how well something is working. Tune in and check out whether you think a sound or a piece of music might be appropriate; then watch like a hawk as you start using the sound. Of course, this is for both yourself and for anyone you are working on.

As previously mentioned, there are several main components of sound and music that contribute to a relaxed state.

First, there is the consistency and flow of the sound and music that can put you "in the zone," so to speak. This state is the same as the coherent heart rate state where your heart rate goes up and down in a smooth s-curve. It is an active state where you are at peace. Crystal bowls and drums are especially effective at creating this state. However, when we look at a Galvanic Skin Response monitor, that monitors tension in the body, the person may not actually be relaxing.

Soft warm sounds and sweet melodies seem to bring us into more of a relaxed state based on tension in the body. Low frequency sounds are also extremely effective– low strings or a soft murmur.

Steven Halpern has pointed out (and researched) the fact that certain musical intervals, like the musical fifth, create tension by "wanting" to resolve to the home note. However, other intervals, like the musical fourth, actually don't have this need to go home and thus can actually create more of a relaxed floaty feeling.

But, most importantly (and as mentioned many times throughout the book), the key component for bringing people into a restful state of mind is to end with a slow fade on the home note. The slower and smoother the fade in volume, the more effective and profound is the state of peace. The effect is even more enhanced when there is a large amount of bass in the song or instrument.

Having had thousands of people on our sound tables (massage tables with speakers mounted on the bottom), I have come to believe strongly that they are the most effective stress relief devices in the field. The bass is exceedingly powerful and when the music is flowing with the right intention the effect is beyond profound – particularly as it fades to perfect peace.

However, when played in the right way, there are many sounds and instruments that can and do take people into the most amazing states of peace ever. Again, consistency is key – consistency in the sound, the rhythmic flow, the chord changes, and the intention. Generally a certain amount of repetition tends to help us get rid of stress. Sounds with many changes are more activating, and though excellent for learning and productivity they often do not create the consistency associated with peace and stillness.

Anxiety Relief
There is nothing better than sound for dealing with anxiety – particularly panic attacks. Anxiety and panic could just as easily have been addressed under the section on Emotional Healing, but I have found that once the anxiety builds up enough to become a panic attack, it has normally gotten to the point where there are toxins in the body that take awhile to clear out even if the emotional issues have been dealt with or resolved.

Having had many panic attacks years ago, this has become one of my specialties. First, I believe very strongly that for most panic attacks, love is the antidote. One of the simplest techniques you can do is tune into the energy of love as much as you can. Then listen for the sound of that love – high or low. Make the sound and send that love with the sound to your own heart. Generally, it comes out as a really soft sweet sound – sometimes even a song.

When helping others with this technique, I will actually sing along with them softly. If someone is too embarrassed to sing out loud, I will do it for him or her and invite him or her to join in if they like.

To really help anchor this energy of love, so it can be easily accessed, I will sometimes listen for what note the person goes to when they start singing. This is most likely the key of love for that person. I then make them a CD in that key (I have a few of my songs in every key). I tell them to sing along with the CD and send love to their heart whenever they are feeling anxious.

This technique also works amazingly well for anyone who is dealing with a loss – whether it is a breakup or a death.

I have also found that using sound on chakras will get rid of a panic attack completely. Let me say this again a little bolder:

Using sound on chakras gets rid of panic attacks

I would like to go on the rooftop and announce this to the world. There are so many people who are suffering intense fear and anxiety and the only help they know of is drugs. And sadly, the drugs ultimately create a deficiency in the system that then makes the panic attacks worse.

I explain a technique in detail for doing a sound treatment on the chakras in Chapter 42, "Harmonizing Chakras with Sound."

Meanwhile, there are so many things you can do for anxiety relief using consistency, home notes, slow fades, and intention. Instruments placed directly on the body are also effective as they help bring you back into your body.

- Play an instrument that sustains. Play a crystal bowl daily (even a few times a day). Tone with it if you like. Be sure and hold the silence for at least five minutes after the bowl fades out.

- Use tuning forks on the spine. You can also use tuning forks on the chest and head.

- Do at least 10 minutes of toning, chants, and mantras per day. Ultimately 10 minutes three times a day is ideal.

- Listen to relaxing music. Seek out music that really does it for you. Take time in your day to stop and give 100% of your intention to the music you are listening to. You can also put on music while working or doing odd jobs around the house.

- Get on a sound table. Sound tables with the right music are extremely effective for getting rid of the anxiety that leads to panic attacks, however the sound table can be too activating during an actual panic attack.

Fibromyalgia
There are a wide range of physical issues that result from stress. Some of the most common are digestion issues, fibromyalgia, and muscle tension. The National Institute of Health has actually done a study on the use of sound tables to treat fibromyalgia and results have shown their effectiveness.

Chapter 27 – Healing Organs, Body Parts and Body Systems

Sound is more effective on certain parts of the body than others. We haven't done scientific research to prove this, but I have been paying close attention over many years.

Based on my experience, these are the primary areas where sound is really effective, in order of the most effective to least effective.

1) Endocrine Glands – As previously discussed many of the endocrine glands are either constructed similarly to the ear, or have crystals inside of them, so it seems that they have consciously been designed to receive and be affected by sound. In my experience they are very easily affected. I have found that simply transmitting a sound to the gland (even silently), easily calms it down such that the gland begins resonating at its own natural frequency again, which means that it again begins functioning normally.

Again, it is nice if you can find the resonant frequency of the gland; however most importantly is that you transmit a consistent frequency with a good intention. As usual, the voice is the most powerful tool, however you can focus the sound of a tuning fork, crystal bowl, Tibetan bowl or even a tone generator right on the gland.

We also have frequencies based on some research by the Germans during World War II that are extremely effective. There are 6 frequencies for each gland (therefore a timbre) that seem to massage the glands quite effectively.

Don't forget that you can also do a frequency sweep and find a gland's frequency. And remember, even if this seems beyond your sensitivity at the current time, I have seen many, many students develop this capacity over the years when they thought it was not possible. Simply practice over and over and there is a good chance that you will start to develop this sensitivity.

As you can well imagine, being able to help or even heal endocrine glands is huge. Thyroid problems are a huge boon for the pharmaceutical companies, and the thyroid is so easily affected by a simple "OM," or "AH." Similarly, the adrenal glands are wiped out in many people due to the overwhelming amount of stress that we take on in our lives. Imagine being able to simply harmonize the adrenals with a sound. Then there is the thymus gland, which is known for being the portal to Universal Love – and who doesn't need more love in their lives? A healthy thymus has also been associated with a healthy immune system.

Some say that if you don't use your pituitary and pineal glands, they atrophy and die, so it is also critical that we get them activated – and sound is an amazingly powerful tool for this. As we'll discuss in Chapter 42 on chakras, you can also activate these glands energetically by focusing on the energy of each chakra.

2) Bones, Ligaments and Tendons – Two separate research projects have found that the frequency of a cat's purr actually regenerates bones. The core frequency is 45 hertz. We

have also had incredible results using the Cymatics frequencies on broken bones. One woman had broken her leg in 6 places and it was healing in just two weeks. The doctors said they had never seen bones start receiving calcium after a break in less than one month.

It seems that the bones require sounds over a long period of time (at least 10-20 minutes), which is difficult to do with the voice. Therefore, it is often best to use instruments, electronic devices or CD's.

3) Muscles – Muscles are also easily affected by sound. Low frequencies are the most effective. Technically low frequencies transmit more energy than high frequencies (and it takes more power to create them). Again, it is like a deep tissue massage.

The voice works quite well on muscles. I like to get right on the muscle with the mouth and make a loud and powerful vibration. "Uuu" as in "who" is one of the easiest sounds to make powerfully. (It's much harder to make the sound "Ahh" with a lot of power).

Sound is especially effective if you can apply it immediately after a muscle gets strained or twisted. If you can start toning or get some sound right on the muscle within 2 or 3 minutes it is like the muscle never gets the message that something bad has happened, and it doesn't tighten up. I know this for sure as I have twisted my back a few times in a way that would normally be painful for a few days or a week. However, when I was able to apply a vibration to it – even by simply moving my fists briskly up and down on the spot – then it was fine within an hour or so.

4) Digestion – Digestion seems to be especially susceptible to stress and tension. We've had really good luck with using frequencies on the stomach, small intestines, and large intestines. We've also had some good results working on the kidneys and bladder.

The digestive track especially responds well to the Cymatics frequencies and tuning forks, although I've seen a miracle recovery on nausea using the voice. A friend had been vomiting for 3 days and I did a voice healing on her. Within 10 minutes she felt 100% back to normal and even wanted to go dancing. I've never seen such a dramatic transformation happen so quickly.

5) Cells – When you transmit the resonant frequency to a cell it feeds the cell energy. However, again, if you turn up the volume or hold the volume for a sustained amount of time, the cell can be destroyed.

Of course, it is much trickier to find the exact frequency of a cell intuitively. Therefore, I often try the frequencies in the charts first. Sometimes, if you are really tuned in and in the zone, you just might be able to hear the right frequency – it can seem as though Spirit simply whispers it in your ear. I find it much more effective to do the frequency sweep in my mind, instead of out loud. It seems that the energy used to make a sound out loud, and all the resulting resonances in the other parts of the body, distract you from the subtle sensitivity you need to tune into something as small as a cell inside your body.

6) Body Cavities – Resonating the chest and/or abdomen cavities can help facilitate flow and healing in all of the organs in the cavity by simply feeding the area energy and the accompanying internal massage. Same with the head cavity – resonating the cavity will activate the entire brain and will feed energy to each of the endocrine glands within.

As mentioned, finding the resonant frequencies of body cavities is really easy. If you put your hand on that part of the body you can feel when it vibrates the most as you zone in on the correct frequency.

7) Organs – Finding the precise frequency for organs is sometimes difficult, however there are many frequencies in the frequency charts that you can try. I actually find it quite easy to find the frequency of my own organs and I must say it feels so good to resonate any particular organ. However, I have a hard time feeling most organs – particularly the pancreas and spleen.

You can use any instrument, but the voice is almost always preferable because of its direct connection to Spirit. Remember, the precise frequency is not critical (though nice). A consistent frequency sent with a good intention is the most important and still extremely powerful.

8) Skin – Skin is especially receptive to sound treatments. I believe this is due to the fact that it is so malleable and consists of so much water. I saw a workshop at a Sound Healing conference, where they had developed a whole protocol using specific frequency tuning forks for a complete facial.

I saw a person who had burned her fingers on a wood burning stove. She actually got burnt twice. She applied tuning forks immediately to the first burn. The second, she did nothing to. The first burn was practically gone in two days. The second burn turned into a large blister and took about 2 weeks to heal.

Later we'll explain how you can also send the frequency of love or other higher energies with sound directly to any organ or part of the body.

Again, the order of the above list (based on which parts of the body are the most receptive to sound work) is not based on scientific research and it is likely that we will find that other parts of the body are even more affected by sound – particularly when the appropriate frequencies, timbres or music is applied. Ultimately, you should be able to heal everything from a fingernail to a wart – it's all frequency!

Chapter 28 – Sound on Disease

Of course, we (or you) can never claim that something as inexpensive as sound could actually cure a disease. However, there are so many stories to share from people that have had cancer completely disappear, or had a disease go into remission and never return.

I believe that the true miracle stories are more commonly a combination for physical, mental, emotional (especially emotional) and Spiritual transformations that happen as a result of the sound – when the person is open and ready to allow the transformation to happen.

As previously mentioned, you can use sound to explode cells by transmitting a sound at a loud volume to the cell. Even though this technique is murderous, so to speak, if I had cancer, I would not hesitate to bring out the big sound guns.

For this approach I believe that the best technique is to create binaural beats around the core frequency of the disease in order to break it up or destroy the cells. This is precisely how a wine glass gets broken with the voice.

You would think that the glass breaks by matching its resonant frequency with a loud volume. However, a research study (that a student brought to me) showed that you need to make the sound at the resonant frequency of the glass ten times louder than the human voice is capable of making. In the research project, they actually found the resonant frequency of a wine glass and then played speakers at its frequency. The volume that it took to break the glass was way beyond what the human voice is capable of.

You can actually break a wine glass with the voice and there is a YouTube video where a woman does so.

Woman breaking a wine glass YouTube video
http://www.youtube.com/watch?v=eTWDEsGlPO8

So what is going on? Here's how it works. You first sing the frequency of the wine glass to get it humming. You can do a frequency sweep to find the frequency, but it's easier to simply tap the wine glass or run a wet finger around the rim and listen for the note. Then, sing the same note. Then, go up and down in pitch ever so slightly just above and below the resonating frequency of the glass. You can also do this with the voice's natural vibrato. Vibrato in the voice naturally goes up and down in pitch ever so slightly.

You now have two different frequencies: 1) the frequency of the glass vibrating, and 2) your voice, a little off pitch. When you have two frequencies very close to each other a third frequency is created, which is the difference between the two frequencies. In this case, this difference frequency is going to be less than 5 hertz, normally around 1 cycle per second. Well, the wavelength of 1 cycle per second is about 1,130 feet physically in the air. This is a huge and powerful waveform that can easily knock over a house (with enough power), and it has no trouble at all exploding the wine glass.

I believe this concept is one of the most powerful healing techniques there is. There are many reasons why I believe this to be so.

One of our previous instructors had a tumor in her breast that was about a millimeter in diameter. She decided to go to the woods for a month and work on the tumor. She said that she focused her voice on the tumor and when she hit the right frequency she could actually feel the tumor heating up. She then intuitively moved her voice up and down, above and below the frequency that was causing the tumor to heat up. She also had her friend play the didgeridoo right on her tumor. The didgeridoo also has a frequency that goes up and down a bit – particularly when the player does a "growling" sound.

A couple of months later she went in for surgery. Before surgery they did another x-ray. Then, the doctor told her that something was wrong with the x-ray machine and they had to do another x-ray. The doctor came back and said there was no sign of the tumor – the tumor was completely gone. As of the date of writing this book, the tumor has been gone for over 7 years now.

I used to get treatments from a psychic who was really powerful. She would mentally go inside my body and take out stuck energy. One day I asked her, "What the hell are you doing in there?" She said that she could see the stuck energy as a frequency, and that she would "rock it" loose. Again, it occurred to me that she was doing a small frequency sweep up and down, above and below the frequency of the stuck energy.

In Cymatics, the treatment normally oscillates slightly above and below the frequency of the specific issue.

Therefore, we have 3 pieces of evidence (counting the science on how sound explodes a wine glass with binaural beats) that point to binaural beats breaking up diseases and stuck energy.

Therefore, the key is to first find the frequency, and then simply go up and down in pitch, above and below this frequency. If you can sing with vibrato that will work also (in fact, the actual speed of the vibrato might also have to do with it). And, don't forget to ask for help from higher powers (if appropriate) and set your intention for the treatment to work. When it does, please email me about it. The more we can prove this works, the better chance that we will finally be able to get it into the mainstream (both homes and hospitals).

Another well-known sound healer in the field claims that simply playing each of the notes in an octave will break up certain diseases. He says that cancer cells are very brittle because they have lost their elasticity and flexibility. Therefore, the sound frequencies simply break up the cells as they hit the resonant frequencies of the cells. He also has photographs of cancer cells being destroyed by these sounds.

John Reid has discovered that each cell has within it a Cymatic pattern.

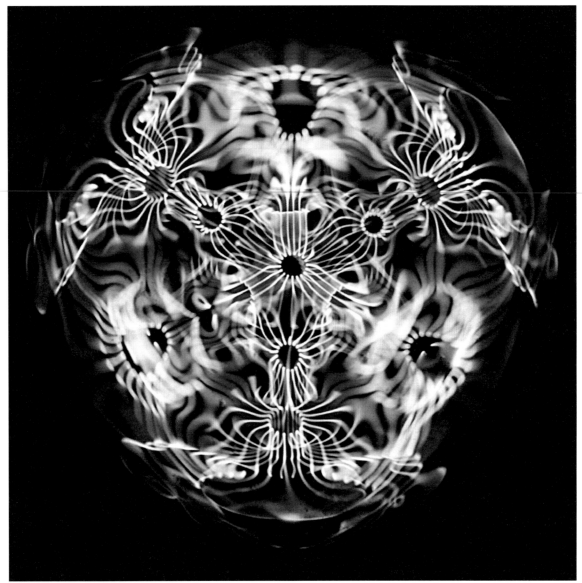

Cymatic visual

He has come up with a treatment plan that starts by doing a biopsy on the offending cell. You then find the frequency that creates the same cymatic pattern. You then can explode the cells by simply playing the frequency on the cells at really loud volumes. And, since only the problem cells will resonate at their own particular frequency, no other cells in the body will be affected. I really believe this is the future of medicine – 100% effective treatments without side effects.

However (and a really big "however"), we are still using the warfare model of healing, and many people believe the body just doesn't go for that. Alternatively, the goal is to use techniques to transform rather than destroy cells. Using the iso-principle you can resonate (or meet) the cell where it is, then slowly change the frequency to transform it.

Ultimately, I believe all healing will focus on raising a person's consciousness so that the diseases do not happen in the first place.

Parkinson's
Results using sound on Parkinson's have been quite astounding. We have done research at the Sound Institute with 12 Parkinson's patients. We placed each person on the sound table and played a song for 20 minutes. All but one of the patients got complete relief from their tremors and it also freed up frozen muscles. The results lasted an average of 24 hours – which means no meds for a day and a good night's sleep. Several patients have the sound table and say it has completely changed their lives.

My song Unconditional Peace even works in headphones without the sound table. One patient uses the CD, "Journey through the Matrix," with Qi Gong daily and is reporting a 70% reduction in symptoms.

Chapter 29 – Releasing and Overcoming Pain

Sound is so consistently effective for relieving pain that it is amazing. It is just wrong that sound is not a common protocol for pain relief in hospitals. I have seen people's pain (including my own) go away over and over – never to come back. And, there are no side effects in the least.

Quite a few years ago I fell in the shower and broke some ribs. I found that as long as I kept screaming that I felt no pain. I screamed for almost an hour, which was great except for the fact that no one else could be in the room with me.

Then, in 2010, I had surgery and I again used the technique whenever the pain was too much. However I was quite a bit more limited now because I was not alone. Not only did I completely annoy my roommates and the nurses, but also I was told I was upsetting the patients in other rooms down the hall. Finally, a doctor came in and I explained to him that when I make loud sounds I have no pain. He said the reason is that

Our pain receptors can only handle so much information,
and when they get filled up with sound,
there is no room left for the pain.

The voice is unbelievably powerful for getting rid of pain, and the amazing thing is that often the pain doesn't come back. This technique is more effective when you do it on yourself than when you do it on others (but still does work on others).

The technique is this:

1. Set sacred space and visualize an octahedron around you and the room. Or, simply ask for help protecting the space. This step is especially important for this technique because

when you make the sound of pain, it can attract in negative energy.

2. Simply make the sound of the pain in your body. You might have to actually play with making different sounds until you really match the feeling of the pain. You will know when you hit it. Not only does the pain go away but you might find that tears well up. Make the sound as long as you need to.

3. Then make the sound of what that part of the body would be like if there were no pain in it. This one is a little trickier to find – particularly if the pain is still present. In order to find the healing sound, you might focus on another part of the body that is not experiencing pain. Play with different pitches and tones until you find one sound that seems to fit the harmony that is present in the body part that is pain free. Then use that sound on the body part that is experiencing pain.

You can do this technique as often as you like (you are also welcome to edit, leave out or add any other technique or energy you would like).

Another proven and powerful tool for getting rid of pain is tuning forks. I have had a seriously sore back and had the pain go away within 10 minutes.

I did a tuning fork treatment on a guy who had a broken neck. He'd had surgery on his neck and the doctors had to break his neck in order to get it realigned. He was wearing a neck brace and could not move his neck at all. The man returned the week after his tuning treatment, and not only had the pain been diminished by 80% but he had regained movement in his neck. He said that when we were doing the tuning fork treatment he mentally went back into the moment of the trauma when they broke his neck. He said he was able to release the fear associated with the trauma, which allowed his neck to release the tension holding it stiff. He was grateful and in tears over the transformation.

You can simply place the tuning forks in the area of the pain. Normally, you don't place the forks right on the pain; however after I had surgery for appendicitis I found that the forks did help when placed directly on the painful area.

Depending on the type of injury and where it is in the body, different pitch and frequency of forks might be helpful. Again, try and come up with the right frequency intuitively. Also, you may just simply try different forks to see which ones are the most effective. Remember to also use your intention to help get rid of the pain. In this treatment, the primary goal is to get energy flowing again through the painful area. Therefore your main focus is to visualize the energy flowing through the section of need, totally connected to the rest of the body.

Other instrument sounds might also work quite well. For the most part, sound or music that is emotionally powerful enough to take you into higher states where you are no longer focused on the pain, can be quite helpful. This could be as simple as listening to or singing along with a crystal bowl. Even something like Pink Floyd could do the trick.

Chapter 30 – Using Sound to Create Nutrients

Sound has been shown to actually create a wide range of nutrients out of thin air. As incredible as it might sound, it is true.

First, Alfred Tomatis has shown in research that all frequencies are nutrients. If you are missing a particular frequency it can affect a particular organ or create very specific types of learning disorders.

Based on our previous assumption that all matter in the Universe is born out of the information carried within a sound pattern, it follows that every vitamin and mineral can also be created.

Jeffrey Thompson has done research on the frequency that creates oxygen in the blood stream. Kae Thompson-Liu has laid out the frequency of hundreds of nutrients. Ultimately, you can simply tune into the frequency of what you need, set your intention to receive the nutrient's vibrational value, and intuitively make the sound to bring the nutrient into the body. (Some might use sound to just create something like chocolate.)

This, I believe, is how we will heal ourselves in the future as we become more advanced and tuned in. Just the fact that this is possible might open some horizons for some of you.

They say that Sai Baba in India used sound to create any object he wanted. He created so many things such as gold rings and the like, that the government started taxing him on his creations.

SECTION VIII – Emotional Healing and Expansion with Sound

"It has been found that musical vibrations make their impact upon the entire body, being picked up by the nerves, spinal column, and even by the bones. This is why people who are deaf can react to music. It has also been demonstrated that music affects the pulse, respiration, and blood pressure; but its deepest effects, and those from which most of its curative properties are derived, are mental and emotional."
- Doren Antrim (Music Is Medicine) current

"Today, like every other day, we wake up empty and frightened. Don't open the door to study and begin reading. Take down a musical instrument."
- Rumi (1207-1273)

Introduction – Eradicating 50% of the Cause of All Diseases

Many believe that stuck emotions cause around 50% of all disease. If this is true, then learning how to release stuck emotions could save your life. It could also reduce our health care costs by 50%!!!

Deep emotional issues are also commonly the roots of much of our unhappiness. Also, subconscious negative beliefs are strongly resonating vibrations beneath the surface that are keeping us in stuck patterns and blocking opportunities to expand our wealth, and harmonize our health and relationships. Just as importantly, most of us would love to be able to get off the roller coaster of emotions and simply live in peace.

In this chapter emotions are explained as sounds and music. You will also learn eight different voice techniques for releasing and harmonizing emotions and emotional issues. I will then explain a powerful technique for accessing and transforming negative beliefs that might be holding you back. Finally you will learn how to prevent emotions from getting stuck in the first place.

Chapter 31 – The Sound of Emotions

"He that divines the secret of my music is freed from the unhappiness that haunts the whole world of men."
- Beethoven (1770-1827)

Based on the hierarchy of sound, emotions can be equated to frequencies, tones, music and energy. Generally, emotions correspond more to timbres and music, than to an actual frequency or pitch. Emotions also correspond to the flow of music. Stuck emotions are like a broken record; flowing, healthy emotions are like a song that ends on the home note.

There are two general types of emotions: Those that break down our system physically, and those that support our system, creating more health. Even though many say there are no negative emotions, there are ones that are negative for the body. For example, anger, fear and anxiety are not good for your heart, digestion and nervous system. On the other hand, gratitude, compassion and love not only support your physical health, they can cause spontaneous healing.

So from the body's perspective there are positive and negative emotions. In the world of sound, we have the exact same varieties – there are sounds that are not good for us physically and others that totally support and enhance our health.

The Frequency of Emotions

Overall, many people refer to gratitude, love and joy as higher emotions, and anger, fear and anxiety as lower emotions. However, are they really higher and lower in frequency? I think not. You could easily say they are higher or lower in energy or quality of energy, but not necessarily frequency. In fact, when I have groups make the sound of compassion, they often make a very low frequency sound. And, anxiety often seems to correspond to a high-pitched squeal.

However, it is interesting that the higher emotions do seem to have their own frequency hierarchy. When I have people make the sound of compassion, gratitude, love and joy, the frequency gets higher and higher – Compassion being a lower note and joy being the highest note (weeeeeehhh!!!). It seems that Spirit has the highest frequency of all.

You might also say that the sound of depression would be a lower frequency than the sound of anxiety.

However, it seems like emotions correspond much more closely to tones and timbers than frequency or pitch.

The Tone of an Emotion

When we were born we would naturally and spontaneously make the sounds of emotions as they arose. Sadly, we then learned to be "normal." Still, when someone is frightened they often emit a sound similar to "agh." In the extreme case, we scream. When someone is angry they often growl. When someone is hurt they sometimes whimper or cry. Even cats, dogs and other animals often express their emotions with very particular sounds.

We often think of emotions as being grating or annoying, or beautiful and harmonious – just like we refer to different instrument sounds or timbres. In fact, we can easily associate particular sounds to particular emotions.

Negative emotions tend to be inconsistent or distorted sounds that affect our bodies quite negatively. They do not support the body's physiology. Think of how fear or anxiety might sound (perhaps something like *"sccccccqqqqkkkkk"*). The sounds of both fear and anxiety are not good for your heart or nervous system, or any other part of your body. In fact, research shows that they actually break down our blood vessels and nervous system.

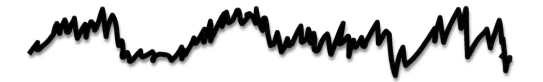

Waveform of Negative Emotions

In Chinese medicine they say that the fear is stored in the kidneys. Imagine being a kidney and having someone right next to you screaming in fear for a couple of hours… or for days (or God forbid… for months or years). If I were a kidney I would give it up. And, kidneys do!

Just for fun let's look at what might be the corresponding sounds for many of the so-called negative emotions:

Grrrr - Aggravation, irritation, agitation, annoyance, grouchiness, grumpiness

Hmph - Exasperation, frustration, dismay, disappointment, displeasure

Aghh!!! - Anger, rage, outrage, fury, wrath, hostility, ferocity, bitterness, hate, scorn, spite, vengefulness, dislike, resentment

Ergh - Disgust, revulsion, contempt, loathing

Icckk - Torment, agony, suffering, hurt, anguish

Ugh! - Depression, despair, hopelessness, gloom, glumness, sadness, unhappiness, grief, sorrow, woe, misery, melancholy

Mng - Guilt, shame, regret, remorse

Eeek! - Alarm, shock, fear, fright, horror, terror, panic, hysteria, mortification

Ghgzzzz - Anxiety, nervousness, tenseness, uneasiness, apprehension, worry, distress, dread

Almost no Sound - Depression, helplessness, alienation, isolation, neglect, loneliness, rejection, homesickness, defeat, dejection, insecurity, embarrassment, humiliation, insult

Notice that hardly any of the sounds that you came up with for any of these emotions are sounds we like. Just about every sound is inconsistent, oscillating, or distorted. Sometimes the sound jumps around from one frequency to another and sometimes has noise scattered throughout the harmonics. They might be interesting and fun, but these sounds are definitely not ones that you want to hang out with all day long. They would make a really bad radio station, and most importantly they are not good for you physically.

Here are some negative emotions to play with. It is important to get to know the sound of an emotion, so you can recognize it when it is in your body. We have become so accustomed to these negative sounds in our system that we often let them go untended.

Fear - Make the sound of fear out loud (if you can't do it out loud at the moment, make the sound in your head). If you listen really closely to the sound as you make it you might notice that it is like two sounds oscillating back and forth really quickly. It is not one pure note. Also notice the feeling that the sound gives you when you make it. In particular notice your heart and nervous system.

Worry - Now make the sound of worry (come on, don't be shy – just play with it). I think of worry as two sounds: the sound of a good outcome, "Ahhh," and the sound of a bad outcome, "Erggg." However, the sound of worry is actually these two sounds oscillating back and forth – *"AhhhErgggAhhhErgggAhhhErgggAhhhErggg"* – as we go back and forth between the good and bad outcomes. So worry is also two sounds, not a pure tone. Again, notice how it feels in your body when you make this sound.

Anxiety - It is not a good idea to make the sound of anxiety, however you can imagine what it might sound like. It is definitely not good for your nervous system or any other part of your body.

Anger - Now make the sound of anger. The sound does have some power to it, but it is also not a pure sound. It is a sound that is not supporting your health for you. It is particularly bad for your veins and your nervous system, and can cause strokes and heart disease.

On the other hand, whenever people make the sound of positive emotions like gratitude, compassion or love, they never make a sound like "scccccqqqqkkkkk". They always make a vowel sound. Positive emotions tend to be pure consistent frequencies like each of the vowels (uu, oh, ah, eh, ee). These sounds totally support our physical body in every way and can even open higher states of consciousness that can transform our lives.

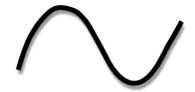

Waveform of Positive Emotions

Music of Emotions

Just like music, emotions are feelings that naturally flow through us. Healthy emotions pass through us like a free flowing river. In fact, the biggest problem with emotions is when they actually become static – when they get stuck and no longer flow on through.

A stuck emotion is like a song that gets cut off in the middle of the song. It's like this:

a song that gets… |||||||||||

…. It leaves you hanging. As previously mentioned, our whole system naturally wants to go home to a fundamental root note. So a stuck emotion is simply one that hasn't resolved to the home note.

Even worse is when it keeps repeating in our head and body… again and again. It's like a skipping record – sometimes over an entire lifetime.

It's like this…. a song that gets…

gets…

gets…

gets…

gets…

stuck.

Not being able to come home creates anxiety and diminishes our mental capacity. In the worst case, it manifests in the cells of our physical body as disharmony, which then can even transform the cells negatively (based on Transformative Resonance). Our body tenses ever so slightly, our heartbeat is interrupted a bit, and our nervous system is distracted from the normal clarity that happens when a song ends naturally.

There are two types of emotions that require different approaches: emotions that happen once and are hard to get out of, and emotions that get stuck and keep coming back. An example of a one-time emotion is a car that almost hits you and you go into fear and start shaking. In this case, you can use a sound to simply calm down your nervous system and return to a centered place. It's not like you need to face and feel the emotion. You are already in it completely, and it doesn't feel good.

The second type of emotion is one that keeps repeating itself. Sometimes a previous unresolved experience of a trauma can be reignited with even the smallest trigger. A really minor conflict triggers a huge unwarranted response.

It seems that our deepest being knows that we must come home. Therefore, when we have a really strong experience that is left unresolved our psyche does whatever it can to re-resonate the previous experience so that we can finally resolve it. Often we will unconsciously use the laws of resonance to attract these "second chances" into our life until we figure out how to resolve it to a home note – where we finally return to our natural state of peace – from which all other joyous states blossom effortlessly.

Insanity is the rebellion of a person against certain experiences over which he has no control. The conscious mind center in the cortex (upper brain) is the area where mental disease becomes established. The seat of feelings and emotions is in the lower brain. The latter it appears, is not involved in mental maladies. Music affects and influences a patient through this lower brain center. Musical therapy meets NO barriers in mental derangement cases, as does the written or spoken word that works through the upper or conscious area.
- Dr. Altschuler (1942)

The Worst Emotion of All – By Far
Resistance to emotions is generally the whole problem that makes emotions get stuck in the first place. When there is resistance, the emotion never has the chance to complete. If you simply feel the emotion, with no resistance, it naturally dissipates and moves on through and out of your system. In psychotherapy, one of the first steps when working with emotions is to feel them.

Imagine what "resistance" would sound like – perhaps something like "Nunt-a." Imagine yourself avoiding something, doing everything you can to not turn and face it, while saying, "Nunt-a." Technically, you now have two negative sounds going on, "Nunt-a" (which is a really bad sound itself) and the sound of the other negative emotion being held at a distance. We are now so far from a peaceful home note, it's ridiculous.

In the worst case, we shut down altogether. Some go to a place of no sound at all – a place devoid of feeling altogether.

Others use distraction to avoid emotions. Entertainment and amusement are common ways of avoiding emotions. Some use addictions to avoid emotions. There are many ways to run away from our feelings.

> Don't runaway from emotions
> They always run faster.
> Sit with them
> and they leave on their own.

Some people are not even running away from emotions – they are just so scattered that no emotion ever has time to fully complete its song. It's like there are many sounds jumping from one to another erratically. In fact, scatteredness should be on the list of emotions since so many people live so much of their lives in this place. The sound of scatteredness is like continually switching from one radio station to another. It is also a sound that is not good for any part of the body. The heart especially finds it difficult to cope with this extreme case of inconsistency.

Addiction is an extreme case of resistance to emotions. We believe the key to addiction is that people are just longing for Spirit. People are bored to death with the mundane world. Of course, some people are just trying to avoid the pain and sadness. Many just have no way to go to a state of peace and are just running away from their anxiety and fears.

When it comes to addiction, sounds and music on the sound table have been amazingly effective (now being used in several addiction centers). The songs "Water of Life," "Unconditional Love," "Unconditional Peace," and "Anti-Depressant," are the most effective. They work on headphones but are even more powerful when played on a sound table. I believe the most important keys are music with intention that is imbued with love, is relaxing but also interesting enough to hold one's attention, and resolves to the home note at the end with a slow fade – leaving people in a state of complete peace and stillness – a place we are all longing for.

Sadness – The Most Misunderstood Emotion
Many people believe sadness to be a negative emotion. In fact, it normally falls into lists next to other emotions like depression and hopelessness. I have come to believe (very strongly) that sadness is not a negative emotion by any means. The emotion itself does not break down the body. It is the resistance to sadness that breaks down the body.

The proof is in the sound. Make the sound of sadness. Come on... go for it. Sadness is not an incoherent, gritty sound like the other so-called negative emotions. Sadness is a beautiful sweet sound. In fact, we normally love sad songs – at the right times. The sound and music of sadness are actually good for our whole system.

We believe that one of the biggest problems in our society is the fear of sadness. Perhaps this is because depression is not very far from sadness. Fear of sadness is rampant throughout our society. We are told by friends and the media that we should be happy all the time. Boys are told to grip up and stop crying. "Only girls cry."

Sadness is important because it allows us to feel the reality of a sad situation and move through it. In fact, we believe that unless you spend time in sadness (when appropriate), true happiness will elude you.

> If there is something that makes you sad, be sad.
> Then it will complete on its own
> and you will be able to be totally present
> with any happiness or joy that comes your way.

> *"It's OK to get down,*
> *Down to the ground,*
> *Tomorrow we'll be laughing"*
> *- Song by David*

Some feel that sadness has some bad friends that you have to watch out for: Addiction, Loss of Self Esteem, and Self Destruction. However, I strongly believe that each of these is simply a reaction to the avoidance of sadness.

The key to healthy sadness (and all emotions) is to not stay too long – the ultimate goal is to move through it. However, what is the right length of time? And who is to say? If someone in your family dies, grief and sadness may be appropriate for a very long time. Some cultures have been known to grieve for months. In some cultures "wailing" is done in public.

Some people who have been abused their whole childhood might think that they cannot cry enough to release all of the pain. The extreme example is when a whole culture is wiped out. The pain can seem so deep. Just imagine the intensity of the sorrow after the bombs fell in Hiroshima and Nagasaki.

> Often people think that sadness or grief is too much to handle.
> However, the sound that is too hard to handle is "resistance"
> Relish in the sweet sounds of sadness.
> It is your sweet friend or parent
> holding you and nurturing you.

Sadness is like a ladder you climb back up to the positive emotions. The good news is that when you let go of the resistance to sadness, it can feel so good. Sad songs make up at least 1/3 of all hits on the radio.

Grief

There is good grief and there is bad grief. Although I have now come to believe that the bad grief is only "resistance to grief." When you allow the grief to flow through your system, it may not feel as good as sadness, but it does not break down your system!

In many cultures they spend weeks, even months grieving. They wail and cry, then ultimately, celebrate.

The big difference with grief is that it takes a much longer time to resolve than probably any other emotion. And, people commonly do not give it enough time! It is so common for people to go back to work or continue on with their busy life, without having given sufficient time for the song of grief to play through their system. Unresolved grief remains within as an unresolved song and it is hard to be totally present and feel complete again – much less be fully happy.

Recently, my cat Joy died. This might not sound like that big of a deal for those of you who have lost a close loved one, however I really loved my kitty. I actually canceled classes and took off an entire week. I especially listened for music that seemed to help me – and I found they were all sad songs. I was not up for going dancing or listening to any happy songs. And because I had no resistance to the sadness, I actually ended up feeling more peaceful and grounded than I had been in a really long time.

Take the time to be in the sound of Grief
when necessary.

Of course, grief can take years to completely resolve its sad song. You cannot rush the song of grief. Don't resist it and it will resolve quicker.

Combinations of Emotions

The most difficult emotions to deal with are when there is more than one emotion at the same time – particularly when two emotions conflict with each other. For example, someone you love very much treats you really badly or actually abuses or hurts you. You then have both anger and love, and often it is difficult to fully feel either one.

When you consider the emotions as sounds or songs, then the two do not sound good together. In fact, rarely can a CD or mp3 player play two songs at the same time. Even if they could, it would be extremely confusing to listen to and feel.

The key is to simply feel the emotions one at a time. And, feel them completely. Hold the other conflicting emotion at bay, while feeling the first completely.

Ultimately, a whole new song emerges when you step back or zoom out and see both songs at once. This new song is one of peace, often laced with a bit of sadness or compassion.

One of the most extreme examples of conflicting emotions is suicide.

Dealing with Suicide
Recently I've been helping someone whose daughter killed herself.

The tricky part about suicide is again, the problem of dealing with several conflicting emotions. First, there is grief. Second, there is anger. Sometimes it is hard to feel sad and allow the grieving process to complete because of the anger. Sometimes it is hard to be angry because of how much you miss the person. Then there is the nagging guilt – what might I have done differently? Might there have been something I could have done? And, what might other people be thinking?

Again, each one of the emotions must be dealt with individually.

Actually, the suicide of someone close to you takes the longest time of all to resolve. There is no rushing it through. However, the amount of time that one feels guilty about it is totally up to the person. In this case, you set the deadline.

Positive Emotions
Now let's explore the sound of the positive emotions in a little more detail.

First, let's resonate a positive emotion now.

> Tune into the energy of gratitude. Bring up feelings of gratitude for your physical heart (not your heart chakra, but your physical heart) – beating 24/7 keeping you alive. Thank you.

> Let this feeling of gratitude for your heart flow through your whole body – through every cell in your body. Let it surround you like a bubble as it goes through all of your auras. Feel this feeling of gratitude and appreciation for your physical heart completely.

> Now, if this feeling had a sound, get that sound going in your head. Play with it until you find a sound that seems to match the feeling of gratitude for your heart. Is it high or low? Then, when you are ready, make the sound out loud.

The feeling of gratitude is even stronger when you make the sound of it.

**Making the sound of an emotion
creates a stronger resonant field
for the emotion to exist.**

It also brings the energy of the emotion into your physical body with the physical sound waves of your voice.

Now, notice the quality of the sound that you made. As mentioned, inevitably the sounds people make for higher emotions are always really consistent – coherent and beautiful sounds that are beneficial for your health in every part of your body. A coherent sound might look something like this:

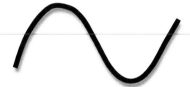

Positive Emotion Waveform

Positive emotions are fluid and stable – supporting health in every way.

If you like, take the time and tune into each of the following emotions. Then, come up with a sound to match. Tune into the energy of each of the following emotions and see what kind of sound you can come up with for each. These are very powerful emotions and the sounds can be extremely healing when you take the time:

Caring
Tenderness
Passion
Cheerfulness
Amusement
Bliss
Satisfaction
Ecstasy
Enthusiasm
Hope
Contentment

Other Emotion Lists
Of course, if you do a search on the web you will find many lists of emotions categorized in different ways. Here are a couple of lists that I like.

Abraham's Scale of Emotions

Esther Hicks and Abraham have the following list of emotions (notice where I drew the line between positive and negative emotions). Abraham says that you might have to move up the emotional scale step-by-step. It might be practically impossible to go from depression to joy in one big jump. But you just might be able to go from depression to anger, which is higher on the scale.

However, many of us are not very stuck and can easily shift out of negative emotions and quite easily jump to very high emotions with the right stimulus. Of course, sound and music can be just the stimulus.

Consider what each of these emotions might sound like.

Joy/Empowerment/Freedom/Love/Appreciation
Passion
Enthusiasm/Eagerness/Happiness
Positive Expectation/Beliefs
Optimism
Hopefulness
Contentment

Boredom
Pessimism
Frustration/Impatience
Overwhelment
Disappointment
Doubt
Worry
Blame
Discouragement
Anger
Revenge
Hatred/Rage
Jealousy
Insecurity/Guilt/Unworthiness
Fear/Grief/Depression/Despair/ Powerlessness

Lisa Rene's List of Emotions
I really like this list because it shows that the best way to gauge whether an emotion is so-called good or bad is based on whether you are equal to a person, or whether you are above or below them. When I check in on an emotion and I'm either above or below someone, I then look for another emotion to shift to that still feels true to me, and leaves me as equal with my fellow human being – as we truly are.

If you listen for and make the sound of each of the emotions within the 3 categories, you will notice a difference in the overall timbre.

Superior Thinking – Intolerance, Impatience, Arrogance, Manipulation, Attack, Anger, Judgmental thinking

Inferior Thinking – Worry, Low Self Love or Esteem, Jealousy, Guilt, Hurt, Fear, Attachment, Martyrdom

Centered Spiritual Self – Self Mastery, Unconditional Love, Confidence, Personal Power, Balance, Integration, Self Love, Cooperation, Forgiveness, Faith, Compassion, Oneness, Unity, Harmony, Surrender, Non Judgment, Humility

The key is to become aware of the sound and music quality
of the emotions within you at any given time
so that if you don't like the sound
you can use techniques to shift the sound
to one that is healthy
and has a sound, melody or rhythm
that feels better.

Chapter 32 – Eight Techniques for Releasing Stuck Emotions with the Voice

"Deeply listening to music opens up new avenues of research I'd never even dreamed of. I feel from now on music should be an essential part of every analysis."
- Carl Jung ((1875-1961)

"We trust that the magic of sound, will contribute to
an ever greater measure to the relief of human suffering."
- Robert Assagioli M.D. (1888-1974) Founder of Transpersonal Psychology

One way to deal with emotions is to simply be present enough to notice when you are resonating the irritating sound and music of lower emotions, and simply change the station to the consistent and beautiful sounds and music of the higher emotions.

However, often the emotions get into our body at our cellular level and it takes some deeper work to transform the cells back into a clear channel for the next wave of emotions to come through unimpeded.

This is serious work and incredibly powerful.

The process can take as little as a minute or up to several hours. If you are working on a minor issue, like frustration with traffic or a person, you can utilize the techniques on the spot. If working on deep-rooted issues, make sure that you have plenty of time to complete the process. If working on something as deep as grief or something like childhood abuse, the process may take more than one session. In any case, be gentle on yourself.

If any deep issues come up that you find hard to handle, don't be afraid to get some help. However, trust that you will make it through – clear, at peace and ready to let deeper levels of happiness and joy in. It's also good to give yourself a ½ hour after completion to process what just happened before continuing with your day.

Now, choose a stuck emotion or deep emotional issue you haven't released yet and would like to work on. Emotions that haven't yet been released will commonly keep popping into your head over and over. Getting bent out of shape over anything is a good clue that there is something which is not flowing. Perhaps there is someone you are still upset with, or you might be worried about something, or perhaps you are afraid of something, or you still have some grief that you haven't processed.

For your first time, we recommend that you choose one particular emotional issue to work on and try all eight of the techniques below on the same emotion. Notice which techniques work the best for you – different people prefer different techniques. However, also note that different techniques might work better on different types of issues. We'll give some suggestions and guide you through each technique.

OK… now think of an issue that you would like to work on at this time.

Set Sacred Space
The sounds of negative emotions are very powerful. They can be really intense, weird and bizarre sounds, such as when making the sound of pain. It's important to remember that when you make the sounds of any negative emotions, the sounds can get imprinted into the room. There is also a danger of calling in negative energies from other dimensions (if this point sounds too "out there" for you…just continue on). Therefore, it is really important to create some protection. As previously outlined in detail in Chapter 24, "Performing a Sound Healing Session," you can simply say with power "I set sacred space now," You can also visualize an octahedron around yourself or the entire room.

The first five techniques are about focusing on the stuck emotion to release it.

1. Make the Sound of the Emotion with the Intention of Releasing It
The technique is especially good for any emotion you might be resisting. The only way through an emotion is to first feel it completely.

Caution: This technique is not good for emotions like anxiety (especially panic attacks) or fear. Resonating these emotions can amplify them in your system making them worse. For the most part, fear and anxiety are useless. They do have the positive aspect of making us aware of a dangerous situation and providing adrenalin so we can run or fight. However, these days there are very few lions, particularly in our cities.

The key to this technique is to stay completely focused on the intention of releasing the emotion. You don't want to simply make the sound of an emotion and create an even stronger resonant field. If you only resonate an emotion you make it stronger in your system. You want to actually have it move on through and out.

Now, simply allow yourself to tune into the emotion. Feel it completely through your whole body. Play with the sound until you feel that the sound you are making is actually matching or expressing the emotion that you are feeling. The sound you make might be really intense. You might find yourself screaming. If the emotion is just too intense and it is overwhelming you, you can also try using the homeopathic method where you make the sound of the emotion softly.

If you are dealing with resistance to the emotion, it might take awhile to actually get to the real emotion behind the resistance. Sometimes, when you find the right sound, it might even shift into a whole other sound. Occasionally, you might find the perfect sound where the emotion actually begins to open up and unravel a whole litany of information behind the emotion. Don't worry if this doesn't happen, as it is pretty rare. You cannot make any <u>wrong</u> sounds when doing this! The key is to let yourself go enough to find sounds that really seem to fit.

Now, make the sound of the emotion with the intention of releasing it.

We'll wait here, until you are done.

There are two places that people most commonly end up when doing this technique. First, many people start crying. If this happens, don't resist the tears. Sometimes people just end up in a quiet state of sweet sadness.

Second, many people come to a place of complete stillness. This might also happen after the tears. And this place may have a tinge of sadness around it. Relish in this peace. Hold it as long as you can.

Whatever happens, just be present with it.

The last step is really important – sit still in silence for at least 5 minutes.

If this technique didn't happen to work, don't worry – we have eight more.

Sadness Exercise – This exercise is only necessary if there is something that you have not yet let go of, or more specifically – something that you have not yet spent time grieving over. This might be about someone who has died. It could be for some abuse of pain you have suffered. It could be for some abuse of pain that you have witnessed. It could be because of the state of the planet and society. Whatever the issue, allow yourself go to the core of that sad- ness and feel it completely, knowing you will be moving through it.

Have no fear that you will get stuck in this place. Then make the sound of what you are feeling. You might put on a sad song if you have a hard time coming up with the right sounds. If so, sing or hum along with the song. The point is that you want to get the sound of this sadness resonating inside you. Then, love the feeling of the sound of the sadness. Even if it is painful, love the feeling. Let the sound of your sadness get louder. Regardless of how bad a singer you are, sing out the pain of the sadness. Keep doing this until you feel complete. Know that this process could possibly take a few hours depending on the depth of the sadness. You'll know the process is done when you can smile again.

2. Make the Sound of the Emotion and Transform it into a Harmonious Sound
In this technique you make the sound of the emotion and slowly transform it into a beautiful harmonious sound. The slower the transformation, the better. Also, the more beautiful the harmonious sound, the better, and the longer you make the harmonious sound, the better. To make the transformation even more dramatic, you can also move your body to the sounds you are making.

In another variation, after making the sound of the emotion to release it, you then fill up the space with the sound of higher emotions such as gratitude, compassion, love, joy or pure Spirit – or any other really positive sound. The concept is that once you have released an emotion, it is important to fill the space with light, so it doesn't revert back to its previous incoherent state.

In these techniques you make the sound of the emotion for a much shorter time, therefore this technique is really good for emotions where you are already in the thick of it – in the fire, so to speak. That is, emotions that you are not holding much resistance around.

Now, try this technique on the same emotion that you were previously working on.

Again, we'll wait here, holding space, until you are done.

3. Make the Sound of the Remedy for the Stuck Emotion
In this technique you come up with the sound that you think will help. The beauty of this technique is that you aren't resonating the negative emotion at all – you are simply making the sound that will help. Using the vocal sounds in Chapter 21, "The Voice," you can simply try different sounds and see how they work or you can intuitively come up with the sounds that you feel might mitigate the stuck emotion.

Even more powerful, is to let a higher power come through you and let it make the sound. If you can, tune into Spirit, get out of the way, and let whatever happens happen. Spirit is much smarter and wiser than we are.

If you have any guides, or work with any ascended masters, archangels, or beings of light, try calling on them to do the work. Again, the key is to get out of the way and let it happen. You can find many lists of ascended masters and archangels if you do a search on Google.

Often when you work with Spirit or Beings of Light, you end up making sounds that you might never ever have imagined (it is a good way to actually learn how to make new sounds). And then, you find the issue has completely resolved throughout your mind, body and Spirit.

4. Make the Sound of the Part of the Body that is Holding the Emotion

In this technique, you also don't make the sound of the emotion, so there is no danger of making the emotion stronger by resonating it. This technique is based on the commonly held concept that emotions are stored physically in the body.

First, notice in your body where the stuck emotion seems to be residing. It may not be completely obvious and you might almost have to guess. Also, when you start the sound, the emotion might seem to move around in your body. You might have to track it down. However, it is often completely obvious where the emotion is located in the body – perhaps a stiff neck or upset stomach.

In Chinese medicine, different emotions are held in different parts of the body. I feel it is best to feel in your body where the emotion is stuck; however, sometimes it is not so obvious. In that case, here is a chart that can help. You can also work with the sound of each of the antidotes below.

Emotion	Body Part	Symptoms	Antidote
Stress	Intestines	Indigestion	Relaxation
Worry	Cervical Nerves	Stiff Shoulders	Easy Goingness
Irritability	Parasympathetic Nerves	Insomnia	Calmness
Perplexity	Autonomic Nerves	Lower Back Pain	Good Grace
Excess Fear	Kidneys	Renal Diseases	Peace of Mind
Anxiety	Stomach	Dyspepsia	Relief
Anger	Liver	Hepatitis	Compassion
Apathy	Spine	Weakened Vitality	Passion
Impatience	Pancreas	Diabetes	Tolerance
Loneliness	Brain's Hippocampus	Senile Dementia	Pleasure
Depression	Blood	Leukemia	Joy
Grudge	Skin	Skin Ulceration	Gratitude
Grief	Lungs	Asthma	Acceptance

Now, let's make the sound that the part of the body wants you to make. Again, you almost have to intuit the sound that the muscle or organ would like to express. If it is not completely obvious, play with different sounds until you come across something that

234

seems to resonate with the particular part of the body. When done, be quiet, and listen to your body in silence.

**Listen for where the emotion is being held in your body,
and make the sound that part of the body wants you to make
to release the emotion.**

Again, we'll be here sending positive energy your way
until you are done.

The following techniques are about focusing on and resonating higher vibrations versus focusing on the specific issue.

Instead of focusing on what is wrong,
focus on what is right and resonate that.

All of the following techniques use the laws of resonance to overcome the incoherence and stress of the negative emotion. As you focus on and resonate positive frequencies throughout your system, these strong resonant fields overcome and harmonize the weaker emotional fields.

These techniques are especially good when simply trying to shift your energy versus trying to release a stuck emotion. For example, say you are in fear from almost being hit by a car, or you are angry over something – it may not be a deep stuck issue, but simply a feeling that you would like to shift out of.

These techniques are also especially effective for emotions that are very destructive to the body – particularly anxiety and fear. Many of the current books on anger say that you shouldn't resonate the actual anger too much – simply because it is so detrimental to the body.

A primary key to getting off the roller coaster of emotions is to simply not identify with the emotion itself. Normally, when we are "in" an emotion, our entire system is controlled by the ups and downs of the emotion. When we focus on another consistent vibration – particularly one that is a part of our own being – we are no longer on the roller coaster. We are a stable frequency with an emotion passing by. Each of the techniques below is based upon this concept.

Instead of being the emotion:

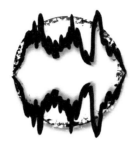

We are a peaceful whole, with the emotions just passing through us:

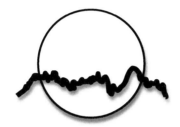

A Centered Person with Emotion Passing Through

5. Be Present in Your Body with the Stuck Emotion

The most powerful frequencies to become aware of in the body are the array of frequencies that make up the body itself. By simply being present in your own body, you are resonating these powerful frequencies collectively. This includes being aware of how all the frequencies around you are affecting your body, and how all the frequencies of emotions are resonating through your body as well. Notice the temperature of the air around you. Notice the sky and sun, moon, or stars. Notice all the sounds around you. When you are simply present in the moment with all frequencies in and outside you as a whole, emotions inevitably dissipate. In fact, emotions do not exist in the moment of pure awareness.

Commonly, when you are simply present with emotions in the body, the emotion dissipates and goes away. Emotions tend to be amorphous feelings that are easily overcome by stronger, more real frequencies. Shining the light of awareness on the emotion in the body is often all that needs to be done.

Though simple, this technique is incredibly powerful.

6. Resonating Your Home or Soul Frequency

The key is to resonate a strong coherent frequency that the rest of your body entrains to, so that it is not at the mercy of wily emotions that bring stress and chaos. The strongest frequency in your system is your home note or Soul frequency. This is the frequency that the rest of your system is based on. It is also the place where you are at peace. Again, when you get off the roller coaster onto a stable and still frequency you are at peace regardless of where the emotion goes.

We will go into detail on how to find your signature frequency in Chapter 46, "Connecting to the Soul with Sound." You can use a CD in your key, play a crystal bowl or tuning fork, or use an instrument or guitar tuner to tune into your frequency once you know it. Toning your frequency is especially effective. The emotion might still be there, but you are not it! You are yourself, a frequency separate from it, and it is just passing through.

7. Send the Sound of Love to the Emotion or Body Part where It Is Stuck
First, simply resonate love. Bring love into your heart. You can either send this love to the emotion itself to help harmonize it, or you can send love to the part of the body that is holding the emotion. Don't underestimate the power of love. It is one of the strongest resonant fields on the planet – capable of not only harmonizing your entire system, but also transforming the frequency of inharmonious emotion to a higher and more harmonious frequency.

When you resonate any higher emotion you get off the rough sounding roller coaster, and you have more energy to use to help you relax the resistance you have to the emotion.

8. Harmonize Higher Emotions and Resonate Consistent Coherent Frequencies
Simply "be" the higher frequency of gratitude, compassion, love or Joy – or the most powerful one of all – Source. When you are one with the Universe, nothing can affect you. Negative emotions often dissolve completely when subjected to such powerful resonant frequencies

Releasing All the Issues in Your Life
You can see how powerful these techniques are (especially if you did the exercises). As mentioned they can be used at various times to release minor emotions or to work on deep emotional issues.

Now, if you are ready and willing – and seriously want to change your life – make a list of all of the emotions that might still be stuck inside. These might be large emotional issues from childhood or even a past life.

Then, over the next few months or year you can begin working through each issue – one by one. Spend as much time on each issue as is needed.

Choose the techniques that resonate the most with you. You might try different techniques for different issues. You might even use combinations of techniques. Feel free to combine these techniques with any other modalities that you might know of.

Just imagine – being free of all the issues in your life that are keeping you from living a happy and fulfilled life.

Helping Others to Release Stuck Emotions
All of the above techniques can also be used on someone else in a therapeutic setting.

First, set sacred space in case the sounds get intense. Ideally, it is best to have them make the sounds for themselves. Guide them through the process as I have done for you. Often it is helpful to make the sounds with them. This often makes them feel more comfortable and allows them to go deeper with their own sounds. However, occasionally a person is simply too shy or unable to make such silly sounds. In this case it is normally just as effective to make the sounds for them.

It is normally easier to get someone to make positive sounds like love as opposed to the dark sounds of some emotions. Therefore, you might help them do the releasing, and then get them to help with the sounds of love and light.

It is also really nice, to have them practice these techniques at home on their own. It is always more important to empower people than to just do a treatment.

Again, feel free to modify these techniques to make them your own, and don't hesitate to add them to treatments that you might already be familiar with.

Moving to Higher Levels of Consciousness in Relation to Emotions

> *"Emotions of any kind can be evoked by melody and rhythm;*
> *therefore music has the power to form character."*
> *- Aristotle (384-322 BC)*

Depending on your level of development there are various ways to deal with emotions. As you progress on your path you might move from one level to another.

Level 1 – Face the Emotions
For many people on the planet the first step is to feel their emotions in the first place. Many are actually stuck in resistance to emotions. Some people have completely shut down and are not feeling anything – nothing at all.

As mentioned, if you are resisting an emotion, you are creating a second negative sound ("Nunt-a"). Exercises 1 to 4 above are designed for you to get in touch with the emotion before transforming it. If you simply bypass some emotions they will come back to haunt you later. Based on the laws of resonance, you will attract the same situation over and over until you finally are able to resolve the sound of the broken record.

Level 2 – Moving Through Emotions
The next level after being present with an emotion is to move through it. All of the exercises above can help you do this in one way or another.

Level 3 – Being in Your Center or Soul Frequency
This is the beginning of getting off the roller coaster of emotions. The biggest problem with emotions is when we become the music of them. That is, we are completely enveloped in their sound. When you are able to separate yourself out from the emotion and return to your own harmonious sound, you break the attachment to the roller coaster ride. You still feel your emotions, but you are not them. This makes it easier to let go of them.

Level 4 – Not Letting Emotions Get Stuck in the First Place
This is one of the most important steps in emotional maturity. In order to explore how to do this let's differentiate between emotions and feelings in this way: Emotions are caused by thought. Feelings are movements of energy through the body. Since emotions are caused by thought, *they can be undone by thought*. There are several techniques that can be used to undo emotions or stop them from getting into the body in the first place.

You've probably had the experience of getting upset over something that previously didn't bother you. Or, the opposite – you don't get upset over something that bothered you before. What is it that makes the difference? Some say it is your level of stress, which is true. However, when a person is not stressed they are often able to put things in perspective – up front before the situation elicits an emotion.

There are two powerful keys to put so-called negative emotions in perspective and nip them in the bud – compassion and gratitude. Both of these techniques require a "zooming out" to be able to put the situation in perspective. They also require some presence of mind in order to remember to do it while in the thick of it. Finally, it also requires that the tempo of your thoughts slows down, so that you have time to think before you react.

Compassion – Compassion is especially helpful for any type of frustration no matter how big or small – from full blown anger down to a simple "hmpf."

Instead of creating a negative sound in the world in reaction to any situation, the trick is to react with compassion – then we are bringing a really beautiful sound to the situation and we end up with it resonating through our Soul. Compassion can be brought to a situation in many ways (we'll go into much more detail in Chapter 49, "Using Sound to Deal with Challenges and Conflicts."

First, if we simply look at what has brought this person to be doing what they are doing, it can mitigate the negative emotion. Often it is parents or society that brings people to do uncaring things. Sometimes it is just a matter of being tired or stressed. Another compassion technique is to tune into that place where we are all one (more detail later). Again, compassion is a wonderful tool for averting a stuck emotion in the first place.

Gratitude – If we can have gratitude for challenges, no matter how intense, then the sound of gratitude (which supports our entire body physiology) becomes the #1 song we are singing internally throughout the day. Remember how nice the sound of gratitude feels? We can be grateful for every challenge because it makes us stronger (and gives us an opportunity to learn compassion). When we learn to be grateful for every challenge in our life our entire inner sound landscape changes drastically.

Again, the key here is to be present enough to remember that you have an alternative to reacting, and then to remember the technique. Then you won't need techniques 1 to 4 of the eight above at all – the emotions never get inside in the first place.

Level 5 – Dropping the Emotional Body

This requires a high level of enlightenment and awareness. It is not necessarily an easy state to attain; it can take a lot of work – some say many lifetimes (but things are really accelerating these days, and we have no limits as far as expansion goes). Dropping your emotional body does not mean ignoring emotions; it just means that there is no resonant chamber inside you for them to be triggered. The key to this state is to resonate such a consistent and powerful state of love and light that there is no room for any negative emotions to ever get in. Love and light means just about any of the higher positive emotions previously listed.

Another key to living in this state is to see all emotions as frequency and vibration. At this level emotions are just frequencies. There is no judgment, except to be aware of the difference in the vibrational level so you can catch yourself whenever you fall below the line.

Some say that this might be boring – not living in the world of emotions. However, you are still surfing the waves of positive emotions. When living in love and light, negative emotions seem so useless. When living in love and light, the level of ecstasy is so high, you are never bored. The soundscape is always incredibly beautiful.

240

Joy Meditation

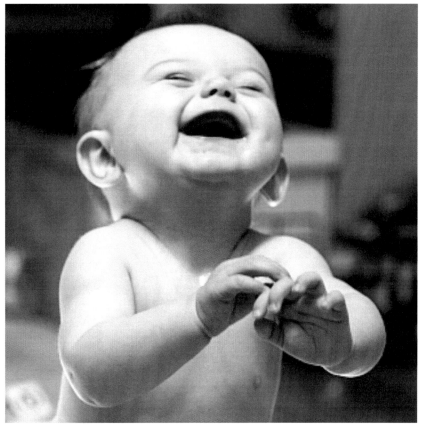
Joy

I would like to end the chapter with a meditation on Joy, so you can really enjoy these higher vibrations yourself.

Joy is an unusually powerful vibration and the sounds that go with it are especially infectious. It is difficult to not be entrained by the frequency of someone that is in a state of pure joy.

To help us get going, here is a quote from the *I Ching* on joy:

> A joy that is shared is symbolized by a group of friends playing, or a carefree young girl singing to herself while engaged in her work. Happiness is rising within, and spreading out into the world.

> Joy arises through gentle means, but springs from a solid inner base. The power of pure joy should not be underestimated. The enjoyment of learning and discovery, for example, has led to great innovation and much material progress. Accordingly, that which brings the most joy into the world – love – is the source of life itself.

> If happiness is supported by personal stability, it will eventually wear down the stiffest barrier and win over the hardest heart. True joy is a beacon in the world, and

though it is indeed rare, its presence is an indication of great good fortune, both now and in the future. How could it be otherwise?

Think about the last time you were in a state of joy. Joy is like extended happiness. It seems that joy is not something that happens over a short span of time. Joy might be brought about by an experience with friends, groups, nature, babies and love to name a few. Sometimes joy seems to come for no reason.

Now go back to that time where you were in a state of pure joy and feel it to the core of your being again. Let it encompass your whole body. Let it expand until it surrounds you like a bubble. Now think of all the people on the planet that are also sharing joy at this moment. Who knows…but I would say there is at least a million (especially if we count the babies and kids). While resonating your own joy, let your field of joy connect with that on the planet. Now…if joy had a sound, get that sound going in your head. In fact, get it going in your head really loudly (although silently). Now, make that sound out loud, resonating the pure joy inside of you.

Remember this sound of joy. It can help you return whenever you like. Your homework for the rest of your life is to now resonate joy in the world as much as you possibly can – and make the sound out loud whenever you can. As previously mentioned, when you make the sound of an emotion, it creates a stronger resonant field for that emotion to exist at even a deeper level within you.

The key is to now be present
with the sounds and music of your emotions
throughout the day.

Whenever you find that you don't like the music
or you find that it is stressing you out
use these techniques to change
the sound and music inside your head
to higher and more consistent
beautiful sounds and music.

In Chapter 50, "Living with Sound – Using Sound in Your Daily Life," we share some daily sound meditations you can do be more present with the music of your own emotions.

Chapter 33 – Transforming Negative Beliefs

"Some of our beliefs are received from the group consciousness or dominant paradigm, such as the belief that "the earth is round" (whereas in the past it was commonly believed to be flat), or that a certain disease is incurable. Other beliefs, such as cultural beliefs, have been passed on genetically through our parents. Genetic beliefs are a reflection of the experiences and worldview of our ancestors, and may include things like prejudices, or beliefs such as "I have to feast before the famine". We also form our own core beliefs based on how we view or interpret our own life experiences. These beliefs tend to be on the conscious level, and may include things such as "I'll never be good enough" or "I have to put others first". Our beliefs impact our day-to-day lives in ways we may not realize, and can manifest as physical or emotional conditions, blocks and fears."
- Gregg Braden

Negative beliefs make up one of the strongest resonant fields within our mind – a powerful frequency controlling our lives. The strength of their resonance can be so strong that they not only determine the way you are, and how you are in the world, but also how you affect other people. These beliefs often predetermine your wealth and abundance, the types of people you hang out with and the quality of the relationships, and the health issues that you manifest.

Using the laws of resonance many people practice the law of attraction in order to attract what they would like to be and have in their lives. The basis of the law of attraction is to resonate the energy of what it would be like to have the things you need or desire. Many people work quite hard at being above the line in the higher emotions to attract what they want.

However, people are still not getting what they want. The problem is that our negative beliefs keep attracting many things that we don't want.

The truth is, based on the laws of resonance we are attracting exactly what we are resonating in our subconscious – and these resonant beliefs can be extremely powerful resonant fields that have been built up over time and strongly reinforced by friends, family and our society.

Many of us are often completely aware of our negative beliefs, but we just don't know how to change such strong patterns. However, sometimes we are not even aware of these negative beliefs – they are vibrating below our conscious level. Sometimes they peak their heads out, but then go back into hiding. Other beliefs never peak their heads out and remain completely hidden. If hidden, the first step is to become aware of our subconscious beliefs that are holding us back.

Finding Your Negative Subconscious Beliefs
They are actually easy to track down if you just become aware of your thoughts. You can

also try and reverse engineer the situations you get into. Ask yourself, what could be the belief that got me into this mess in the first place?

Another way to track them down is to look at the list below and see if any of them resonate with you. The beliefs in the list might also remind you of others that you are resonating that aren't on the list.

Self
- I am not good enough (probably the most common negative belief on the planet)
- I am not smart enough
- Good things never happen to me
- I don't deserve good things because of what I have done
- Life is never easy
- I am an incompetent person or a bad person
- I am not good looking enough
- I am not tall/short enough, the right body type, athletic enough, correct weight, etc.
- I am not spiritual enough
- I'm too emotional / not emotional enough
- I am a simple person incapable of great things
- I am not worthy of Spirit or enlightenment
- I'm not pure enough to help heal others

Relationships
- I am not caring or loving enough
- I am not lovable
- I don't deserve to be loved
- I cannot trust anyone
- I am always exploited by others
- People are often jerks or assholes
- I'm so afraid of being judged by others all the time
- I always screw up relationships once I start to get close
- People don't see my value, I'm invisible

Wealth
- Money is the root of all evil. If I have a lot of money, others will have less. It is wrong to have a lot of money when others are starving.
- I don't deserve to be rich
- I need to compete with other people to succeed in life
- It's tough to make money
- I'm not clever enough to run my own business
- Whenever I make a lot of money I always lose it
- Rich people are bad

Health
- I always have some health issue going on, I'm never completely healthy
- I don't deserve to be healthy

- I don't have it together enough to be healthy
- I'm an emotional mess most of the time
- Life sucks…You just grow old and die
- I am not capable of healing myself
- I am not pure enough, or of high enough consciousness to help or heal others
- I don't deserve it all – health, wealth and harmonious relationships

Transforming the Beliefs – Making the Sound of the Opposite
This procedure is quite simple, but incredibly powerful. You simply flip around the negative belief into a positive statement, hold the statement in your mind, and make the sound of it. Again, just play with it until you find a sound that seems to fit the positive affirmation.

Here are some examples of opposites:

Self
- I am good enough
- I am smart enough
- Good things happen to me
- I deserve good things regardless of what I have done
- Life is easy
- I am a totally competent and wonderful person
- I am really good looking
- I am tall/short enough, the right body type, athletic enough, correct weight, etc.
- I am spiritual enough
- I am emotionally balanced and I feel or accept my emotions
- I am capable of great things
- I am worthy of Spirit or enlightenment.
- I am pure enough to help heal others

Relationships
- I am caring and loving enough
- I am lovable
  I deserve to be loved
- I can now trust anyone
- I will never be exploited again
- People are often pure loving spirits
- I am no longer afraid of being judged by others. I am secure in my own way of being and doing things.
- All my relationships are harmonious no matter how close I get
- People respect me 100% of the time

Wealth
- The more money I have, the more I can help others
- I deserve to be rich
- I don't need to compete with other people to succeed in life

- It's easy to make money
- I'm totally clever enough to run my own business
- When I make a lot of money, I will not lose it ever again. I will save and spend wisely.

Health
- I can be perfectly healthy from now on
- I deserve to be healthy
- I have it together enough to be healthy
- I'm emotionally stable from now on
- Life is wonderful, an adventure to treasure
- I am 100% capable of healing myself
- I am perfectly able to help others with healing and raising consciousness
- I totally deserve it all – health, wealth and harmonious relationships

As you can see, just reading the opposite makes you feel good. However, when you make the sound, it reinforces the positive statement and brings it into every cell of your body – transforming the belief at a cellular level.

It is extremely important
to make the opposite of the negative belief
be believable.

If you say some thing like, "I am always loving," your subconscious mind might be thinking, "Yeah, right." You need to craft the statement in a way that makes sense. Perhaps you might say something like, "I am a loving being. I do my best to be loving most of the time."

Now, try it. Pick some negative beliefs that you may have lingering in your subconscious, and make the sound of the opposite. Make the sound as long as you feel comfortable (the longer, the better).

Also, whenever you come across a situation in life where you notice that a negative belief has reared its head, immediately make the sound of the opposite. Often negative beliefs are behind the negative emotions that you might be experiencing. For example, a negative belief about not being good enough can easily lead to fear in a particular situation.

There are other techniques that can be quite helpful that are good to be aware of.

Emotional Freedom Technique (EFT)
EFT involves tapping on acupuncture points while expressing the negative beliefs in order to desensitize your reaction to them. You then tap on the same points while expressing the positive affirmation in order to bring that energy into your system.

The tapping on the acupuncture points happens at the rate of about 5 taps per second, which is within the theta brainwave state. This allows you to access the subconscious, which they say can be accessed when in the theta state (just as in Hypnotherapy).

This technique is about getting energy to once again flow through your meridians and your system so that the stuck emotion or belief is not hampering your life giving flow.

Techniques of the Future
Ultimately I believe that we will be able to use sounds on acupuncture points to do the same type of releasing of emotional issues and negative beliefs. There is a website at www.acupuncture4themind.com that has a similar technique. I believe that in the future we will ultimately have a system to clear out the entire emotional body so that we can simply resonate higher emotions and consciousness more consistently all the time.

We are currently working on such a system within our virtual reality system. You can check out some information about it at www.soundhealingcenter.com/inside.html

Imagine
being clear of all of the emotions and beliefs
that keep us imprisoned

so that we can then
be present within our own Soul
connected to Spirit and Source
living in love and light
all the time.

Just imagine!

SECTION IX - Mental Expansion with Sound

"Music can minister to minds diseased, pluck from the memory a rooted sorrow, raze out the written troubles of the brain, and with its sweet oblivious antidote, cleanse the full bosom of all perilous stuff that weighs upon the heart."
- William Shakespeare (1564-1616)

Introduction – Brainwaves and Brainwave Entrainment

There is a lot of definitive clinical research on how sound and music can be used to activate the brain and memory, and create more mental clarity (including the Mozart effect). We know that high frequencies activate the mind. We also know that sounds and music that are changing all the time also activate the mind. Brain plasticity and health is based on the creation of new neural pathways when there is new information being received.

On the other hand, low frequencies calm the body, and repetitive sounds and music allow the left brain to go to sleep. The right brain then takes over and we are able to go into deeper or higher states of consciousness.

Then there is the frequency of the brain. As previously mentioned, different parts of the brain vibrate at different rates: delta, theta, alpha, beta and gamma. There have been many clinical studies using EEG to measure these brainwave rates, so the science is very definitive. Science has also proven that when you create a frequency or rhythm that falls within one of these brainwave states, your brain will entrain to that frequency within one minute.

Using low frequencies to entrain the brain can help with stress and pain reduction, ADD, ADHD and is helpful for relaxation, meditation, sleep, learning, enhanced creativity and intuition, being more present, telepathy, remote viewing, lucid dreaming, out-of-body experiences and connecting to Source.

When the frequencies are played on headphones they also synchronize the left and right hemispheres of the brain.

Here is a list of rates of vibration for each of the brainwave states (in cycles per second).

Deep Delta	< .5	Deep meditation.
Delta	5 – 4	Deep sleep (about 1.5 hours of the night).
Theta	4 – 7	Dream state. Creativity. Portal to subconscious and Oneness.
Alpha	7 – 12	Relaxed attention. Creative problem solving. Presence.
Beta	12 – 30	Normal day to day thinking and processing.
Gamma	30 - 100	High state of meditation.

Entraining the Brain with Rhythms and Binaural Beats

Whenever we experience a vibration within any of these brainwave states our brain will be entrained into the same frequency – normally in less than a minute. In science this is referred to as "the frequency-following response." Just about all rhythms fall into the brainwave range. Therefore, almost every rhythm in the music we listen to entrains our brain. Our brains are commonly entrained by the rhythms around us.

As discussed earlier (in Section IX on binaural beats) you can also create these subsonic frequencies by using two frequencies that are detuned a little bit from each other. When these two frequencies are played into the left and right ears separately they are called "binaural beats." Binaural beats were discovered in 1839 by a German experimenter, H. W. Dove. Binaural beats are the generic term for these low frequencies. Technically, when played through speakers they would be called monaural beats. However, many companies have come up with their own trademark names including hemisync and holosync.

Because these frequencies can be somewhat annoying to listen to, the frequencies are often placed at a low volume in a mix of other sounds or music. People often use pink noise, nature sounds and a wide range of music. Sometimes I will listen to the binaural beats completely on their own to receive the maximum effect.

If you would like to try this for yourself, you can see a free tone generator (Mac or PC) at

Free online version (site that is selling Sound Healing Tinnitus treatment):
http://www.audionotch.com/app/tune/

Free software for Mac or PC (two week demo, then about $35)
http://www.nch.com.au/tonegen/index.html

In the ToneGen program, choose "Stereo" under "Tone" menu. Select the frequency you want to modify by highlighting it and then select "Edit Value" under the "Tone" menu and type in the frequencies. Then hit the green "Play" button.

If you put in 100 hertz and 104 hertz, the frequencies are so close together that your ear can hear both of them. Your ear actually makes up 102 hertz. The two frequencies also cancel each other 4 times per second, which causes the volume to go up and down 4 times per second (the difference between 100 and 104). It is just the same as if you were to turn the volume up and down on your stereo 4 times per second. This oscillation of volume going up and down will entrain your brain into a high delta state because delta is between .5 and 4 cycles per second.

This works whether listening on speakers or headphones. Many believe that you must wear headphones to entrain the brain but this is not true – your brain will be entrained even by a rhythm on a drum.

There is an additional effect that occurs when listening to headphones. When you place one frequency in the left ear and another in the right ear, the two frequencies don't actually meet and cancel out each other because your brain is in the way. Therefore, in order to keep reality consistent your brain makes up the 4 hertz (in this example). In order to do that, the brain has to connect the left and right brain. The tone in the left ear actually goes to the right brain and the tone in the right ear goes to the left brain. The two tones get connected across the corpus collossum, the part of the brain that connects the left and right brains. And when the corpus collossum is lit up you are in the zone. Left and right brain synchronization is the ideal state to be in, and it rarely happens throughout the day.

To get a little more technical: Synchronized brain waves have long been associated with meditative and hypnogogic states, and audio with embedded binaural beats has the ability to induce and improve such states of consciousness. The reason for this is physiological. Each ear is "hardwired" (so to speak) to both hemispheres of the brain (Rosenzweig, 1961). Each hemisphere has its own olivary nucleus (sound-processing center), which receives signals from each ear. In keeping with this physiological structure, when a binaural beat is perceived there are actually two standing waves of equal amplitude and frequency present, one in each hemisphere. So, there are two separate standing waves entraining portions of each hemisphere to the same frequency. The binaural beats appear to contribute to the hemispheric synchronization evidenced in meditative and hypnogogic states of consciousness. Brain function is also enhanced through the increase of cross-colossal communication between the left and right hemispheres of the brain.

This is major – to be able to synchronize the left and right brains within a minute.

As mentioned, all rhythms also entrain the brain. Four cycles per second is actually the same as 60 beats per minute tempo.

Here's how to figure it out mathematically, in case you are interested.

You can figure out the rhythm that equals a brainwave state by multiplying by 60 to get beats per minute (BPM) and ocatavizing the BPM down until you get a usable range (between 40 and 200 BPM). For example, using 4 cycles per second:

$4 \times 60 = 240$ (But 240 is too fast)

½ = 120

½ again = 60

Both 120 BPM and 60 BPM would fit the 4 cycles per second rate (depending on whether you play ½ notes or ¼ notes)

Every rhythm within a song
actually entrains your brain into a specific brainwave state.

Different tempos of songs create different states.
Love songs are typically entraining you into Delta or Theta.
Dance music normally puts you into Theta or Alpha.

Shamanic trance drumming or journey work is practiced at a tempo of around 110-150 BPM, which ends up being between 4 and 5 cycles per second – right on the threshold between delta and theta. People commonly go out of their bodies into higher realms and reportedly access their Spiritual and animal guides.

Not only does music entrain you into brainwave states, but also any consistent rhythm can do it. Fans and motors commonly take us with them. The washing machine is a powerful delta entrainer. The dryer is normally still delta, but is approaching theta.

You can also get the same effect with flashing lights. When you drive by a row of equally spaced trees, the flashing lights coming through the trees can easily entrain you into a brainwave state. In fact, there are units you can buy that are generally called, "brain machines" that use flashing lights to entrain you.

Isochronic beats are frequencies that are panned from ear to ear at the specific brainwave state. Some claim these to be even more effective than normal binaural beats.

Tuning Brainwave Frequencies to You
Every body vibrates at a different frequency within each brainwave state. For example, the exact frequency of delta that you go into when in deep sleep is slightly different from the frequency I naturally go to while in deep sleep. In each brainwave state we have our own natural rate of vibration within that particular state.

There is now good evidence to show that the particular frequency that your brain vibrates at in each of the brainwave states is based on your overall resonant frequency or "Soul" frequency. Binaural beats that are tuned to you are much more effective.

There are a large number of companies that create CD's with embedded binaural beats, but they are not necessarily tuned to you (unless you get lucky). This explains why the effectiveness of CD's that are tuned to a specific frequency can vary dramatically. (At the Sound Institute, we can find your home note and create CD's tuned to you for each of the brainwave states.)

Now, let's look at each of the brainwave states in more detail, and how they can be used to help you and your clients.

If you research brainwave rates, you will find that they vary as to the threshold between one state and the next. This is because everyone has a little different threshold as to when they transition from one state to the next.

Chapter 34 – Delta State – Sleep Enhancement and Direct Connection to Source

Again, delta is .5 – 4 cycles per second.

Delta brainwaves occur when you are in the deepest, dreamless sleep, which happens a few times through the night, normally in 1.5 hour segments. It also occurs during unconsciousness.

Deep sleep is when you are one with Source or God!
This is where you get replenished.

It is interesting that just about every animal on the planet is required to go back to Source every night to be replenished.

Therefore, this is one of the most important brainwave states, particularly when we are interested in raising our consciousness. However, as we'll discuss later, higher consciousness requires a combination of brainwave states throughout the body.

Another interesting thing about delta is that when fully entrained, we disappear and have no memory. We never remember those 1.5 hour segments in the night when we are in deep sleep. Whether asleep or in a deep meditation, it is like we become one with the Universe. It actually requires another part of the brain to be active and recording the experience for us to remember the state. When the brain is entrained to delta frequencies and awareness is maintained, a unique state of consciousness emerges. This state is often referred to as hypnogogia – "mind awake/body asleep." People report that there is no mental imagery or awareness of our bodies. Some talk about being aware of a point of awareness, but most speak of being one with all of the frequencies around them.

As with all brainwave states, remember that there is one small range of delta that your brain vibrates at when in deep sleep. Be aware, that if you get lucky, and the CD you are listening to happens to have binaural beats in your particular frequency, it can knock you right out!

Because of this
it is extremely dangerous to drive or operate heavy machinery
while listening to binaural beats in delta.

Things that Create Delta
You can use two tone generators to create delta. Most crystal bowls oscillate at the tempo of delta. This is why the crystal bowl can be so effective in bringing us into deeper states of meditation. Larger Tibetan bowls also naturally have delta oscillations in them (some smaller ones do too).

You can also use two crystal bowls that are the same note but tuned a bit differently. The oscillation in volume up and down is intense and can easily take you out. Generally, crystal bowls are not tuned to specific frequencies (unless you pay extra), so you have to just get lucky to get two that create this beating.

About the only way to know the precise delta frequency would be to use tone generators and adjust the frequencies until the binaural beats created by the tone generators match the binaural beats created by the bowls. You could also find the beats per minute (BPM) using a metronome and then divide the BPM by 60 to get the actual cycles per second.

The oscillation of a singer's vibrato is normally in delta.

You can also use two tuning forks. Tuning forks normally are labeled with their frequency so it is easy to simply figure out the difference between the two frequencies, which is the binaural beat frequency.

Elephants put out a low frequency of 3 cycles per second. Perhaps they use it to lull any animal around them into a deep sleep. Or perhaps they are somehow resonating with a deep frequency within the earth.

My favorite delta entrainer of all is the purr of a cat. Cats purr at 25 hertz (with a prominent harmonic around 50 hertz). However, this purr frequency goes up and down in volume as they breathe – entraining you into delta.

Delta Uses
There are several key advantages to this state:

1. Relaxation – It is a very relaxing state. You may have noticed this while listening to the 2 cycles per second example.

2. Meditation – Delta can take you into a very deep state of oneness with Source where you are completely regenerated. When combined with other brainwave states you might even remember where you went.

3. Sleep Enhancement – When you listen to binaural beats and get entrained into delta it is like you have taken a nap. Delta is especially helpful for insomnia. There are many companies (including ours – www.soundhealingcenter.com/music.html#sleep) that have CD's to help you sleep. Many people swear by them, and of course, there are no side effects. Some people leave the CD's on all night long to help them stay asleep.

4. Breaking up wily cells – As mentioned in the section on physical healing, delta frequencies are such long wavelengths (as long as 1500 feet) that they can easily shatter a brittle cell like cancer. Again, this is how a wine glass is broken – by the powerful low delta frequencies.

5. Breaking up stuck energy and blockages – these frequencies and rhythms create a dissonance that can be really effective for breaking up stuck patterns.

Chapter 35 – Theta State – Enhanced Creativity and a Portal to Oneness in the Universe

Theta is generally 4 – 8 cycles per second

Theta is typically thought of as the dream state (whether asleep or awake). When you start getting sleepy and drowsy you are entering theta. Most of the night we are in theta. We also are in theta when daydreaming (in that floaty dreamlike space). It is a state where we are nearly unconscious. In fact, when someone is given anesthesia, doctors monitor their brainwaves and don't start the surgery until the patient stabilizes in the theta state.

Most people do get groggy when in this state, however, if other parts of your brain are in more active states such as alpha or beta, then theta can be a very creative state. Many report getting creative downloads and this state is associated with intuition and fantasizing. Therefore, theta is a good state to access if you have a creative block while working on a project. As with dreams, it opens up your internal world. Since it is common to access mental imagery, theta often gives you a plethora of creative material to work with.

Theta also houses the emotions. It is a state that seems to open up access to the subconscious. When you are hypnotized you are in theta. Therefore, the key component of hypnotherapy is to bring you into this state with guided meditation. Because of this capability, the theta state can be used to re-program your habitual tendencies. It is also effective to accelerate learning – specifically deep transformational work (versus absorbing information mentally).

On the negative side it is believed to reflect activity from the limbic system and increased activity is observed in anxiety, behavioral activation and inhibition.

Portal to a State of Oneness with the Universe
You go into theta whenever you tune into more than one thing at a time. This happens when you look at sparkles on the water. As your eyes de-focus and you start to see waves of light moving across the sparkles you have entered theta. It commonly happens in that state while listening to music where you "become the music." Some explain it as "the music goes inside of me." Theta commonly happens in many artistic endeavors when the artist becomes immersed or one with the project. It also easily happens in nature when looking at a panoramic view of a sprawling landscape or a beautiful field of grass.

Your logical mind (alpha and particularly beta) shuts down when you access multiple things at once. This is not the same as multitasking – when multitasking we are normally jumping back and forth from one focus to another. True theta is a very peaceful state where you disappear. You simply are the experience. There is no awareness of your body.

This state is the same that people report when they are one with the Universe. People who can access this state say that they disappear and are simply one with every thing they perceive. People who have had near-death experiences say the same thing – "I was one with everything in the Universe – with God." Therefore, theta can be used as a portal to access the ultimate state of oneness.

You simply tune into more than one thing at a time. In Chapter 47, "Connecting to Spirit and Source with Sound," the chapter on "oneness," we will share a guided meditation where you tune into all the frequencies in the Universe simultaneously to access this state. In the chapter on Chakras (Chapter 42), we will also share a technique for tuning into all of the chakras simultaneously. Both of these meditations will take you out of your body into the altered state of awareness – where you can also access the rest of the frequencies in the Universe.

Theta Healing is now a popular technique where this high state of theta is used to access these higher levels of consciousness; then the energy of Source is accessed to help others with their own healing. Practitioners are simply using the theta portal to access oneness. They claim instantaneous physical and emotional healing.

Therefore, it is important to not ever discount the theta state as simply that place of drowsiness before we go to sleep. I have come to believe that the theta state has some of the largest potential to bring us into higher states of consciousness – particularly what I believe to be the highest state of all – Oneness with Everything in the Universe.

And, the sounds that create theta states are very relaxing to listen to.

Things that Create Theta
Again, you can use two tone generators, crystal bowls, or tuning forks to create theta (technically, any two instruments, including two voices can create any binaural beat). The oscillation of a singer's vibrato is sometimes in theta.

Individual Tibetan bowls commonly have a theta oscillation going on when you strike them. The difference in frequency between the two bells in tingshas is almost always in theta. And, of course, you can always play drums at a tempo that will put people into theta states.

Whales actually put out a low frequency of 8 hertz, which is right on the threshold of theta and alpha. Some say this frequency is very important in holding together the earth matrix. It seems to be tied into the earth's root chakra.

Later, we'll discuss the Schumann resonance, which is also right on the threshold between theta and alpha.

Theta Uses
Here are the key advantages to this state:

1. Relaxation

2. Aids in falling asleep

3. Help accessing a creative state where you can access new information – especially unusual visuals (as in visual imagery).

4. To access the subconscious in order to reprogram, make changes, or heal

5. As a portal to a state of Oneness with everything in the Universe.

6. Resetting your brains sodium/potassium ratio in theta – Your brain cells reset their sodium & potassium ratios when the brain is in theta state. The sodium & potassium levels are involved in osmosis, which is the chemical process that transports chemicals into and out of your brain cells. After an extended period in the beta state the ratio between potassium and sodium is out of balance. This is the main cause of what is known as "mental fatigue". A brief period in theta (about 5 -15 minutes) can restore the ratio to normal resulting in mental refreshment.

Chapter 36 – Alpha State – Help with ADD, ADHD, Mental Clarity and Memory

"Music is the mysterious key of memory,
unlocking the hoarded treasures of the heart.
Tones, at times, in music,
will bring back forgotten things."
- Lord Edward Bulwer Lytton (1803-1873)

Alpha is generally 8 – 12 cycles per second.

I believe the best term for this state is "relaxed attention." If you are listening now, you will notice that it is a pretty active state. Alpha is relaxed mind. It is not about conceptual or detailed thinking, major body sensations, or having strong emotions. It is more about seeing the forest instead of the trees – the overview.

Alpha is often associated with creativity, but it actually happens when information to resolve a situation simply comes to you, instead of you mentally figuring out the answer to something. You might know the various bits of information that contribute to the solution, but they don't all come together by way of a logical process. It's like the answer just pops into your head. However, as you have probably experienced, the answer does not come to you until you relax. This is alpha. Because of this, alpha is often associated with learning and is used to enhance accelerated learning.

The same happens with memory. The more you get stressed trying to remember something, the more you remain in beta. The radio station (so to speak) of the memory is commonly in low alpha (often right at the threshold of theta), so you have to relax your mind in some way so you can access the right address. Often, I will go do something else and then the memory will easily pop into my head.

Alpha is actually quite a common state. Some have associated it with daydreaming as with theta. Alpha waves generally happen in the occipital part of the brain responsible for our visual world, therefore it is much easier to access alpha with the eyes closed. Visual stimuli and pain (or physical pleasure) generally take you out of alpha.

Probably the most important aspect of alpha is that it is associated with calm alertness. This is really the essence of "presence." You are in your body and aware of everything around and inside of you. It is associated with body/mind coordination required for things like dancing and sports.

Things that Create Alpha
Same as before, you can use tone generators, two tuning forks or two crystal bowls – or any two instruments. I've noticed that some Tibetan bowls actually have oscillations in alpha.

Alpha Uses
1) Stress Reduction – Since the state brings calmness and alertness it is especially helpful when dealing with a chaotic situation.

2) Accelerated Learning – Particularly learning that is based on seeing things from a higher perspective.

3) Creative Problem Solving – Often we try and figure things out (beta) instead of relaxing and letting the answer come to us.

4) Being Present in the World – Relaxed attention – Ready for whatever is to come.

5) Mental Clarity – Entraining the brain into consistency with alpha can bring your thoughts into order.

If you have been listening to the alpha frequencies while reading this chapter, note how you feel.

Chapter 37 – Other Higher and Lower States – Gamma and Deep Delta
We address many other brainwave states in this chapter.

Beta - 12 to 20 cycles per second.

Beta is our normal day-to-day thinking and processing. If alpha is about seeing the forest, beta is about seeing the trees – it's more detail oriented. Accountants and lawyers work in beta most of the time. It is also associated with intense emotional and physical experiences.

Low beta, 12-17 cycles per second is normal information processing and mental activity; high beta, 17-30 cycles per second happens when we are in a heightened state of alertness fight or flight, tension, fear, or anxiety. It is interesting to note that even though beta is technically a consistent frequency, it is associated with emotions that do not produce consistent sounds.

The positive aspect of beta is that it is also associated with a high degree of alertness and presence. Since this is the most common state of mind of most people, we are easily entrained into it by the people we are around throughout the day.

Beta Uses
1. Some people with ADD/ADHD cannot access beta frequencies. We do a treatment at the Institute where we play beta frequencies in each key while a person tries to read and study something very complicated. It always amazes me that when we happen to hit their home note in beta, they can immediately focus on the material. We then make a CD with those particular beta frequencies for them. The results are nothing less than miraculous.

2. Very good for serious mental processing – particularly mathematical calculations, figuring out your schedule, and how to make a living.

It is generally a state that we want to get out of.

Gamma - 30 to 100 cycles per second
(Sometimes referred to as "super high beta")

University of Alabama discovered gamma around 40 hertz. It is called the binding frequency and is increased under heightened perception and specific types of meditation. It also occurs during the process of awakening and during active rapid eye movement (REM) sleep. It also happens when bursts of precognition or high-level information processing occur. It does not occur under anesthesiology.

This state has been found in people that are in really high states of meditation. It also happens when our left and right brains are synchronized.

Super high gamma states (sometimes called hyper-gamma) between 100 and 200 hertz have been associated with ecstatic states of consciousness. Kundalini experiences and out-of-body experiences come with these super high brainwave states. Moments of extreme inspiration come at around 100 hertz.

You can think of higher brainwave states as having more moments of reality. It's like having better resolution with more dots in the picture. To the observer, it actually makes the outer world slow down. Perhaps you have had the experience of being in a car accident or falling down, where everything goes into slow motion. This is because your brainwaves have sped up.

It has been found that boxers (especially the best ones) have extremely fast brainwave states. As a result, they see the glove coming at them in slow motion. In the same way, the common house fly has an extremely fast brainwave state, so they see your hand coming at them in extreme slow motion, and have no problem flying away before your hand gets to them.

This is an interesting concept when you think about it.

The higher our brainwave state,
the slower the world around us becomes –
essentially the more peaceful and still the world appears!!!

Deep Delta – Less than .5
(Sometimes called Epsilon)

Recent physiological studies of highly hypnotizable subjects and adept meditators indicate that maintaining awareness with reduced cortical arousal is indeed possible in selected individuals as a natural ability or as an acquired skill.
- Sabourin, Cutcomb, Crawford, & Pribram, 1993

Deep delta is associated with out of body experiences, spiritual awakening, and moments of epiphany.

Research from the people at HeartMath has shown that your brain vibrates at a frequency of .1 cycles per second when your heart is in a state of coherence, or when you are in most high states of bliss. This is also the state of ideal heart coherence.

This frequency actually matches the rhythm of a slow breath. It is well known that when in a deep state of meditation, your breath, heart and mind all synchronize their rhythms.

Chapter 38 – Using Brainwave Entrainment to Access Higher States of Consciousness

Many people in the field now feel that higher consciousness is not necessarily about raising your vibration, it is actually about going higher and lower at the same time (I have come to believe that it is not only higher and lower, but resonating all of the frequencies in between as well). In the area of brainwaves this is especially true. When we monitor the brainwaves of people in high states of meditation and bliss, we see they have brainwaves in both gamma and deep delta – they are going both directions at the same time.

It is also interesting to note that the purring frequency of a cat is in gamma (25 hertz with the second harmonic at 50 hertz); however, those frequencies also go up and down in volume based on the breath of the cat. The breath of the purr is in delta, so cats are also taking us in both directions at the same time.

Brain Maps

The truth is that our entire brain is rarely in one state or another. One part of the brain might be theta, while another part is delta, and yet another part is humming in alpha. In fact, if we were solely in delta we would be totally asleep and unconscious of any bliss we might be experiencing. If we were in theta, we would be quite spaced out. We actually need the alpha to be able to remember and hold our consciousness together. However, even alpha is missing the direct connection to Spirit that comes with delta and theta.

Dr. Jeffrey Thompson used an EEG to monitor the brainwaves of some Dalai Lama trained meditators. He found that when they were in extremely high states of meditation they had a full range of brainwave states spread across their brain. He then took this "brain map" and used binaural beats to create each of the frequencies present in these meditators. His CD, "The Awakened Mind," was at the top of the new age charts years ago.

This opens up a whole world of possibilities. We should be able to do brain maps for each of the higher emotions and easily entrain people out of the lower emotions. Though, quite possible in the future, there are currently a few problems with this thinking.

First, when you enter coherent emotional states the heart and brain must synchronize their rhythms. It is possible that your brainwaves can trigger your heart to then synchronize. Or, the brainwaves could actually induce the emotional state and your heart falls right into alignment. In the future, this might very well be possible. However, I like to think of brainwave entrainment as an adjunct to other more potent aspects of sound and vibration. For example, I believe that flowing music actually has way more emotional power than static binaural beats.

This leads us to the other problem with binaural beats – they don't breathe like us. Normally binaural beats are set to an unchanging frequency. However, nothing in our body is that stable (except maybe some cells and the frequency of some of the materials in our body (bones, muscles, etc.). Most of our system is breathing and changing up and down in frequency ever so slightly. Besides our breath, our heart rate is fluctuating. Our hormones are making adjustments every second. Every part of our body is a living, breathing piece of flowing music and energy. Ultimately, I believe that binaural beats should be more musical, just like the essence of our system.

Again, in these high states of consciousness a full range of brainwaves are spread across the brain in very specific locations. When you play the entire brain map of binaural beats into the ears they are all mixed together, **and all frequencies go to all parts of the brain.** How could the brain possibly know to divide up all of them and send them to the correct locations in the brain?

Meanwhile, there has been some research on Parkinson's patients where they actually attached electrodes to different parts of the scalp and transmitted different frequencies to various parts of the brain. This makes sense and has much more likelihood of getting the heart and the rest of your system to follow and fall into synch.

Ultimately, we hope to use sound, music, energy and light within a Virtual Reality system to provide as many different stimuli as possible – all with the same intention of resonating us into really high states of love and direct connections to Source. All of this with the intention of teaching a person how to access these high states on his or her own. We don't want anyone addicted to technology – we want to empower people to use their own personal power.

Flowing through All of the Brainwave States
Another system that is quite interesting is the Roshi System. This system was created by Chuck Davis who used to work at the Monroe Institute where some very interesting binaural beat research was done for the purpose of exploring a wide range of states of consciousness.

Chuck took off and developed his own brain machine using flashing red LED's instead of sound. Just about all of the "brain machines" on the market actually flash at a consistent rate entraining you into one or more of the brainwave states. Instead, the Roshi System quickly moves the brain from one brainwave state to another –so quickly in fact, that your brain never has time to entrain to any one particular state. But, here's the key: The system changes tempo from one brainwave state to another based on the Fibonacci curve that is found in nature. It goes from deep delta to gamma, speeding up and slowing down based on the spiral found in the conch shell and throughout nature.

I have seen depression completely transformed in people within one week. It is also extremely effective for post-traumatic stress disorder (PTSD). As mentioned, using EEG, stuck emotions and PTSD can actually be seen as looping theta waves in the brain. It is an incredibly powerful system.

Again, this is evidence that flowing frequencies and music are more powerful than static frequencies and timbres.

Detecting Consciousness
It is interesting that music does somehow have the capability to entrain our brain into very specific states of consciousness. The truth is we don't really know exactly how this

complex mechanism works. But, we're definitely getting closer.

In fact, the latest research (discussed in detail in the movie "The Living Matrix") is now talking about the fact that our consciousness may not even be located in our brain. It is actually located in a "field" that some say is around the brain and others say is partially located in the electromagnetic field of the earth. On its own, even the scientific evidence supporting the phenomenon of remote viewing is sufficient to show that mind-consciousness is not a local phenomenon (McMoneagle, 1993).

As crude as this may seem, certain EEG patterns have been historically associated with specific states of consciousness. It is reasonable to assume, given the current EEG literature, if we see a specific EEG pattern it is probably accompanied by a particular state of consciousness.

The truth is that brainwave frequencies are a really simple way to look at the immense complexity of consciousness that we are capable of experiencing. There is no objective way to measure mind or consciousness with an instrument – yet. New equipment is being developed that is giving us even more detail – as we speak (or write). There is already equipment available that monitors the energy of chakras.

I hope that the information in this chapter will one day inspire someone (or many) to take the use of binaural beats to a whole new powerful level to help us all be healthier and able to expand our consciousness with ease.

Chapter 39 – Nature's Entrainers

The Schumann Resonance
The Schumann Resonance is a frequency that is resonating in our atmosphere. It entrains every brain on the planet into a brainwave state right on the threshold of theta and alpha. It is actually a resonant frequency between the earth and the ionosphere.

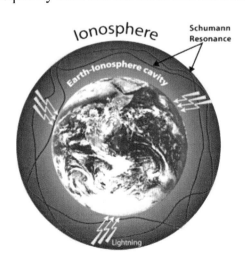

It is triggered by lightning strikes, which occur every second on the earth. It's like the lightning is ringing a bell –actually, it is ringing the space inside the bell to be more accurate.

This resonance is named after physicist, Winfried Otto Schumann. It is an average of 7.83 hertz – a wavelength equal to the circumference of the Earth. It varies slightly throughout the day as the ionosphere fluctuates (+ or - .5 hertz). There are harmonics at 6.4 hertz intervals. The harmonics are not the normal mathematical multiples (1x, 2x, 3x, 4x, 5x, etc.) because of the spherical shape of the cavity around the Earth. The harmonics average around 14.3, 20.8, 27.3, 33.8, 40.3, 46.8, 53.3, and 59.9 Hz. You can actually see these frequencies for the last month at www.glcoherence.org/monitoring-system/live-data.html

The main frequency of 7.83 hertz is right on the threshold of theta and alpha, and it has been shown to entrain our brains. In fact, every brain on the planet (including those of animals) has always been, and is always being entrained by this frequency. Even though the fundamental frequency is not that strong, it is has been consistent over millions of years. Therefore, you could say that we have become addicted to it – in a good way.

Herbert König, who was Schumann's successor at Munich University, demonstrated a correlation between Schumann resonances and brain rhythms. He compared human EEG recordings with the natural electromagnetic fields of the environment (1979) and found that the first five Schumann resonances, 0-35 Hz, to be within the same frequency range as the brain waves in a human EEG and the 7.8 Hz signal to be very close to the brain's alpha rhythm frequency.

In fact, we actually need the Schumann Resonance. NASA has discovered that astronauts are healthier if they receive this frequency while in outer space. Therefore, astronauts now have electromagnetic devices attached to their bodies, which transmit the frequency into their system when outside our atmosphere.

Essentially, when we resonate at this frequency we are in tune with nature. The problem is that the electromagnetism in a city obscures this frequency. Some people report that they can actually hear the frequency when out in the countryside (even though this is an electromagnetic frequency – not sound).

Research has also shown that fluctuations in this frequency (based on fluctuations in the ionosphere) can dramatically affect moods and energy. There is also evidence that these fluctuations correspond to international conflicts and wars.

You can actually buy electronic devices built into watches and amulets that put out this frequency consistently. One of our instructors has a watch that is pulsing at the 7.83 hertz frequency all the time.

We currently sell a device that embeds this frequency in water that you drink. You can check it out at www.SoundHealingCenter.com/GIA. We also sell the frequencies by themselves on a CD – go to www.SoundHealingCenter.com/music.html

Ocean Waves

The average time between 2 waves in a series of waves in the ocean is around .1 cycle per second. This is the same as the frequency that HeartMath has discovered that our brains go to when transmitting love. Therefore, the ocean is entraining your brain into a state of love!

The Binaural Beats in Sound and Musical Intervals

When you play any two frequencies at the same time, and the two frequencies are close enough to each other, you will get binaural beats. Therefore, every musical interval creates binaural beats. In fact, it makes sense that the binaural beats in musical intervals are the most important component of how that musical interval affects us – and creates various states of consciousness.

It also follows that ancient tuning systems that are based on the natural harmonic series found in nature are creating binaural beats that are more in tune with our own natural system.

Additionally, the musical intervals found within the harmonic structure of a sound are also creating a specific combination of binaural beats – akin to a brain map! Different timbres actually create different brain maps!

Even though many of the harmonic musical intervals in most music don't have enough time to create a coherent brainwave state because the notes are too short, most of the notes in Sound Healing music are much longer and do have the capacity to entrain.

Also, based on the concept of the Roshi System above, maybe it is not critical to entrain to a particular brain state. Just maybe the flow from one brainwave to another is the most important part, and that's why music is so powerful.

~~~~~~~~~~

There is a large number of sites offering brainwave CD's. Here are some of our favorites:

• Globe Institute (mine) – www.SoundHealingCenter.com/music.html
• Acoustic Brain Research – Tom Kenyon – www.TomKenyon.com/store/abr
• The Monroe Institute (Hemi-Sync) - www.MonroeInstitute.org/resources/hemi-sync
• Centerpointe – Holosynch - www.Centerpointe.com
• Brain Sync – www.BrainSync.com
• Jeffrey Thompson – www.NeuroAcoustic.com/BrainFitnessKits.html

Chapter 40 – Sound Therapy for Learning Disabilities

Sound Healing has been a part of mankind forever. But in the past 70 years the field of "listening therapies" has expanded greatly. The field began in Denmark when Christian Volt launched his work with frequency-enhanced recordings. As an early sound healer he understood the continuum of the effect of sound on our being. He used a simple assessment tool for determining which frequencies his clients were "tuning out." He then had them stand on a wooden box between two large speakers and played the appropriate (missing or tuned out) frequency enhancements until the body "tuned in" to these frequencies again. From physical ailments to learning challenges to raising consciousness, his frequency enhanced records had great anecdotal success.

In 1944, Dr. Alfred Tomatis applied his genius to the idea and became the father of this field when he developed the Tomatis Method. The primary component of the Tomatis Method is the use of the machine he called the Electronic Ear that delivered psychoacoustically modified music to retrain and enhance the auditory-vocal loop, thus improving speaking, singing, acting as well as learning disabilities, communication disorders and a number of other challenges people faced. Dr. Tomatis is best known for his discovery that "The voice can only reproduce that which the ear can hear". This is called the Tomatis Effect. His lesser known laws are gaining more recognition since the publication of Norman Doidge's book "The Brain that Changes Itself" because they speak to the neuroplasticity of the brain.

The second law states: If the missing frequencies are presented to the ear there is an instantaneous and unconscious restoration of the frequencies in the voice. The third law states: If there is sufficient auditory stimulation there will be a lasting improvement in the ability to listen and reproduce these sounds. Tomatis says, "Once an individual is able to accurately hear the sounds of another language and this listening ability is imposed on the individual through the electronic ear, the individual over time and practice of his own vocal emissions is able to retain and repeat those foreign language sounds with minimal accent."

Tomatis began his work with singers, actors, musicians, and those wanting to modify their accent, but it soon became evident to him that those with learning challenges could benefit greatly. Those who had dyslexia and a whole host of developmental challenges then searched him out and began using the Tomatis Method.

The field then expanded with new researchers, practitioners, programs and equipment. There are a great number of "listening therapies" available now with varying components for varying populations but they all have a connection with the fundamental concepts of Dr. Alfred Tomatis.

Here is an overview of these fundamental concepts:

1. All frequencies are nutrients.
Our brain especially needs high frequencies (this is part of the basis of the Mozart effect).

Our body needs low frequencies. Tomatis actually believed that the spine is mapped to the full frequency spectrum. If you are missing a frequency in your system it can affect you physically, mentally and emotionally. There are several ways in which you lose out on frequencies.

First, your ear has several bones, which laymen call the hammer, anvil and stirrup. These bones are connected to muscles, which have the capability to "tune out" the annoying frequencies around us, in order to protect us – because our ears don't have eyelids! There are many causes of frequencies that the ear and brain see as a threat to our well-being. These include: exposure to a sudden loud noise, constant loud noises, illness, injury, allergies, or emotional threat.

The unconscious part of our brain takes charge in the protective approach and will tune out frequencies that are perceived as threatening.

As well, if you have a parent that has an annoying critical twang to their voice, your ear will simply turn that frequency down. If you happen to grow up with a particularly annoying refrigerator motor blaring into the room all the time, your ear simply turns down that frequency. When you then move out of the house, the annoying frequencies are no longer present. The problem is that your ears do not readjust and now you are missing those annoying frequencies, which are actually healthy nutrients when you don't have too much of them.

Different cells need specific frequencies to flourish. These missing frequencies can also affect perception, organs, emotions, learning, creativity and spiritual awareness. The key is to shift into a loving or growth oriented approach to re-awaken the perception of all frequencies, restoring them to mind, body and spirit and thereby restoring health and well-being.

It is also possible to be born with physical disabilities that make it so you don't hear normally – deafness being the extreme case.

2. You don't make sounds that you can't hear.
Of course, you <u>can</u> make these frequencies with practice, otherwise Helen Keller wouldn't be able to speak at all. However, naturally, your voice will drop out frequencies that your ear has either turned down or does not hear at all.

Therefore, you can use the voice to tell what is going on with your hearing – and the amount and detail of the nutrients that are getting in.

This basic concept also translates into the whole field of voice analysis that we spoke about earlier.

Assessment
There are several ways that you determine what frequencies are missing and to what extent.

a. Intake Questionnaire – A good one is usually enough to determine if there are any sound sensitivities or fight or flight behaviors.

b. Voice Analysis – The test shows what frequencies (harmonics) are coming through your voice.

c. Audiogram – This is a simple hearing test. It shows what frequencies you are not hearing.

d. Movement – Our instructor, Elizabeth Grambsch has created a detailed system for watching the way people move in order to assess disabilities that have come from missing frequencies. The basic concept is that the different frequencies activate different types of motor skills.

Treatments

a. Choosing the right sound or listening therapy is important with sound protection issues because if the therapy triggers more sound protection the situation can actually get worse. The Listening Program plays classical music and then rolls off the low frequencies more and more until you only hear the highs. It then slowly brings them back in. This simply reactivates each of the frequencies. Research has shown these low pass filters to facilitate emotional regulation, relieve anxiety and PTSD and help people feel more grounded in their body.

The program also introduces chaotic frequencies, called "gating," which serve to exercise the muscles as well as the hairs within the inner ear. The Listening Program is the most well known resource for doing this.

b. The most basic treatment is to simply play the missing frequencies back to the person so these nutrients can be reestablished in the body.

c. Tomatis felt that a person should get at least 3 hours of high frequency stimulation per day. Mozart's music is used because it contains a large amount of high frequency sound.

d. Listening to your own voice with the missing frequencies turned up.

3. When certain muscles in the ear don't move freely like they are supposed to, it can cause problems similar to missing nutrients.
There is one main muscle in the ear particularly associated with learning disabilities and even autism, called the Stapedius muscle. When functioning properly it can make adjustments 100 times per second. In fact, it is the fastest and most agile muscle in the body.

When the Stapedius muscle is not working well or is a bit lethargic from overuse, or because the acoustic reflex is chronically active, the sound is not accurately processed and the frequencies going into the inner ear and brain may be distorted. This distortion can be associated with learning disabilities and those on the Autism Spectrum.

Assessment

Assessment
This can also be assessed by the same methods above since the Stapedius muscle also affects the distribution of frequencies going into the inner ear and brain.

Treatment
The key treatment is a therapeutic listening program. There are several psychoacoustic modifications made to the music that help a person exercise their middle ear muscles. A modification Tomatis called "gating" is one of the most important for exercising the stapedius muscle.

4. Active listening can be challenged when the hair cells of the cochlea are not functioning properly.
Tomatis learned to use a hearing test similar to the audiogram we use today. He became especially interested in very low volume hearing perception; that is, sounds that are just above the threshold of hearing. He became adept at using the audiograms to discern physical or emotional challenges the person may be facing. In these very quiet ranges lay the secret of observing the dynamic process of "tuning in" and "tuning out" – what we call listening.

Tomatis also learned that active listening is based on how the inner ear reacts to sound and energy that return to the ear – once sound has passed through the brain, electrical sound impulses are sent back to the ear. It has been discovered that if this whole feed-back mechanism is not functioning properly then a person has a difficult time with active listening.

The Tomatis Method is meant to exercise, energize and revitalize these sluggish hair cells and their responses to sound.

Assessment
Special reading of the standard audiogram. A number of other audiologic assessments are helpful; e.g., SCAN-A or SCAN-C test for auditory processing.

Treatment
Sweeping the frequency range in order to activate each of the hairs in the cochlea.

5. Anything that gets in the way of the natural flow of the sound nutrients while in utero can dramatically affect the physical and emotional growth of the fetus – and therefore affect a person's entire life.
The key nutrients come from the mother's voice through bone conduction as it is transmitted down the mother's spine into the head of the baby. There are physical things based on the positioning of the fetus in the womb that can get in the way, but also invasive technologies can completely interrupt this important flow of sound into the baby.

Assessment
a. Audiogram or Voice Analysis.
b. A psychological exam to determine emotional issues.

Treatment
a. Playing sounds and music that simulate the sounds that a fetus hears inside the womb.
b. Having the client speak into a microphone; the sound is then filtered and fed into his or her own ears. Again, the filtered sound simulates the sound of being in the womb.

Both of these techniques are meant to re-frame any trauma that occurred while in the womb or during the birthing process.

6. A healthy person has a nice balance of hearing from the left and right ears, and from bone conduction versus the ear.
The key aspect of this concept is that the right ear goes to the analytical left brain, and the left ear goes to the emotional and feeling right brain – and we need a combination of both to give us a clear picture of reality.

If one ear is deficient in hearing overall or in specific frequency ranges, then all kinds of imbalances can happen in our system. For example, if you are left ear dominant, you will hear in a person's tone of voice more than what they are saying, which can lead to mis-understandings. This can especially be a problem when someone's tone of voice is not in alignment with the message. Even if it is in alignment, those that are left ear dominant might easily react emotionally based on their emotional perception of the information they are receiving.

Tomatis also believed that there is an ideal balance between what we hear through our ears and through the bones in our head, so he would test for good bone conduction through the head.

When both ears and bone conduction are functioning normally, it's like the brain gets a 3D version of reality instead of a 2D version. In the realm of consciousness this means that we are functioning with a better balance of the physical and Spiritual realms. Ultimately, it means that we are able to "zoom out" and see reality from multiple per-spectives instead of being on the roller coaster that comes from a limited perception of tunnel vision. Essentially, we see the forest and the trees at the same time.

Assessment
There are two techniques: one low tech and one high tech.

a. Place a tuning fork (around C 256 hertz) on the right side of the head and notice whether or not you hear the sound on the left side. Then, place the fork on the left side of the head and note whether the sound is audible on the right. If the tone played on one side is not audible on the opposite simultaneously, you are not getting full left and right transmission of sound into both ears through the bone conduction of the skull.

b. Karl Johannson from Denmark has an electronic device that does the assessment in much more detail. It is called a Binaural Audiometry Test.

Treatments

a. Binaural Beats played in headphones synchronize the left and right brain.

b. In the Listening Program the practitioner can change the balance so the right ear is getting more stimulation and so learns to become the lead ear.

c. Any number of movement programs that foster crossing the midline can facilitate integration of the hemispheres and improve whole brain listening.

d. Use of headphones and microphones to enhance the perception of your voice through air conduction.

There are several main books we recommend in this specialty area:

• "The Ear and The Voice" by Alfred Tomatis

• "When Listening Comes Alive" by Paul Madaule

• "Healing at the Speed of Sound: How What We Hear Transforms Our Brains and Our Lives" by Don Campbell and Alex Doman

• "Listening for Wellness – An Introduction to the Tomatis Method" by Pierre Sollier

• "The Power of Sound – How to be Healthy and Productive Using Music and Sound" by Joshua Leeds

• "Sound Bodies through Sound Therapy" by Dorinne S. Davis

SECTION X – Spiritual Enhancement with Sound

"The prime objective of all Initiatory music in the Temples of Antiquity was to bring about physical purification and renewal, mental stimulation and alertness, spiritual exhilaration and Illumination."
- St. Ambrose, 340-397 AD
(he brought the diatonic scale of Pythagoras to the Church)

Introduction – Clearing out Negative Vibrations vs. Resonating Positive Vibrations

This chapter focuses on creating various states of "bliss" with sounds that harmonize your whole system – including the frequency and music of love (self love, social love, and Universal Love).

Spiritual Healing, Awakening, and Reconnection

Sound and music have been used since the beginning of time in cultures all over the world to help bring us into states of Spiritual Healing, harmony and awakening.

Most people see Spiritual Healing as a physical, mental, and emotional clearing process, which works by clearing out negative and incoherent vibrations within us that are simply getting in the way of higher and purer vibrations.

It is difficult to resonant higher vibrations of Spirit and Source when we are not healthy or when we are in pain. When we do the work to harmonize our physical body we then have a clearer vessel through which Spirit can vibrate. We have already covered how to use sound physically in Section VII, "Physical Healing with Sound."

It is also important to get our mind clear so that it doesn't keep leading us into stressful roller coaster rides fraught with anxiety and dead-end thought patterns. It is also helpful to get our mind humming at a vibration where we are able to remember the lessons we have learned in order to move forward. But most important is learning how to bring the mind to a place of stillness so the buzzing sound of our thoughts is no longer the only thing we hear. We have already discussed how sound can help with such mental issues in Section VIII, "Emotional Healing and Expansion with Sound."

Even more importantly, it is hard to move to the next level Spiritually, when we have negative emotions, deep emotional issues and negative belief systems resonating us back into disharmony. One of the most difficult tasks of all is to clear out these discordant vibrations so we can more clearly resonate love and light. Ultimately, we use sound to get us off the roller coaster of emotions so we can be present with each moment while staying connected to Source. Again, we addressed many techniques on how to do this in Section VIII, on emotional healing.

Now once we have all of the non-harmonious vibrations cleared or harmonized the key is to resonate with higher vibrations. First we can harmonize our chakras and auras, which are our link from the body to the Spirit world. We can also resonate with higher energies such as gratitude, compassion, love and joy. And, we can resonate a direct connection to our Soul, which then provides information as to our Soul purpose and where we are on the path to enlightenment. But most importantly, we can use sound to reconnect to Spirit and Source where we are one with everything in the Universe.

Many believe that we need not deal with the clearing and harmonizing aspects of the physical, mental and emotional bodies. Instead of focusing on the "stuff," the belief is that we simply open our hearts more fully to life and experience Spiritual harmony. People of this belief have reported that diseases and physical issues often fall away entirely, emotional issues sometimes resolve on their own, and mental clarity seems to ensue out of the blue (or white light).

Regardless of this outcome, as we resonate these higher vibrations we again come into alignment with our own natural essence and its relationship to Source, which includes everything in the Universe. When we recognize that our Soul development and awakening happens at its own natural speed without interruption or impediments, we again fall into alignment with that natural flow of ease where we are meant to be, and everything falls into place.

Definitions
We are now moving into an area where the very definition of Soul, Spirit and Source has been defined quite differently by many cultures, traditions and religions. Therefore, let us establish how we are using the terms. This is not to say that the way we define these terms is right or even the best way. But, it is simply necessary so we are on the same page.

It seems that we generally agree (though not always, of course) on the basic layout of the Spiritual world, but we use different terms to explain it. For example, people have drastically different interpretations for terms Soul, Spirit, and Source.

Here is how we will be using the terms – from a vibrational perspective.

Soul – The Soul is our divine essence, which is also connected to Source. Since everything is vibration, the Soul must also be a frequency. It is a frequency (or harmonic structure) that carries all the information about us from lifetime to lifetime.

Spirit – Many people use the term Spirit to mean the same as Source. In fact, we have been doing exactly that throughout the book so far. From now on, in alignment with the teachings of Alice Bailey, we will be using Spirit as the "enlivening energy" from Source. It is the life energy that flows through our whole system. When Spirit leaves our body the physical body dies.

Source – Same as God, All that Is, etc. Source is all frequencies in the Universe. Many believe we are a hologram or reflection of Source.

Higher Emotions of Gratitude, Compassion, Love, Joy, etc. – These are simply rays of energy that come from all the frequencies of Source. It is like a prism that splits light into multiple rays. Each ray is a particular frequency, which is an aspect of Source – All That Is.

Chapter 41 – Using Sound to Achieve Presence and Mindfulness

Many now believe that presence and mindfulness are the ultimate ways to be in the world. The concept is that our true essence is a "point of awareness." This is who or what we truly are. This is the focus of the "non-dual" movement. Eckart Tolle, Adaya-shanti, and Ganga Ji are some of the leaders in this area. The movement goes all the way back to the teachings of Ramana Maharshi (1879-1950). Thich Nhat Hanh also talks a lot about presence. There are many Buddhist traditions about mindfulness teachings that have been around for a very long time.

Presence or mindfulness has been defined as being 100% aware without judgment. There are many components of presence and mindfulness, and there are many portals that sound offers to help us enter these states.

First, the question is what are we being present with? What is the essence of the world when we are simply a point of awareness? Ultimately, the world is simply vibration. At a more detailed level, it is a hierarchy of holograms of frequencies, musical intervals, timbres, chords, rhythms, music, and energy vibrations.

Commonly, our experience of the world is based on whether we "like" or "dislike" something. The world "as it is" becomes something "it is not:" a relationship for better or worse for our own needs or desires. In one way, this judgment process can be helpful for our survival and can make us more comfortable. In another way, this categorization of the world takes us one step away from the intrinsic reality of "all that is," and traps us in a world of stress. When we don't get what we want, it feels bad. When we do get what we want, it is never enough and we often fear losing it. But more importantly, it leaves us in a reality that is disconnected from the true nature of the world – nature and Spirit. We then begin to lose contact with that Source energy that naturally feeds us all. We become tired, lonely and sometimes anxious and desperate.

Therefore the ultimate goal is to see the world as it is – vibrations and combinations of vibrations.

When you want to be present, you can begin by focusing on one thing. The flame of the candle, the pull of gravity on your body, the temperature in the room, your own breath, the warmth of your lover's body, the light in the room. However, ultimate presence is an awareness of multiple things at once. This could be as simple as two things at once, or all of the above. Or, it could be as complex as being aware of reality at all dimensions of time and space, including dimensions of no time and space. Ultimately, it is a place of presence and mindfulness of being one with everything in the Universe.

However, in this case just knowing where you are going – to a place of awareness of all as frequency – does not necessarily get you there.

The key is going to a place of peace.

One of the best aspects of sound
is its ability to bring us into a place of
absolute peace and stillness.

And yet again…

Peace is a frequency consistently humming.

As we have discussed previously, a slow fade of volume on the home note leaves you in a profound state of stillness as the frequency continues to hang in the air. This consistency of frequency that we feel inside is the peace we are all longing for. And, in this peace and stillness we find we are present with everything around and inside us.

The point of awareness that we are, is a peaceful point, where frequencies are not jumping around chaotically. They are simply humming consistently.

A consistent melody and rhythm can help you hold that consistency. However, the ultimate presence is simply one note humming consistently in your head – as if forever. As the note fades out it remains with you in the present.

This is a simple and profound portal to presence and mindfulness. As mentioned before, crystal and Tibetan bowls are wonderful for this. Tuning forks and songs that simply fade out slowly on a home note are also amazing (particularly those that contain a large amount of bass frequencies in them).

Another difficulty is having the energy to hold that place of peace with 100% focus when there are so many distractions from the world around us. Often we are simply too tired to be present. We relax into whatever vibrations seem to be around or inside us. However, the energy of judgment is rampant in the ether. We are so easily led down the path of disconnection – even by the patterns and rhythms of habit that play through our own mind.

Therefore, the question is how do we get more energy? Of course, one answer is living a life where the sound and music you have around you and within you are not draining you. The food you eat, the exercise you do, the way you treat yourself, the people you spend time with, etc., can all drain or feed you.

However, the ultimate answer is to connect to Source energy.

When you are connected to Spirit or nature, you get fed pure energy. There are many that live off it – and never eat. Connected to Source with the energy of Spirit flowing through you gives you plenty of energy to hold a consistent frequency forever. In fact, when connected to Source you are naturally present.

Chapter 42 – Harmonizing Chakras with Sound

"In the etheric body are centered the forces animating man's physical vehicle, so disease is evidenced in the etheric before it manifests in the physical. The etheric, composed of finer, more attenuated substances than the physical, is corresponding amenable to vibratory influences. It is upon the former that harmony and rhythm have the most potent effect. Good music readjusts its molecular structure in accordance with the original divine plan, the archetype, and refines and accentuates its vibratory currents. All forms of beauty and harmony increase this regenerating process."
- Corinne Heline (1882-1975)

Each celestial body, in fact each and every atom,
produces a particular sound on account of its movement, its rhythm or vibration.
All these sounds and vibrations form a universal harmony in which each element,
while having its own function and character, contributes to the whole.
- Pythagoras (569-475 BC)

Chakras are energy centers in the body. These energy centers have been described in detail in many cultures as relating to specific pitches and sounds. The most common and accepted descriptions are from Sanskrit. Although there is no scientific evidence on chakras, there are now technologies that measure the resonance of chakras.

Each chakra has been associated energetically with an endocrine gland in the body. The basic concept is that when you resonate the energy of a chakra it then triggers the associated endocrine gland, which then puts out a chemical or hormone, which makes you feel a particular way. In addition, each gland also functions energetically. In fact, each gland actually has two parts – one dedicated to creating the hormone, and one dedicated to energetics.

For example, when you are resonating love, the thymus gland is activated. It then puts out a hormone that helps to create a certain type of white blood cell that is critical for a healthy immune system. It also activates the energy of Universal Love throughout your whole system.

Chakras not only affect us physically, but they are also directly linked to our emotions. Both emotions and mental stress and anxiety can throw them out of balance. Balancing the chakras can also harmonize our emotions and create more consistent brainwaves. When in balance, they allow the natural smooth flow of energy for resonating higher vibrations of Soul and Spirit, and they actually provide a clear channel for connecting to Source.

We actually communicate with each other by resonating chakras with each other – creating resonant fields.   We connect at each chakra whether sexually, through power struggles (or sharing), through love, communication, intuition or Spirit.

Over millennia chakras have been associated with frequencies, pitches, sounds (timbres), music and energy (again, we see the Hierarchy of Sound, Music and Energy from Section II).   Here's a chart showing the various chakras at different levels of vibration as explained in different books.

CHAKRA SOUNDS, PITCHES, AND FREQUENCIES

		TIMBRES						PITCHES		
	SANSKRIT NAME	JONATHAN GOLDMAN	SANSKRIT	KAY GARDNER & GARDNER-GORDON	TIBETAN WARRIOR	DAVID GIBSON		SANSKRIT	CHINA	TIBET
7th	Sahasrar	EEE	OM OR SILENCE	EE		SILENCE		B	B	G
6th	Ajna	AYE (as in 'say')	OM (OHM)	MM	A	EEE		A	E	F
5th	Vishudda	EYE	HUM (HAHM)	UU	OM	AH		G	A	E
4th	Anahata	AH	YAM (YAHM)	AH	HUNG	MMMM		F	D	D
3rd	Manipura	OH (as in 'go')	RAM (RAHM)	AOM		WOA		E	G	C
2nd	Svadhistana	OOO (as in 'you')	VAM (VAHM)	O	RAM	OOO		D	C	B
1st	Muladhara	UH (as in 'huh")	LAM (LAHM)	E	DZA	OOM		C	F	A

		FREQUENCIES					COLORS	
	SANSKRIT NAME	DAVID HULSE SOMA-ENERGETICS	BASED ON PLANETS	CYMA-THERAPY	DAVID GIBSON		TRADITIONAL COLORS	TIBETAN WARRIOR
7th	Sahasrar		172.06 (Platonic Year)	944	5000-20,000		VIOLET/WHITE	
6th	Ajna	213	221.23 (Venus)	1321	1000-5000		PURPLE	WHITE
5th	Vishudda	185.25	141.27 (Mercury)	312	600-1000		BLUE	RED
4th	Anahata	159.75	136.10 (Earth Year)	1125	400-600		GREEN	BLUE
3rd	Manipura	132	126.22 (Sun)	816	200-400		YELLOW/GOLD	
2nd	Svadhistana	104.25	210.42 (Synodic Moon)	359	60-200		ORANGE	RED
1st	Muladhara	99	194.18 (Earth DaY)	673	20-60		RED	GREEN

Chakra Chart

The Energy of Each Chakra

First, for those of you who are not familiar with the energy of each chakra (and for those who would like a refresher), let's take a look at each one.   There are a very large number of books that go into detail on each.   Most of the books speak about having a balance of energy in the chakra. The energy of the chakra can be sluggish or stagnant, or no energy at all.   The chakra can also be over amped, blown out, or simply buzzing uncontrollably.

1. Root Chakra
Associated Gland – None (I often think of the earth as the associated Endocrine Gland)
The energy of the root is grounding. On one level this about being 100% present in your body and in 3D reality around you – both physically and sound-wise. Notice how your body feels. Notice the space you are in, the temperature, the light, the smell, etc. And, notice all of the sounds in the room you are in (or around you if you happen to be outside at the moment).

The root chakra is also about survival and money issues. When we are worried about such things, we often lose our grounding. When we are too grounded, we feel sluggish and some become overweight.

More importantly, the root chakra is about our connection to the Earth. We can actually feel the earth under our feet. We also often feel grounded when working with the earth – when we get our hands in the dirt – particularly planting and growing things.

But, the most basic connection we have to earth is gravity. Every one of us is now being pulled directly to the center of the earth. We often take gravity for granted. Feel gravity in your body now... pulling you to the center of the earth.

2. Sacral or Naval Chakra
Associated Gland – Sexual Organs
I often think of this chakra as the emotional chakra, and the sensual chakra. When this chakra is stagnant, we have little libido or sexual energy. Often unprocessed emotions get stuck in this area.

3. Solar Plexus Chakra
Associated Gland – Adrenal Glands
This chakra is about your power and will. It can go stagnant when our self-esteem is low – particularly when we have been criticized, or demeaned (especially over long periods of time). On the other hand, this chakra commonly gets over-activated whenever we get upset or angry. I can actually feel it leaking energy from my body when I'm upset over something. Many people commonly relate to the world from this chakra – seeing people as either above or below them. Also, seeing how we can get an advantage.

When balanced we are in our power, but still equal with everyone around us. It is also the place of personal power from which we manifest things – whether relationships, business or health.

4. Heart Chakra
Associated Gland – Thymus Gland
Of course, this chakra is about love. Some say that we actually have two heart chakras: The lower one is about personal love. The higher one is where we connect to Universal Love.

5. Throat Chakra
Associated Gland – Thyroid Gland
This chakra is about expression – particularly sound created through the voice. It is also about listening to sound – the thyroid gland actually has follicles exactly like those in the inner ear that are designed to pick up sound.

Women sometimes have trouble with the throat chakra, likely because the way men have not allowed women to express themselves over many lifetimes. Even today it is hard for both men and women to speak their truth because so many people are resonating the power and competition of the 3rd chakra.

6. Third Eye Chakra
Associated Glands – Hypothalamus and Pituitary Glands
This chakra is about our intuition, and our laser-like mental clarity. It is also about vision, and being able to see things from a higher perspective. People with their 3rd eye open can see inside another's body and do healing work on it.

7. Crown Chakra
Associated Gland – Pineal Gland
This chakra is about our connection to our Soul and our connection to Source. The pineal gland is actually made of crystals so it resonates a very specific frequency.

Pitches of Chakras
As previously mentioned, there are many charts that cover the frequency of just about everything in the body and the Universe, and no two people seem to agree on anything. However, when it comes to the pitch of each chakra there is more agreement than anywhere else in the field. More than 50% of people on the planet subscribe to the C to B chakra system.

7th - B
6th - A
5th - G
4th - F
3rd - E
2nd - D
1st - C

However, in Tibet they used A as the root.
7th - G
6th - F
5th - E
4th - D
3rd - C
2nd - B
1st - A

In parts of China, F is the root. In the Chinese system, the notes go up by musical fifths instead of whole notes, like this:

7th - B
6th - E
5th - A
4th - D
3rd - G
2nd - C
1st - F

At the Institute, after many years of research and experimentation we have come to believe that each person has their own particular root chakra note.

Although the system of C to B is so well accepted, it seems to have a few problems. First, just about everyone uses equal tempered tuning, and there is nothing in nature that is tuned this way. There is no way that our chakras could be tuned to a piano, which is almost always in equal tempered tuning.

The other problem is that it seems that all of the chakras should sound good if they are all playing at the same time. When each note is a whole step, as in the Sanskrit and Tibetan system, **they do not sound good when all played at the same time.** Next time you are around a piano or keyboard try playing 7 of the white notes at the same time. It certainly does not sound harmonious like a person should be when all their chakras are humming at the same time. We'll address this in more detail in the next section.

Frequencies of Chakras
Of course, as you can see from the chart at the beginning of the chapter, different people have come up with different frequencies based on their own research and intuition.

I generally think of the each of the chakras in these frequency ranges.

7th - 5000-20,000
6th - 1000-5000
5th - 600-1000
4th - 400-600
3rd - 200-400
2nd - 60-200
1st - 20-60

I have come to believe that the frequencies of the chakras should span the full frequency spectrum from the lowest to the highest frequencies. It just makes sense that the root is an extremely low frequency, and that the crown chakra is an extremely high frequency. This is also in alignment with the school of thought we mentioned earlier in Chapter 2, whereby every frequency is a nutrient, and we need the full frequency range to be healthy, whole and complete.

There is yet another problem with the traditional C to B Sanskrit system. C to B is only one octave! It just makes no sense that our chakras would only cover one octave <u>and</u> sound horrible when all played at the same time. Some people actually try to get around this problem by starting with C, going up an octave and over to D, then up another octave and over to E, and so forth. Then, you do cover the full range of frequencies, however the 7 sounds still don't sound good when played all at the same time.

The Chinese system does sound harmonious when all the musical fifths are played at the same time, but they still only cover a few octaves of the full frequency range.

It makes sense that the chakras would actually be based on the natural harmonic series found in nature, but even this would only cover a few octaves.

I often like to do meditations with each Chakra at its own octave. Therefore, we cover the full range of sounds – 7 octaves. It is so nice when all of the sounds for each chakra are completely harmonious with each other, and they cover the full range of frequencies.

I have created 2 CD's that are based on 7 octaves
Go to www.SoundHealingCenter.com/music.html
and look for "Chakra Journey" and "Chakra Guided Meditation"

Now, this is not to say that any of the other systems are wrong. We definitely don't want to throw out any babies with the bath water. The truth is that so many people have been resonating with their chakras based on the C to B system for so many centuries that it has created a very powerful resonant field you can easily tap into. However, you now know of other options.

Timbres and Tones of Each Chakra
There are sounds we can make with our voice and particular instrument sounds that seem to resonate each chakra.

<u>Vocal Sounds</u>
First, let's look at the sounds that are commonly made with the voice. The key is to find which sounds work best for you when resonating the particular chakra. Tune into each chakra one by one, and try each of the sounds below to see which one works best for you (see the chart to identify who to attribute each sound to).

Remember, sound works the best when you actually make the sounds out loud. Tune into each chakra and make each of the following sounds (make each sound for at least a minute or so). Try saying the sound at different pitches until you find a pitch that works for you. Also, try saying the sounds in different ways with different accents and durations.

1st Chakra - LAM, EH, DZA, OOM
2nd Chakra – VAM, OH, RAM, UU
3rd Chakra – RAM, AOM, WHOA
The sound "WHOA" is best made extremely loudly and with full power. Imagine that a lion is attacking you and you have the power to stop it with your voice. On 3 stop the lion

1, 2, 3, WHOA!

Try this until you can do it with full power. If you are having a hard time, try it at a different pitch.

4th Chakra – YAM, AH, HUNG, MMMM
5th Chakra – HAM, UU, OM, AH
6th Chakra – SHAM, OM, MM, AH, EEE
7th Chakra – OM, EE, SILENCE

Again, find the frequency or note that works best for you. I have my favorites, but I have also found that some sounds work better for me on different days. Don't hesitate to try to create sounds of your own.

Instrument Sounds for Chakras
1st Chakra – The most basic component is instrument sounds that have a lot of bass in them – particularly the bass guitar and large drums (actually just about any large instrument). The Japanese Taiko drum is one of the most grounding. The main aspect of low frequencies in grounding is that you can simply feel them in your body.

The didgeridoo is also quite grounding for most – especially when it is played right on the body. Large gongs are grounding for some, but can be ungrounding for others.

People often ask me, "What's up with Rap music?" From one perspective, the huge bass is extremely grounding. Listening to Rap is simply like getting a massage, and allows one to feel something in a world that might not often be so warm. They simply want to be touched and are using the sound to do so.

Often, I find that classical music does not have enough lows in it to help me ground (although some do). Choral music tends to be a little lacking on the low end as well. Of course, these styles of music have other purposes for which they work perfectly.

The most grounding animal sound is the whale, although elephant sounds are also quite effective. Just about any nature sound is normally grounding – even the sound of water.

Some like to associate the instrument sound with the element of the chakra. Since the root chakra's element is Earth, instruments that are made of clay or other earthy materials can resonate the root really well.

2nd Chakra – When working with the emotions or sexuality I feel that it is important to have low mid-range frequencies. It seems that the cello and violin (including string sections) seem to work well. Of course, the guitar (especially the electric guitar) can also get the emotions going. Sometimes even the saxophone can be quite effective.

For those of you who are into recording, there is nothing like a flange to simulate the floaty feeling of the emotions.

Water is the essence of the 2nd chakra so water sounds are most appropriate. A rain stick, which simulates the sound of rain is quite effective. The howl of a wolf is incredibly effective for releasing emotions.

3rd Chakra – Contains sounds that are powerful without being overwhelming. Powerful vocals seem to be the most effective for activating this chakra. Horns are often excellent for activating this chakra, particularly the French horn. Those long Tibetan horns are also quite activating for the solar plexus. It's said that the Jewish elk horn was used to bring down the walls of Jericho. Seashells can also be powerful.

Some people like distorted rock guitars (especially powerful lead guitar solos), however sensitive people are often overwhelmed by the sound of a rock guitar.

Animal sounds include the eagle and lion. Since fire is the essence of the 3rd Chakra, the sound of fire can be quite effective.

4th Chakra – The voice is the most powerful by far, for opening the heart – particularly a soft whisper. The harp is most likely second. This is probably why it is used in hospice so frequently. I would say that violin and cello are next because they are the most similar to the sound of someone crying. I especially like whole string sections. The electric guitar can also seem to cry. However, even the saxophone, oboe or flute do it for others. Other sounds like crystal bowls can bring people to a place of peace where their heart opens.

It seems to be more the energy that someone is putting into the instrument than the instrument itself, although sounds with too many odd harmonics tend to not work as well.

Since the essence of the heart chakra is air, soft wind sounds can be quite effective, or any woodwind instrument.

5th Chakra – The voice is the main instrument for the throat chakra, and again, there is no instrument better than the voice. Most of the instruments that are played with the breath (the woodwinds) are quite good. Especially any sounds that have a real breathiness to them, like the shakuhachi flute.

The "hoot" or "who" of an owl seems to be especially effective for the throat.

6th Chakra – Sounds that are very high in pitch are quite good at activating and opening the third eye. This includes all types of bells, chimes small Tibetan bowls, Tingshas, Triangles, and Peruvian whistles.

Many high-pitched bird chirps and songs, as well as crickets seem to be very good for activating the 6th chakra. There is a particular type of frog, called the Cokie Frog that also seems to be right at the frequency of the pituitary gland.

7th Chakra – Many of the high tinkly sounds that open the third eye often also work for the crown. I have found that string sections and angelic female choirs do it for me. Again, my favorite sound of all for the crown chakra is silence.

The Music of Each Chakra
Take these recommendations with a grain of sand – think about the music that really works for you in each area – and develop your own collection of music and sounds that really work for you.

1st Chakra – Any type of heavy drum music – particularly Japanese Taiko drumming, even Rap can be quite grounding in its own way.

2nd Chakra – Emotions are often muddy and unclear, so I feel that music that takes you through a transformation from unclarity into clarity is the best.

For making love, I probably don't have to tell you. Of course, slow rhythms that match the breath and movement of the body seem to work the best. No excessive high frequencies, focusing mostly on warm mid-range and lows.

3rd Chakra – I actually like Pink Floyd. The power of David Gilmore's vocals and electric guitar gets me going. Also, Loreena McKennitt does it for me with her powerful voice. For some people there is nothing like the power of opera.

4th Chakra – Love songs do it for many people, but often enmesh us in the emotional world of love and loss. It is interesting how most love songs are so sad, when the true essence of love is not sad at all.

5th Chakra – Listening to Tuvan overtone singing and throat singing are especially powerful for activating the throat.

6th Chakra (Third Eye) – Particularly the sound of crystal bowls or Tibetan bowls.

7th Chakra (Crown) – My music, and the music of Snatam Kaur and Deva Premal are my favorites.

Chakra Sound Meditations
I have come to believe that a Chakra Sound Meditation is one of the most powerful types of Sound Healing you can do. I believe this is because the chakras are so receptive to sound and they are directly linked to each of the Endocrine Glands, which then use hormones and energy to control and affect the rest of the organs in the body.

As mentioned, I've also found that this type of meditation can get rid of a panic attack completely. It's also a very good way to find where you have emotional blockages.

There are many ways that you can do chakra meditations based on the information already provided in this chapter. The key to the effectiveness of any chakra treatment has to do with simply focusing on that part of the body energetically.

You could use each of the notes from C to B using any instrument and simply imagine focusing each note in each of the chakras. You can also simply tone each of the notes with the intention of harmonizing each of the chakras.

Another common technique is to use the sounds from the chart on page 282. Try the various sounds and see which ones work the best for you. Focus on each chakra and simply bring those sounds into it energetically.

One of my favorite chakra meditations is to bring a frequency into each chakra – using the full range of frequencies. Here is the technique in detail.

<u>Frequency Chakra Meditation</u>
I prefer to do this silently (particularly for the root chakra, since it is normally a frequency below what the voice can make). I often get distracted by other resonances in my body when I make sound out loud. However, many people prefer to do this meditation by making the sound for each chakra aloud. For some people, it is quite difficult to hear frequencies in their head. Regardless, both audible or silent sounds can be equally effective.

1st Chakra - The first step in this process is to check in with the chakra and see where it is at energetically. Is it humming nicely, or is it stagnant or even over-activated? Being a creative type, I often have to find my root chakra in order to feel my body at all.

Tuning into the energy of the 1st chakra, resonate the energy of grounded-ness and being connected to the Earth. Feel gravity at the base of your spine pulling you to the center of the earth. The element for the root chakra is Earth.

Now, do a frequency sweep up and down to find what frequency or note feels like it fits your root the most. Some people (particularly musicians) might find that you can go right to the right note for that chakra. What you are looking for is a note that just feels good for this chakra – a note that feels grounding and feels like home! Once you find the note, send the sound energetically (or out loud) to the base of your spine. I often visualize the sound as a sphere surrounding the base of my spine. Simply feel the frequency as if it is harmonizing the base of your spine. Do this for as long as you like. Even one minute can be effective.

You can also add in the color of the chakra if you like. Red is the traditional color for the root. However, you can also do a frequency sweep of all the colors to see which one the root might need at this time. Perhaps a deep blue might be better for you today. I often prefer solid gold!

2nd Chakra - Check in with the 2nd chakra. How is your sensuality lately? How is your digestion lately? Are there any emotions that have gotten stuck in the sacral or abdomen area?

Then focus on the energy of 2nd chakra – flowing emotions. The element for the second chakra is water so I like to feel the flowing water energy there.

Now do your frequency sweep, or go right to the note that seems to resonate the 2nd chakra the best. If you need to, play with different notes until you find one that feels like the right fit. Now resonate that sound around the abdomen (below the belly button) with the intention of harmonizing the chakra.

If you like you can add the color orange around this area. You can also try other colors.

3rd Chakra - Check in on the 3rd chakra. Have you been upset or frustrated with anything lately? Have you taken in any criticism lately that has made you feel insecure or not good enough?

Now bring the energy of being in your power in a balanced way so that you are not above or below anyone. The element for this chakra is fire.

Next, do the frequency sweep until you find just the right sound for this chakra. Resonate it around your solar plexus as long as you like. Add in a yellow light if you like.

4th Chakra - Check in on your 4th chakra. How open is your heart lately? How much love do you have in your life?

Now bring the energy of love into your heart area. This chakra element is air.

Do the frequency sweep or simply listen for the note that resonates love in your heart the most. Resonate this sound of love around your heart as long as you like. Add in green or pink if you like, or try other colors.

5th Chakra - Check in. Have you been able to express yourself freely lately? Can you speak your truth without fear? Are you able to make sounds easily?

Bring the energy of free flowing self-expression into your throat area and find the sound that resonates it the best. Add in an aqua color or light blue if you like.

6th Chakra - How is your intuition? How is your clarity of mind? Is your third eye open?

Bring in the energy of clear vision into your third eye and feel it completely. Now, find the sound and resonate it with the intention of harmonizing this energy in this area.

Add in purple or indigo if you like.

7th Chakra - How connected are you to Source and the pure energy of Spirit? Do you have a Spiritual practice and if so, how is it going lately?

Bring the pure energy of Source into your crown and listen for the sound of this chakra. Add in white or clear light if you like. Resonate it as long as you like.

Now, do a frequency sweep from the highest frequency to the lowest and then back up to the highest. Do the sweep slow enough so that you can feel the energy of each chakra as the sound moves through each frequency range. However, do it fast enough so that you feel the smooth flow of energy up and down the chakras. The key is to visualize the Kundalini energy moving up and down through the chakras. You might notice difficulty getting the energy to flow in a particular chakra. If so, you can stop and go back; do a little more sound work on that specific chakra to get it humming harmoniously. Then, continue the sweep.

This process is especially effective to do before you get out of bed in the morning. When done, you will hop out of bed with your whole system completely activated... ready for the day. However, it is effective at any time.

You can also do this whole process on someone as a treatment. I will actually do 15 minutes of intake at the beginning and ask each of the questions for each of the chakras to see where they are. You are looking for whether there is an issue with that chakra, and whether it needs to be calmed down or activated. It's also nice if you can get the recipient to join in making the sounds with you, however it is not necessary.

You can also add in other instruments besides the voice. With a complete chakra set of crystal or Tibetan bowls, you can use a bowl for each chakra. You can actually use just about any instrument or combination of instruments to do this treatment.

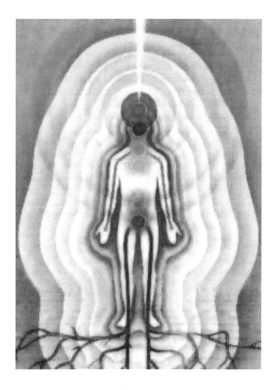

Auras

The exploration of Auras (more commonly called Subtle Bodies) is a little tricky because there isn't much agreement as to how many Auras there are, what each does or their names. Barbara Brennan's version of the Auras is probably the most well known and accepted. This version is similar to hers. Here's the outline first.

Etheric Body
Emotional Body
Mental Body
Astral Body – Octave above the Emotional Body
Etheric Template – Octave above the Etheric Body
Celestial Body
Causal Body (Ketheric Template) – Octave above the Etheric Template

All of the descriptions below are from Barbara Brennan's book, *Hands of Light*.

Etheric Body
One quarter to two inches beyond the physical body, pulsating at about 15-20 cycles per minute.

The etheric body is composed of tiny energy lines "like a sparkling web of light beams" similar to the lines on a television screen. It has the same structure as the physical body including all the anatomical parts and all the organs. This is the body that responds to homoeopathy, Reiki, and other alternative treatments – particularly sound.

By observing the shoulder of someone in dim light against a plain white or plain black or dark blue background, you may be able to see the pulsations of this etheric body. The pulsation rises, say at the shoulder, and then makes its way down the arm, like a wave.

Emotional Body
Extends one to three inches from the body.

The emotional body is associated with feelings. It roughly follows the outline of the physical body. Its structure is much more fluid than the etheric and does not duplicate the physical body. Rather, it appears to be colored clouds of fine substance in continual fluid motion. It contains all of the colors of each chakra. Clear and highly energized feelings such as love, excitement, joy or anger are bright and clear. Confused feelings are dark and muddy.

The Mental Body
Extends from three to eight inches (7.5 to 20 cm) from the body.

The mental body is associated with thoughts and mental processes. This body usually appears as a bright yellow light radiating about the head and shoulders and extends around the whole body. It expands and becomes brighter when its owner is concentrating on mental processes.

The Astral Body
The Astral Body extends out about one half to one foot (15 to 30 cm) from the physical body. The chakras are the same octave of colors as the rainbow of the emotional body, but each is infused with the rose light of love.

The Etheric Template Body
Extends from about one and one half to two feet (45 to 60 cm) from the body.

The etheric template contains all the forms that exist on the physical plane in a blue-print or template form. It is the blueprint or the perfect form for the etheric layer to take. It is the level at which sound creates matter. It is at this level that sound is the most effective.

It allows for the possibility of higher templates again – the doctrine of resonances, of an octave of grades of being, with the lower depending on the one above it, and in turn on the one above that. Just as the Physical Etheric Body contains various channels and meridians, in the Spiritual Etheric are found the drops or bijas. When activated, as in Tibetan Buddhism, these produce blissful meditative states.
Celestial Body (Higher or Spiritual Emotional Body)
The Celestial Body extends about two to two and a half feet (60 to 75 cm) from the body.

This is the emotional level of the spiritual plane, called the celestial body. It is the level through which we experience spiritual ecstasy. We can reach it through meditation and many forms of transformation work. When we reach the point of "being", where we know our connection with all the Universe, when we see the light and love in everything that exists, when we are immersed in the light and feel we are of it and it is in us, and when we feel that we are one with God, then we have raised our consciousness to the sixth level of the aura.

It is the location of higher spiritual emotions, such as the unconditional and Universal Love for all life, as opposed to the Psychic Body, which here is the locus of pure interpersonal human love, and the Physical Emotional body, which is concerned with individual feeling.

The Ketheric Template or Causal Body (Seventh Layer)
The Ketheric Template extends from about two and one half to three and one half feet (75 to 105 cm) from the body.

When we bring our consciousness to the seventh level of the aura, we know that we are one with the Creator. The outer form is the egg shape of the aura body and contains all the auric bodies associated with the present incarnation an individual is undergoing.

When "tuning" into the frequency level of the seventh layer, Barbara Brennan perceives it as beautiful golden shimmering light that is pulsating so fast that it seems to be "shimmering!" One can almost hear a sound when looking at it. I'm sure a sound could be heard if one meditated on such a picture.

Fabien Maman says that each of the auras is based on the harmonic structure of sound. If this is the case, then perhaps the harmonics might look something like this:

Root	Physical Body
2nd Harmonic – Octave	Etheric Body
3rd Harmonic – Musical 5th	Emotional Body
4th Harmonic – 2 Octaves	Mental Body
5th Harmonic – Musical 3rd	Astral Body
6th Harmonic – Musical 5th	Etheric Template
7th Harmonic – Musical 7th	Celestial Body
8th Harmonic – 3 Octaves	Causal Body (Ketheric Template)

However, there are some other correlations that seem to make sense from how different auras seem to be octaves of other auras. Based on the available information on auras, I would say the following makes sense.

Root	Physical Body
One Octave above Root	Etheric Body
	Emotional Body
	Mental Body
Octave above Emotional Body	Astral Body
One Octave above Astral Body	Etheric Template
	Celestial Body
Octave above Etheric Template	Causal Body (Ketheric Template)

Who knows what the notes of the Emotional, Mental and Celestial Body are. Perhaps the Celestial is an octave above the Astral and the Causal is an octave above that.

Even though this mapping is not coming out perfectly based on harmonics, I have a gut feeling that it should. On the other hand, perhaps it is based on the golden mean?

From the information provided, I would say that the Causal Body is the same frequency as the higher self, which is many octaves above the frequency of the Soul (perhaps seven).

In the books by Alice Bailey, each person has a different frequency for each of the bodies. She says that the Soul frequency is the same from lifetime to lifetime. She also says that there are then particular frequencies (Rays) for the Physical Body, Emotional Body, Mental Body, and Spiritual Body. Benjamin Crème actually outlines the Ray structure for all five of these bodies for just about every famous person since the beginning of time. In this respect, we can look at each person as a combination of frequencies: Soul, Physical, Emotional, Mental and Spiritual. This combination of frequencies makes up a person's particular timbre!

Chapter 44 – Resonating Higher Emotions (Gratitude, Compassion, Love, etc.)

Many say that "higher consciousness" is simply residing in any of the higher emotions. Here is the list again of some common higher emotions. Some of these are technically not emotions. Some are more states of mind. Just imagine, living a life where you go gently from one of these vibrations to another. This is higher consciousness. Imagine what sound would correspond to each of these.

Oneness
Unity
Harmony
Joy
Love (Self Love, Social, or Universal)
Compassion
Self Mastery
Humility
Confidence

Personal Power
Empowerment
Faith
Surrender
Freedom
Integration
Non-Judgment
Forgiveness
Balance
Appreciation
Passion
Enthusiasm
Eagerness
Happiness
Cooperation
Positive Expectation
Believe
Optimism
Hopefulness
Contentment

The key is to simply resonate these higher states of mind as much as possible. Whenever you find that you have dipped into the lower emotions you can then simply revert back to a higher emotion. If you find that you can't let go of the lower emotion then you can use one of the techniques in Chapter 32, "Eight Techniques for Releasing Stuck Emotions." If the emotion has been stuck for a long time, this might take some serious work (although using sound to release stuck emotions can also be quite enjoyable).

Some think that since we live in the world of duality, when we resonate higher emotions, we inevitably bring up the dark side, or shadow side. Sometimes this is true. After being in a really high state it might feel like we "crash" as we come down – the loss of that state can feel like sheer desperation.

Another problem that happens is when we find ourselves really high and happy, and we then come across someone who is not in the light. We often pass judgment – even saying something as simple as "jeez." In so doing, we allow our shadow side to emerge, and we are drawn out of the light. And now that we have been flying in higher vibrations, the darkness looks especially dark. We might even spiral down further as we go into fear or resistance. But once again, we use our sound and vibration techniques to get back on the roller coaster of light.

The key is to be present enough to know when we have dipped below the line, and then to remember the multitude of techniques that we have to get back up in the consistent light.

Therefore, much of the practice is about being more and more present with the sounds and songs going on in our head and body.

As we notice where these sounds and songs come from
we can sometimes change our life to tread there no longer.

More importantly, however,
we can simply use our sound techniques to return to vibrational bliss and peace
regardless of the source of the negative entrainment.

Ultimately, we can also come to a place of presence, where we are not on the roller coaster of even higher states of consciousness.

Living in the world of duality, there will always be ups and downs of frequency. However, many of us are now spending more and more time in higher vibrations where duality does not exist. Ultimately, Universal Love and Being One with the Universe have no dark side. The world of Love and Oneness actually encompass the dark side.

Eventually, the goal is to live in these higher states of consciousness all the time. And, as more and more people do so, it becomes easier for all of us to remain there. The resonant field is so strong that it is difficult to ever leave this place of Love and Light.

Just imagine.

Chapter 45 – The Sound of Love – How to Open Your Heart with Sound

"Love is the keynote, Joy is the music, Knowledge is the performer,
the Infinite All is the composer and audience."
- Sri Aurobindo (1872-1950)

Since love is one of the most powerful higher vibrations, emotions or states of mind and body, let's spend some quality time focusing on it.

The first and most important question of all time is, "What is love?"

Since everything is vibration, love must also be a vibration. The truth is that love can manifest as a frequency, pitch, musical interval, chord, timbre (tonality or sound), rhythm, music, or energy.

The energy of love is actually a frequency higher than sound, because one can add love to any sound frequency. However, there are certain tonalities and frequency ranges that are associated with love and are more likely to induce the feeling.

The big interest these days is 528 hertz which is considered the frequency of love. You will find over a hundred videos on YouTube where people are using the 528 hertz to resonate love. As far as pitches, many subscribe to F as the note of the heart chakra. The most common timbre or instrument sounds are the voice, the harp, the cello and the violin (particularly string sections). Actual syllables include "Yam," "Ah," "Hu" and my favorite, "Mmmm." The most common musical interval used to express love is the musical 3rd and the minor 6th. We are quite familiar with the music of love, which often has some sadness and melancholy about it – sadness is often a portal to love.

It seems that the frequency of the energy love is higher than sound. You can bring love to low frequencies, mid-range frequencies, or high frequencies. In classes and in treatments, we often infuse "the frequency of love" into a wide range of frequencies during a session – frequencies that span the entire range of sound.

Let's look at each level in more detail.

Pitches of Love
I have come to believe that there is a Universal pitch of love, and after many years of research and consideration I have some ideas as to what it might be.

I've come to believe that we have three main pitches of love. One is the note of love for your whole system, and this is different for every person. Then, there is the note of love that you use when speaking or singing love. Finally, there is the note of love in the solar system, galaxy or Universe.

<u>Your Own Love Note</u>
The VoiceBio system states that A# is the main note associated with the heart in the body.

Every semester, for many years at the Institute, we have had students find the note of love for themselves. We have them tune into the energy of love and intuitively find the pitch that seems to fit the feeling.

Let's try it now:

First, if you have an instrument where you know what the notes are on the instrument, get it out and have it ready. If not, go to www.virtualpiano.net and pull up the virtual piano on your computer (if this one doesn't work, there are several if you search for "virtual piano").

Now…

Simply, bring love into your heart now and feel it completely. If you have a hard time just naturally doing this, then think of the last time you fell in the love (tune into the essence of the feeling of love and leave the person and any "stuff" around them out of it). Again, feel this love in your heart completely – through every cell of your body, and through all your auras, surrounding you like a bubble – a bubble of love.

Then, if this feeling of love had a sound, get it going in your head. Don't make it out loud yet; just find it in your head. Is it a high note, low note or somewhere in between?

Now… Make it out loud.

Now, go to your instrument (or to the virtual piano on the web) and play each of the notes until you find the note you came up with.

**If you were really feeling it
and it really seemed to feel right…
This is the pitch of love for you.**

If so, please email us the pitch that you found (David@SoundHealingCenter.com), so we can see if there is one main note that people naturally go to, or if everyone has his or her own note.

Based on doing this test with hundreds of students over the last 10 years I have come to believe that the note of love is different for everyone.

Therefore, I feel it is more important you find the pitch that resonates love for you, instead of being told by someone else what it is.

Once you know it for yourself, you can then use it to find the energy of love on your own. And again, when you resonate the energy and sound of love at the same time it creates a stronger resonant field that is much more powerful and enjoyable to bask in. When people find the note that resonates in their heart the feeling of love is enhanced dramatically.

The Note of Love in Your Voice
There is a specific note that each person goes to when they express love with their voice. Normally, this note is different than the note a person finds doing the exercise above (occasionally it is the same). Based on physics, the note of love for your voice is affected by the size of your body and vocal cords. On the other hand, I would guess that the core note of love that you just found is not affected by your size.

This note of love in your voice is important as it enables you to express love with authenticity. It is also the keynote you can use for resonating love for yourself – particularly for sending love to your own heart.

I have discovered that when expressing love, most people go to the home note of the key of their voice. Just as every song has a key or note that feels like home, everyone speaks in a particular key. When we are being authentic we often go to this home note. When someone is stressed or not being honest, the tension in the body makes it more difficult to go to this home note. Politicians (and liars) use this technique extensively.

Getting to know the key of your voice can also help you to express love more authentically.

To find this note of love, you can simply relax and let out an "Ah" with the least amount of energy possible. Most people will actually make the sound of the key of their voice.

You can also simply talk about something that your really love – particularly a person or animal. You really have to go into the emotion completely when expressing your love for the person. For example, when I say, "I really love my kitty," my voice goes to the home note on the word "kitty." Occasionally, some people go to the musical 5th above their home note – you can tell because they don't really seem to go home completely.

Try talking about someone you love immensely. Talk about how much you love them and simply listen to the notes that you use. If you are a musician you might be able to hear the home note. If not, it can be difficult to tell.

I can actually help you find this home note by listening on the phone or Skype. If interested, let me know. Often people also buy tuning forks or crystal bowls tuned to their note of love, so they can bring more love through their voice.

This note is not only good for expressing love authentically; it is also good for toning with the intention of bringing love through your voice – whether it be to resonate love for yourself or to do a voice healing on someone using your voice. If you are a musician, it is the ideal key to use when writing a song about love.

The Universal Love Note
If there is a Universal pitch of love in our solar system, galaxy or Universe, who knows what it really is. If I had to guess, I would say there actually is a "cosmic" note of love in our Universe. However, I certainly don't know what it is for sure, and until multiple people independently come up with the same note I wouldn't believe it. After all, any pitch that someone says is the "cosmic" pitch of love for everyone could have easily been tainted by his or her own personal note (or marketing intentions).

Many say that our Solar System, Galaxy, or Universe is filled with the essence of Universal Love. If so, may we all one day know its keynote.

If there is a specific note of love in our Universe, my guess is that it is a frequency way above our range of hearing. That frequency would be a specific pitch (one of the 12 notes on a scale). Therefore, we can octavize it down – ½, ½, ½, etc., – until it is within the frequency range of sound. When you take ½ of the frequency of a sound it is still the same note at a lower octave.

Many subscribe to the pitch being an F based on the accepted Heart Chakra note. 528 hertz is actually a high C. If I had to guess the pitch I would say that it is D, for a couple of reasons. First, every semester we have students tune into the energy of love and we play various crystal bowls and frequencies, without telling them the notes. More than 80% of the time (over 7 years) people have said that D resonates love the most. Now this research is not scientific, but it is another piece of evidence.

Also, I know a few very high beings (including Joel Andrews, the harpist, whom I really respect) that say that D is the note of love. This also makes sense because Pachelbel Canon is the song that is in more weddings than any other song, and seems to make more people cry than any other song on the planet – and it is in the key of D!

It is also interesting that, more so than any other note, D is the key more people can easily tone and sing in.

Again, who knows for sure? Maybe one day Source will let us all know.

The Frequencies of Love
The frequency of love is similar to the pitch of love, just more specific. There are many frequencies for each pitch. For example, the standard for "A" is 440 cycles per second. However, all frequencies from 428 to 452 hertz are still in the note of "A." And, you can have an "A" that is higher or lower in frequency than this range. Therefore, when speak of the frequency of love we are being much more specific than just the note or pitch.

Over the last ten years, I have noticed that the frequencies that people come up with range from around 60 - 450 hertz.

When expressing love through the voice, I have noticed that personal love is commonly expressed with a really low frequency around 60 - 200 (men 60 -150, women 100 - 200), while Universal Love is expressed with a frequency between 200 - 450 hertz (men 200 - 350, women 250 - 450).

As mentioned before, lately there has been a lot of talk about 528 hertz being the "Sound of Love," as a frequency that unravels the DNA (which I assume is a very positive thing) based on the research of Leonard Horowitz. However, when you look at the science there is no actual definitive research that shows this kind of evidence about 528 hertz.

Many people who are now subscribing to this frequency as the "Sound of Love" are tuning their music to it, and using tuning forks tuned to 528. And, many people are getting good results and getting very high. If interested do a search on YouTube for "528 hertz."

The truth is that 528 hertz is one of the Solfeggio frequencies that do have some auspicious math to them. All of the Solfeggio frequencies add up to a 3, 6, or a 9 numerologically. For example, for 528: 5 + 2 + 8 = 15, and 1 + 5 = 6. Also, there is information that the Solfeggio frequencies just might mimic the mathematical patterns in DNA.

Also, even if the frequency had no meaning at all, the fact that so many people have subscribed to it has created a positive resonant field. When a large number of people tune into the same thing anywhere, it creates its own resonant field, which amplifies the energy of the frequency.

Meanwhile, it is obvious that 528 hertz is certainly not the frequency of love for the voice. For most people, it is very stressful to tone (try toning with the link above and see what you think).

There are many frequencies from Cymatherapy, and other individuals claim to have found the frequency of the heart – although again, the details of the research are unclear. Cymatherapy says the central heart frequency is 1,184 hertz. Others have come up with 6.15, 197, 20, 81, 162, and 5,000 hertz. The frequency of the thymus, which many say is where Universal Love comes into the body and down into the heart has been shown to be 787 hertz.

If you would like to find the exact frequency of love, you can repeat the exercise where you resonate love and find it for yourself using the tone generator.

Free online version (this site is selling Sound Healing Tinnitus treatments):
http://www.audionotch.com/app/tune/

Free software for Mac or PC (two week demo, then about $35)
http://www.nch.com.au/tonegen/index.html

The Sounds or Timbres of Love
When in love, many people often make a soft "coo-ing" sound. My favorite is "mmmm". Mothers (and fathers) often make similar sounds to their babies.

The most common sound for the heart chakra is the sound of "Ah." Try it and see how it feels. The Sanskrit seed syllable that has been used since ancient times is "Yam." The ancient Tibetans used "hung." Today many people subscribe to "Hu" as the best sound to open the heart.

When it comes to instrument sounds, it is often difficult to separate out the energy of a person playing the instrument from the actual sound or timbre of the instrument. Besides the voice, the harp is probably the instrument most associated with the energy of love. Generally, warm "even harmonic" sounds are used to express love (the harp is one of the warmest harmonic sounds). Odd harmonic sounds like bagpipes and heavy metal guitar sounds are normally not associated with opening the heart.

Also, sounds that seem to "cry" or "soar" can trigger the heart. It seems that the violin (especially string sections in an orchestra) and the cello can simulate the sound of crying quite well. Certain drone instruments that play long sustain notes can also instill a sense of peace that helps to resonate love. Many people use crystal bowls to access love or even the drone of a sitar, sarod, harmonium, or shruti box.

Cymatherapy has very specific timbres for the heart. Also Tibetan Pulsing talks about specific timbres for different organs.

The energy of Universal Love might just be a frequency or pitch, however it would make the most sense if it were a timbre. If Universal Love were an actual pitch, then it would actually create some annoying dissonance with certain frequencies or the keys of certain songs. However, if you think of love as sound – a harmonic structure or timbre – then you can apply that timbre to any frequency or pitch and it would always sound completely harmonious. Again, who knows for sure? Hopefully we will one day.

When transmitting love, the heart actually creates harmonics in the sound of the heartbeat that are in golden mean ratios. We have created this timbre using tone generators.

The Music of Love
It is interesting that most love songs often have a bit (or even a lot) of sadness or melancholy in them. Love songs are often in the more sad "minor" keys. However, love in its truest form is not sad. Obviously, the loss of love is sad, or the longing for love can have some sadness to it. However, it seems that when we are feeling love it is a really high consistent hum that is not sad at all.

**Sadness has the ability to get us out of our head
and into our feeling heart
so we can once again access
the love that we are.**

The Musical Intervals of Love
The most common musical interval used to express love is the musical 3rd. The minor 6th interval is also commonly used (it is the interval in the theme song for the movie, "Love Story"). Occasionally, the musical 5th is also used. As some musical intervals are more harmonious than others, sometimes composers will use a progression that goes from more dissonant to more harmonious. Pachelbel Canon, played at more weddings than any other song (in the Western world), has intervals that get darker and darker, and then slowly return to very harmonious intervals. This movement to sadness and back seems to be another pattern that appears to open hearts consistently.

The Rhythm of Love
Of course, slower rhythms around 40-70 beats per minute are commonly associated with

love. In fact, the average heartbeat when at rest is around 55 beats per minute. This is a rhythm that is actually not completely stable; that is, one that "breathes" is commonly associated more with the energy of love. Drum machines do not necessarily connect us to love with their rigid precision; however there are many hit love songs that are based around a drum machine. Often, these songs have other instruments that are creating the "breathing" rhythms with the ebb and flow that is commonly found in nature and Spirit.

Simple rhythms are also more accessible to the heart than complex rhythms.

The actual rhythm of the heartbeat, "boo, boom, pause, boo, boom, pause, boo, boom," also seems to have the capacity to tie into the natural rhythm of the heart when we are experiencing love.

The Musical Flow of Love
It seems like I notice the flow of love the most when making love – that is, making love while completely immersed in love. Based on this observation it seems that pure Universal Love has a flow that is extremely slow and consistent.

Music on the Sound Institute's CD's
"Unconditional Love" and "Unconditional Peace"
are focused on Unconditional Love.

They both have quantum codes embedded in them from Nutri-Energetics that are about the energy of Unconditional Love. The songs were also created while the composer was holding the energy of Unconditional Love.

The Energy of Love
The true essence of love is an energy that can be brought to any frequency, pitch, sound, musical interval, or song. Again, based on the hierarchy of sound, music and energy the most important aspect is simply the energy of love.

The energy of love seems to create two distinct types of effects related to sound and music. First, love is often described as a having a smooth flowing energy. It is not disjointed or grating. It is completely flowing and flexible. Also, the energy of love is commonly described as being the most profoundly peaceful and still energy. When in love, we are at peace. This is in alignment with the concept that the definition of peace is a consistent flowing frequency.

It is almost as if the flow is so slow that it is imperceptible.
This slow flow is the energy of perfect peace and stillness.

May we not get so hung up on the actual frequency of love that we forget to simply love. When someone has a powerful intention of invoking love, the energy is unbelievably powerful.

Most importantly, when you bring the energy of love through any frequency, timbre or music, the love enlivens the sounds and music with the power of Source. The combination is the most powerful healing tool known.

Research

At the Sound Institute we now plan to research the actual frequency of love. Looking particularly at the frequency of Universal Love, we will be doing the research in a major lab with various equipment to identify very fine details of physiological and subtle body changes. We will begin by monitoring a large group of people who say they are accessing love to see what the physiological responses are. We will then use this as a baseline to record when people are actually accessing love in various forms. We will then play the full range of frequencies, timbres, and musical intervals to people to see if the same response is elicited. With enough tests we hope to come up with some frequency that is common to all humans.

Of course, these results could all change as humankind and the planet evolves.

Finally, I have come to believe that there are two main things that bring us into a state of love:

1. Someone else in a state of love – We are often resonated into higher energies by people around us who are holding the energy of love, or who are simply in a state of love.

And more importantly:

2. Finding your own direct connection to Universal Love – Some call it Divine Love, or Spiritual Love. And, when you find this direct connection, nothing is more powerful. You then can access what some call, "The Water of Life." whenever you like.

The Sound of Love is a great tool to help us find these energies of love.

**It is also really powerful to help create a
stronger resonant field that we can swim in.**

**And, most important of all, the Sound of Love
helps create a strong resonant field on the planet,
and when it becomes strong enough
it will entrain the whole planet
into the Sound and Energy of Love.**

The Dynamics of Love

There seem to be several modalities as to how love manifests:

1. Being Love
2. Transmitting Love
3. Receiving Love
4. Resonant Fields

A few years ago I was in Egypt and we were toning in various sacred sites. After 45 minutes of toning the resonant frequencies of the rooms, the ceiling opened up and love and light poured into our hearts.

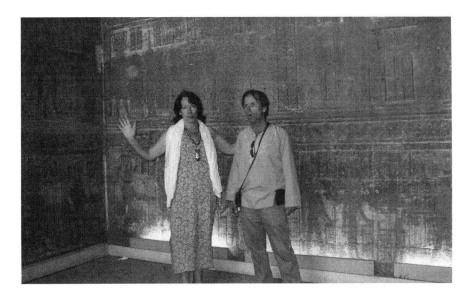

Toning in the Hathor Temple in Egypt

I actually saw the energy of love spiraling into my thymus and down into my heart (I'm sure another person would have seen a different visual). However, the key component was that the love energy was coming from outside of me and flowing into my heart.

On the other hand, many people simply resonate love. As our instructor, Silvina says, "We are love. Every cell of our being is love." In this case it is not necessary to bring love into your heart. In fact, your heart and every cell in your body is love. We only need to simply resonate that vibration that is within us.

When people speak of Universal Love, many do so as though it is everywhere –all around us. Some say that we are fish swimming in an ocean of love.

We can also transmit and receive love from others creating a resonant field around the two of us.

You can look at the frequencies of love in all these ways.

Visually we can look at Universal Love this way:

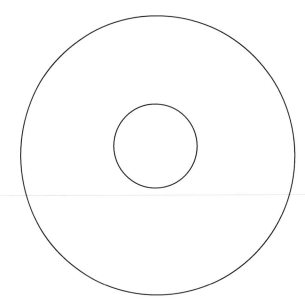

In this case we are the "separate" being surrounded by Universal Love. Some people then feel the energy of Universal Love flowing into them. Others simply resonate love.

On the other hand, we commonly transmit and receive love.

In the following visual a person is sending love to another (or one frequency is being transmitted to another.

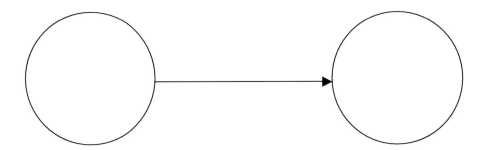

What do you do when you transmit love? Take a second and transmit love to someone. First, you must bring love into yourself – you must access the pool of love before you transmit it. Then you actively move the energy through you and out to the recipient. Again it seems as though it is a river of flowing energy, although the main thing we perceive is the feeling being transmitted and a visualization of the recipient receiving the energy. Therefore, there is a resonance, or sympathetic vibration being setup.

When both parties are sending and receiving love

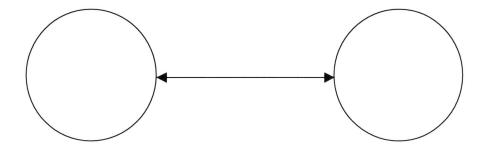

a resonant field is setup. A field of love then seems to surround the two.

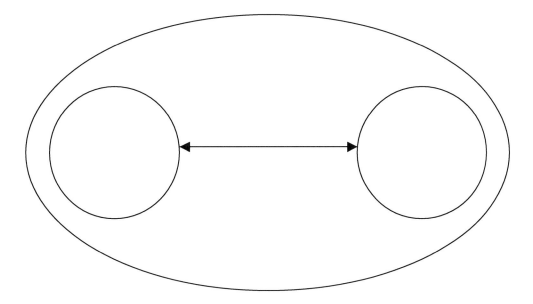

You've probably experienced being around a couple in love, or being in love yourself. The love seems to light up the whole room. You seem to be in a bubble of light everywhere you go – even when you aren't with the person.

This resonant field becomes even larger when there are many people resonating the love. When you have a whole room full of people, or a concert full of people, the resonant field can affect a whole city. Even further:

When you get large numbers of people resonating the energy of love,
the resonant field becomes strong enough
to entrain others across the planet.

Self Love - Using Sound to Resonate Self Love

Based on the above dynamics, I have wondered when you love yourself, "Who is loving who?" I can understand the idea of "my Self" sending love to my physical body or to my own heart. Otherwise, it is hard to conceptualize or visualize.

When you think of yourself as love in the context "I am love," the experience seems to be more of a resonating frequency within us.

For the most part, loving yourself means this: "not feeling bad about yourself; not feeling that you are not good enough; and, not hating yourself." We have already spent a good amount of time on how to release such emotional issues and deep-rooted negative beliefs. Now let's resonate love in ourselves.

As you go through the following techniques, if you find any resistance, or feel that you are not lovable or that you do not deserve love, you might go back to Chapter 32, which describes how to release stuck emotions, so you can release whatever might be stopping you from fully loving yourself.

There are many ways to simply resonate a field of love in yourself with sound.

Tell yourself, "I am Love." – As we described above, simply be love. You <u>are</u> love. Say to yourself, "I am love," over and over, until you are completely humming in a bubble of love.

Tell yourself you love yourself – When is the last time you said, "I love you," to yourself. Anytime you say the words you are transmitting a frequency. Say it now … and say it like you mean it. For extra effect, hug yourself at the same time.

Send love to your own heart – Simply send love to your heart silently. Now, add a sound, so you feel it in your body more. Play with the frequency of the sound until you find one that seems to resonate love the most. Also, play with the sounds (vowels and timbres) to find one that allows love to come through the easiest.

Sing a lullaby to yourself – Sing a song of love to yourself. It could be as simple as an "om," or any other vowel sound. You might just hum softly or sing a whole song. Again, the key is sending love to your self both energetically and physically using sound.

Play with your inner child with sound – Think of that playful side of yourself and notice how present it is in your life. Have you lost that innocence? Can you still be a silly goose?

If your inner child is missing, track him or her down and put him or her back in your heart. See if you can remember how and when your inner child ran away. Then you can use the techniques for releasing stuck emotions in Chapter 32 to release and transform those emotions that came to overshadow your childish innocence.

Or you can simply play. First, try speaking gibberish. Make the goofiest sounds you can. Make silly baby sounds. Play, play, play with sound and reconnect to that precious inner child. Then, use sound to send love to your inner child, and don't forget to take care of him or her in the future.

Each of these techniques helps to create a field of love and harmony with sound in your own system. The more you do it, the more you are resonating the energy of self-love.

The more you love yourself,
the more love you have to give others.

Loving Relationships – Resonating Love in Loving Relationships with Sound
The most important question is, "Why am I not more loving in all my relationships to others?" There are many reasons.

- Being loving makes me too vulnerable. I often get taken advantage of when I am loving. Being loving in the wrong place could actually be dangerous (especially for women).

- I don't have the time. People will want to be around me all the time if I am too loving. Look at what happened to Jesus.

- I don't have the energy. It is a lot of work to bring forth love all the time.

- People might get the wrong impression. They might think that I am being too forward. They might think that I am flirting. In a loving relationship, they might think that I am more committed than I am. They might get the impression I want to take the relationship further than I really want to at this time.

- Being loving in business is not the norm. People will think I am too "woo-woo" and not professional or responsible enough.

Loving family, strangers, business associates/contacts, and romantic partners – all often have different challenges. However, there are many challenges common to them all.

The biggest obstacle to being loving seems to be the fear of being too vulnerable. How can you be loving when people easily take advantage of you? How can you be loving when each person is doing their best to get the advantage? How can you be loving when you are being abused?

Many think that you are either loving or you are defending yourself. And if you don't set boundaries to defend your space, time and money, you will lose out. However, the

305

answer is that you can set boundaries and be loving at the same time. The key is to figure out how to cleanly say how you feel and what you want or need, without fear, upset or anger.

This, of course, is not the easiest thing to do. I sure don't have it down. However, when I am feeling good and not too stressed, I often think of just the right way to deal with a situation. Sometimes, it is a frequency of "this is the way it is." No defensiveness, no energy around it. Sometimes, it involves a camaraderie type of humor. Not a diminutive humor in any way – but a humor that makes us both laugh together; humor that ultimately shows the silliness of the conflict at its core.

Another way to think of it is being grounded in your root chakra in order to not be reactive; being flowing in your second chakra to be able to dance with the negative energy; being in your power in your third chakra in order to be able to set firm boundaries; but at the same time sending or resonating loving energy in the heart chakra.

The key is to notice when the energy you are resonating has dipped below the line into anger, frustration, or even the simplest, "ick" (notice that "ick" has no flow of energy – it is stuck energy). Then, if necessary, transform this non-flowing energy into the flowing energy of love. One simple technique is to simply send the person love energetically. You can also send them a pure tone or vowel silently. If they aren't around you might even send them love with a sound out loud.

Sometimes love flows naturally and every word that comes out of my mouth seems to connect the other person and myself. However, admittedly, it often takes some extra time and consideration in order to figure out just how to be loving in a particular interaction – especially a difficult one. I have found that the more I do it, the easier it becomes. When you get in the habit of being loving, it comes naturally – it becomes who you are.

I have also found that when I am loving, I can sometimes see in a person's eyes that they might be wondering if I am flirting. But as I am consistent with my vibration, they see that I am simply expressing pure loving energy. And, as more people are in this loving vibration, the more we will see it as the norm, as opposed to a flirtatious advance.

Same goes for business. As we all bring more kindness and loving energy to our business relationships, the more it will become the norm. In certain situations I still hold back, but step by step I am weaving in little nuances to get at people's hearts. I know that someday we will begin with the loving acknowledgement of being connected as humans, and continue to hold that energy while doing business.

Love manifests in many ways in relationships. It is recognizable in the frequency of the words we use. Kind words are the essence of love. It can be heard in the tone of our voice – again, "even" harmonics are more loving. It is the musical intervals and music we sing when we speak. This is huge – the amount of sweetness and love in the song we sing when we speak. Love is also visible in the way we move and how we touch someone. It is also evident in the look in our eyes and the flowing consistency of our gaze. And, we can see love in the actions we take. Do we go out of our way to make another person comfortable? Are we kind, considerate and courteous? Do we do things for others – big or small?

All of these things add up to the sum total of how loving we are. We see this sum total of how loving someone else is quite clearly. We all often simply forget or are too tired or stressed to add that subtle bit of sweetness to the sound of our voice.

When we remember to bring more of our love through, we are perceived differently. Doors open to more fulfilling and inspiring relationships and to more smoothly flowing business interactions which in turn leads to more financial flow as well as simple happiness and joy in the relationship. But more importantly, the vibration we are putting out goes into every cell of our own body – including every organ – and we manifest way more health and harmony in our system.

Most importantly, our vibration adds to the overall vibration on the planet: locally in our interactions with every person we come across and also globally through the quantum field.

Loving Relationships
This could easily be a whole book by itself. Here we'll be more concise.

Loving relationships are often the most difficult of all. A very powerful spiritual being once told me that there is no Unconditional Love in loving relationships. If someone doesn't love us back, at some point we normally leave. Also, if someone does not act loving toward us, commonly we are not loving back. The chameleon knows not how to love unconditionally.

The key is to love anyway. However, often we (at least, I...) feel that if I am loving I am condoning the behavior of the other. What if I'm loving all the time, and they aren't? That can't be fair, right? But, of course, when you realize that there is a higher perspective, it is completely fair. Based on the laws of resonance your love can and often does transform the behavior of others.

**Based on the laws of resonance
your love can and
often does transform another's behavior.**

Also, "all the love you give is meant for you." Every bit of love you give goes into every system in your body and creates more health and flow. And, every bit of love you give helps create a resonant field on the planet where we will all eventually be in this state all of the time.

Not loving is not how you change behavior. Sharing your feelings and needs is how it is done. Using requests (knowing you may not get a "yes") and setting boundaries when needed (with love in your heart) is how it is done.

There are several extremely powerful techniques using sound for resolving conflicts in relationships.

Most books say the key to relationships is to get people on the same side. When you are not at odds and instead are working together from a loving and caring position, conflicts often resolve themselves on their own. The best-case scenario is when each person starts arguing (perhaps adamantly ☺) for the other's point of view.

Sound is definitely one of the best tools there is to get two people on the same wave-length and back on the same side.

<u>Making the Sound of Your Feelings</u>
The most profound technique (which is tried and tested) is to simply make the sound of how you are feeling. It is impossible to blame someone with sound!

It is nice to make a pact in advance to use this technique whenever things get a bit dicey. However, I have used it in situations where I have suddenly stopped and said, "I have an idea. You want to try it?" and it has been approved – we're off and running – or rather, off and coming together. Here's the technique:

One person makes the sound of how they are feeling while the other listens. The sounds can be as angry or as sad as the person chooses to make.

Then the other person does the same – expressing how they are feeling, the frustration with the conflict, their sadness with the conflict, their frustration or sadness over the relationship, their frustration or sadness over relationships and conflicts overall. Whatever comes out is all perfect.

Ultimately, it is practically impossible to not have compassion for the others frustration and pain as it is expressed through their voice. This compassionate caring for their pain is the first step to getting on the same page.

Then, both people make the sound of how they are feeling at the same time. It often turns into a dance (in fact, you can even add movement or dance to it if you like). It might get intense, it might get sad, it might get sweet. Commonly, the two end up cracking up. Even more commonly, they both start crying. Sometimes each goes to a place of complete stillness while looking in the other's eyes. Each person's feelings have been heard, and heard without judgment.

Now the healing begins. Negotiating from a place of loving compassion is how it is meant to be. It is our normal flowing way of creating a balanced relationship.

To make the technique even more effective, create sacred space.

Set up candles, crystals, and/or instruments (bowls, etc.) in a nice circle or geometric pattern around you. Then sit cross-legged facing each other. Set sacred space by saying "We set sacred space <u>now</u>." You can ask for any guides, ascended masters, or arch-angels to help, or simply ask Spirit to help. You can set an intention, or do a prayer. Then you can play a crystal bowl or some other instrument, or just do some toning together – all simply to get on the same peaceful wavelength. Out of all of these techniques, do whichever ones resonate with you.

Then, begin sharing your feelings while the other listens. The key is to hold the slow, calm rhythm and energy throughout. Whenever you feel like it, you can also make the sound of your feelings instead of using words. Then, even if you don't agree, everyone is heard.

Resonating Love When in Love
There are also some great techniques to use when you are getting along – to resonate even more love in your relationship with sound.

One is to simply make the sound of how much you love the other person. You might hum, sing or tone using vowels. No judgment…all sounds are completely perfect (how could they not be when they are filled the intention of sharing your love?).

Toning on your mate's body can also be quite effective. Put your lips right on the other's body and do an "ooo" sound. Low frequencies actually work best; however, don't be afraid to experiment with a full range of timbres, tonalities, frequencies, pitches, musical intervals and music.

One of my favorite techniques is to tone inside each other's mouth. Play with different sounds, and you might even do a frequency sweep to find the resonant frequencies within the other's mouth. When you hit the resonant frequency of the other's mouth, it is the most amazing thing. It is as though someone else is making a sound through you. It is also the most profoundly fun experience when you hit the same note or waffle around it creating a wide range of binaural beats.

Toning love on the heart area is my favorite. Many have other favorite areas. Toning on each of the chakras one by one can also be extremely powerful.

The Spiritual Frequency of Love in Loving Relationships
I have come to believe that the purest essence of the love in a loving relationship is that of Universal Love. Often loving relationships are fraught with the energy of fear of loss, attachment and neediness.

Ultimately, the essence of a healthy relationship is when each person is able to resonate the love they need on his or her own. They don't come to the relationship out of a neediness for love, because they each have their own direct connection to Universal

Love. In sacred geometry terms this is the essence of the vesica piscis:

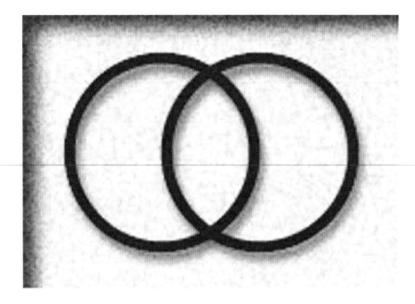

You have two 100% whole individuals coming together and where they overlap is the eye – the eye of God, as some say.

Think of the energy of falling in love or being in love. You sometimes don't need to eat or sleep. It is unbelievably healing. It is like this warm glow follows you wherever you go – lighting up everything and everyone around you.

Being in love also bestows a profound state of peace. There seems to be no time. Just like the timelessness at the end of a slow fade of a crystal bowl. There is also a consistency in every thing you do – including every movement. This essence of stillness is the same found in the consistency of each vowel sound, and the consistent note of a crystal bowl. It is also found in the consistency of Spirit or Source.

When in Love,
I often seem to know
that this is the way I should be all the time.

This is the way we should all be
all the time!

Now, let us honor the pure sacredness of this love that you have experienced in previous relationships. Tune into the last time you were in love. Peel away the person and any story attached to it, and go back into that feeling of being completely in love – and, feel it completely. Feel the warmth, the peace, feel the waves of energy through your body.

Feel the light all around you.

Now, make the sound of this love, knowing it is pure unconditional Universal Divine Love from Source.

Ahhhhooooooommmmmmmmmmmmmmmmm

Keep making the sound of it as long as you like and notice how it feels in your body.

The key is to be able to access this loving energy
of a loving relationship
on your own.

In fact,
you just did.

Imagine, feeling like you are in love, when you are alone. This is the essence of the next section on Spiritual Love.

Spiritual Love – The Sound of Universal and Unconditional Love
Unconditional Love is simply love that is given without any expectation of return or even gratitude. Universal Love (often called Spiritual Love or Divine Love) is a universal energy of love that is present everywhere and is also unconditional. It is free to access for anyone, and most believe that it is unlimited. It is like falling in love with Spirit and being loved back more than you can imagine. Divine Love is the basis of Christianity and is sometimes called Christ's love.

Some say we are fish swimming in a sea of love. Others say Universal Love is within every cell of our body. That it is not outside of us, but within us. Alice Bailey and the ageless wisdom teachings speak of the Ray of Love – Wisdom that permeates our Universe. Spiritual Love is thought of as one of many Rays that come from Source –

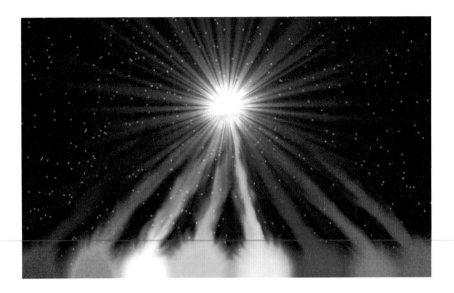

similar to the rainbow colors that come from light.

Some think of Universal Love as being Source itself. I tend to believe that it is just one frequency of many frequencies that come from Source. As discussed previously, it may have a particular frequency, pitch, or timbre, but who really knows for sure.

Over the last seven years I have been polling people in workshops, classes, and events – wherever I go – asking, "How many of you have ever connected to Universal Love before?" About 50% say that they have (admittedly, I often have more spiritually oriented people in my workshops). When asked, "How many of you can connect to Universal Love at will?" about 30% say they are able.

Therefore, I assume some of you reading this have already developed a direct connection and some of you have not.

At the most basic level I would say that I feel a connection to Universal Love as goosebumps and chills. Often they start at the top of my head and move down through my whole body. Sometimes they start in my throat or heart area. Often I feel waves of energy moving through my body. Sometimes the whole room seems to light up. I often feel a comforting sense of warmth as if being held by my mother.

One student said Universal Love is like "an opening."

Again, it is extremely similar to the feeling of being in love, only more powerful – way more powerful when it takes you over completely. Others report being transported into other dimensions of sound and light where everything is completely new and fresh – a place where everything just is.

**Regardless of the details of the description,
everyone seems to agree that Divine Love is just
the most amazingly wonderful feeling
you could ever imagine.**

For those of you who have never felt it, the question is … how do we access it? For those of you who have known the feeling, the question is, how do we access it more? Sound and vibration are unique tools for accessing it.

> For those of you who have never felt it, perhaps you should go to Church. Just kidding. For many, the thought of Church creates the opposite feeling. However, for others, "being saved" is exactly the experience.

We have already done one technique where you tune into the feeling of falling in love or being in love. For many, this has proven to be a portal to the overall feeling of Universal Love. For some, the first time comes when at a sacred place. It happened to me in many of the temples and pyramids of Egypt. For others, it happens after a major trauma, or yet again for no reason at all. Sometimes, tuning in to love is accompanied by angels or apparitions, and sometimes a person's heart is spontaneously blown open with more love than they have ever felt in their lifetime.

One common way that people access it is by sitting with Spiritual leaders – getting it through osmosis. Just being around people that are connected can entrain you into the same vibration. I know many people that use information, music, guided meditations, graphics or videos (especially on YouTube) to access Spiritual Love.

Our basic idea is to use as many techniques as possible. As I always say,

> The more ways you lead a horse to water
> the more chances it will drink.

Some believe certain techniques to be way more powerful than others. However, I have come to believe that some simply work better for certain people. Not everybody is entrained in the same way.

Again, sound and music are extremely potent catalysts in this respect.

It is interesting to look at which music actually invokes this energy of Universal Love. I actually know very few songs. Traditional or pop songs about love can open my heart but they don't put me in the zone of Universal Love where I feel completely enveloped. Om Namo Bhagvate by Deva Premal also works for me. Think about any songs or sounds that do it for you. Or if you don't know of any start keeping track of any that open you up.

Of course, I'm biased, no doubt, but my song Unconditional Love (particularly, the version called Unconditional Peace) does it for me. This song is particularly powerful since it includes quantum healing energy embedded as frequencies (I know that doesn't mean too much to most of you), and every person including myself, held the energy of Universal Love consistently while recording and mixing the song.

Besides using outside stimulus to connect, you can also do your own process. First, think about what sounds might do it for you. For some, it might be Tibetan bowls, for others crystal bowls. For many, the voice is the main catalyst.

First, set your intention to connect to Universal Love. Ask and intend for it to happen. If this fits with your style, also set sacred space and invoke help from higher beings and Spirit.

Sometimes, one sound played or sung the right way with the right intention can trigger an opening and connection to Universal Love. Often though, a long time of doing sound is needed. It commonly takes at least 8 minutes to get in the zone and 15 - 60 minutes before major things start to happen.

There are two ways to go – ecstasy or stillness.

When using the voice toning, chanting or saying mantras for long periods of time ecstatic states often ensue. Often just the deep breathing of doing sound with the voice for long periods of time can get you unusually high. When we were in Egypt it took around 30 - 45 minutes of toning the resonant frequencies of the room before the ceiling opened up.

On the other hand, the deep sense of peace and stillness is also incredibly profound after making sound with the voice for more than a ½ hour. In this stillness many things can happen – particularly when you have set your intention to connect to Universal Love.

Of course, when you know where you are going…it is much easier to get there. Once you have accessed the gem of Universal Love, it is much easier to find. Therefore, it may take you less and less time to join with it. Ultimately, you can do it at will. The first note of the bowl takes you out. One "om" from your lips and you're in! Then, perhaps one day, you never leave.

To explore more, search for "Unconditional Divine Love" in Youtube.
It often works for many.

Using Love in a Sound Healing or Therapy Session

"All You Need is Love; Love is All You Need"
- Beatles

There is no stronger energy than love. Resonating or transmitting love on a sound wave can create miracles – and does so all the time. Simply resonating or transmitting love in any form is already quite powerful. When you add the energy of love to a sound, it is way more powerful and effective. You are creating a stronger resonant field.

You can use love on yourself, or on others.

You can send love to any part of the body by tuning into the energy of love. Bring love into your heart now. And then listen for the sound of it in your head. Do a frequency sweep, or perhaps you have gotten to the point where the sound of love just pops into your head. It may a frequency, pitch, timbre, or even a song. Then, simply use that sound or song to transmit love to any part of the body you would like. You can focus on something as small as a cell, or as large as your entire soul. As previously mentioned sound and energy are quite effective on organs. Sending the sound of love to organs, particularly the heart, can be extremely effective. But, even more effective is sending the sound of love to endocrine glands, particularly the thymus, since it is associated with the energy of Universal Love.

The sound of love is just as effective when performing Sound Healing on a person or a group. First, connect to the energy of love. As you do this over time, you will be able to connect more quickly and get more and more unlimited energy. Then let the energy of love envelope any sound you create. You can bring the energy through your voice or instrument you happen to be playing.

In both cases, you can also use the sound of love silently. Try it. Instead of just sending someone love (whether to help someone in need or for no reason at all) try sending the love with a silent sound – make the sound in your head and send the love on a frequency. The quantum field responds really well to sound.

Regardless of the situation, don't forget to add love.

Creating a Strong Resonant Field of Love to Entrain the Rest of the Planet
Some say there are 3 million Lemurians living in complete love and light underneath Mount Shasta in California. They call it Telos. Regardless of whether this is true or not, imagine being in a room with 3 million people in love and light all the time. How long do you think it will take before you are entrained into love and light also – never to return? Possibly a few minutes - or - Maybe a day or two at the most?

A strong resonant field of millions
will easily entrain
one person.

So… how many people do you think are living in love and light all the time on the planet? Maybe…5? Maybe?

Well, let us not forget the babies. There are approximately 400,000 babies born every day. That means there are over 160 million babies on the planet under the age of 1 and most of them are living in love and light most of the time. There are probably even some 2 year olds living in love and light that have not been indoctrinated yet.

However, I figure that if I am living in love and light 30% of the time, then 3 people like me should add up to a whole person. Fair, right? Even the 5 percenters add up, you know. Even the 1 percenters count and add up.

I would say that the "percenter's" add at least another 200 million people to the total.

This is not even counting all the doggies, kitties, and all animals on the planet. And, it is not counting all the plants and other living things (It is also not counting all the angels, archangels, ascended masters, and positive aliens ☺).

So we easily have close to half of a billion people on the planet living in love and light right now.

When you add in all living things the resonant field is overwhelming.

This is a huge resonant field!

Remember when we imagined the power of just 3 million. The actual resonant field on the planet is way larger. You now have a resource to tap into – you can think of it as your support group.

Ultimately, as we all resonate more and more love and light on the planet, this resonant field will grow stronger and stronger. And then, one day, everyone on the planet will be entrained into the zone.

It happens locally and globally. We see it locally all the time. If I come across just one person happy and beaming, I often get a contact high that can last an entire day. It also happens at the quantum level. We are all connected at the quantum level through entanglement. This is proven science. Therefore, this resonant field of love and light affects everyone, no matter where they are.

Just imagine …
Living on the planet
where everybody…

Everybody
is living in
Love and Light
all the time.

Currently, I have to work at getting back in the zone
and staying there.

Imagine, being in a resonant field so strong
that you never leave.

No one ever leaves.

A planet
with
All Hearts Connected
all the time.

Imagine…

It's easy if you try.

Now make the sound of this intention.

Ahhhhhooooooooohhhhhhmmmmmm

Now here is your homework…

Love Everyone All the Time.

That's all.

Chapter 46 – Connecting to the Soul with Sound

Music sets up a certain vibration,
which unquestionably results in a physical reaction.
Eventually the proper vibration for every person will be found and utilized.
- George Gershwin

"Do you know that our Soul is composed of harmony."
Leonardo da Vinci, Notebooks (1451-1519)

Every single thing in the Universe has its own natural resonant frequency that it naturally vibrates at. Therefore, it makes sense that each of us has an overall resonant frequency.

Every song has a key or home note. The definition of a home note is the note in the music where you experience peace – where you are at rest. In fact, it is practically impossible for a song to not have a home note. Also, every sound or timbre has a "fundamental" root frequency.

Since we are a symphony of frequencies, from cells to organs to chakras and auras, we must have a key or home note. It is practically impossible for us not to have a home note.

It would not make sense that we all have the exact same home note. We are such diverse beings. It makes much more sense that we all have different home notes. In fact, some people in the field of Sound Healing believe that our home notes are specific frequencies, not just specific notes or pitches.

A dozen researchers in the field also subscribe to this concept. Some in the field call this the Super Conscious, the Central Processor, your Signature Frequency, your Resonant Frequency, or your Higher Self. A study at Scripps Hospital in San Diego, conducted by Dr. Jeffrey Thompson, showed that when one finds and listens to their core frequency, the sympathetic and parasympathetic systems come into balance, and the rest of your system comes into a healthy alignment.

I have come to strongly believe that our home note is the note of our Soul.

Everything is a frequency.
Therefore, even the Soul must be a frequency.

Many people talk about the Soul, but there doesn't seem to be much talk about what it really is. The most common idea is that our Soul is our core essence, which is connected to Source or All That Is. It seems that it is commonly accepted that our Soul also contains the memory of all of our lifetimes, and our Soul Purpose.

I think most people don't really know what the Soul is, and don't have any conscious connection to it.

In her books, Alice Bailey says that our Soul frequency is the same from lifetime to lifetime. It is a note that carries our essence from lifetime to lifetime. This makes sense because there must be something that carries the information of our Soul from one lifetime to the next.

Many Spiritual teachings talk about returning to your Soul. Alice Bailey talks about building a bridge between the personality and the Soul. This is referred to as the "Antakarana," in many spiritual traditions. When we listen to the sound of our Soul (instead of our ego and personality), and develop a direct connection to it, we often receive guidance on how to live our lives more fully.

Many people also talk about the "Higher Self." It is interesting that I have never come across anyone who talks about the relationship between the Soul and the Higher Self. I have come to settle on the idea that they are one and the same. However, I believe that the Higher Self is many octaves above the Soul at the same note. I can hear the frequency of my Higher Self about 6 inches above the top of my head (how about that!).

I have also come to strongly believe that your Soul frequency is the frequency of your root chakra.

Just as every sound has a fundamental or root frequency on which all the other harmonics are based, it makes sense that the rest of the chakras would be based on your root frequency, which is the core of your being.

One of the most important aspects of the Soul is its consistency. The Soul is the most peaceful and still place within us; It never wavers or wobbles. No matter what happens in your life, your Soul is never affected. I actually believe that the Soul never needs healing. I believe it is always perfect. This is in complete alignment with the idea that your Soul is the home note of you – your body and your entire Spiritual being.

This frequency is most apparent when a person is centered, grounded or in love. The frequency also naturally emanates from a person when they are in perfect present awareness of the now. And, it is easy to see and hear.

For example, I (and people in our classes) can often easily hear the frequency of Eckart Tolle. In fact, I can often hear the frequency of just about any spiritual leader when they are completely present in the now.

Once you find the frequency of your Soul
you can use that frequency to come home...
to yourself...
where you are at complete peace and
connected to Source at the same time.

The problem is that in the noisy and chaotic world we live in, it is easy to lose track of this "still" frequency within us. In fact, there are so many frequencies that distract us from our own. There are sounds of the city, cars, electricity and electromagnetism, and other scattered people – to mention just a few. It is so easy to lose our frequency.

Finding Your Soul Frequency
There are many ways that sound can help you to reconnect to your Soul frequency.

Nature is a powerful reminder. City sounds distract, but it seems that every sound in nature is helping you to reconnect. Particularly the white noise sounds in nature; oceans, streams, rivers, waterfalls, and the wind. As previously discussed these types of sounds help break up stuck frequencies (mostly emotional) that are resonating a frequency other than that of your Soul. Often, when we are in nature, our natural frequency re-emerges. We might not even notice it as a frequency. However, it is a place where we are completely at ease – totally in the flow – in the zone!

As mentioned, there are many people that focus on this main note: Jeffrey Thompson, Barbara Hero, Wayne Perry, Judy Cole, Sharry Edwards and the researchers at Heart Math – to mention a few. Many of these people focus on the voice to find the frequency. This the technique explained earlier where you simply open your mouth and let a sound come out without pushing or singing. That note is an important note because it is the most natural for your body and vocal chords.

However, after 10 years of helping people to find their note it seems that the actual Soul note is not necessarily the natural voice note. When you focus on the voice you are finding a frequency that is mostly based on the size and physical structure of the body and the vocal chords themselves. I do believe this vocal note is related to the Soul; in fact, it is based on the Soul, but it is not necessarily the Soul note. However, again, it is an important note that can bring much harmony to your physical system.

Some find the note by using the numerology of your name or birth date, or using your astrological sign, or they base it on the key that you speak in. Although each of these is important, I don't believe that they are necessarily your Soul note. Jeffrey Thompson actually uses a heart monitor to determine when your whole body goes into a balance of your sympathetic and parasympathetic systems.

At the Institute we find the note by putting you on the sound table and vibrating the person at each of the 12 notes. Being vibrated so powerfully, it becomes obvious which note it is that brings you into a state of peace and stillness. In the classes, all of the students watch the person on the table and about 80% of the observers come up with the same note for the person.

The first thing you notice in a person is how consistent their frequency is.

The second thing you notice if you simply tune into it...
is the rate that they are vibrating at...
their frequency.

We also do an assessment online (with a webcam). After years of practice I can generally see the frequency when I look at a person while playing each of the 12 notes. I often see the frequency below the chin. Some students see it at the heart; some at the solar plexus. Some see it by detuning their focus and scanning the whole body. I also notice it when the frequency of the breath seems to match the note itself.

You can find it yourself by simply going to an instrument and playing each of the 12 notes. If you don't have an instrument, go to www.virtualpiano.net to access the virtual piano. Simply play each note one at a time and close your eyes and feel it completely – listening to see which note feels the most peaceful to you. It's often good to play each note several times. Let the frequency go through your whole system.

I normally find a note that is a person's "happy" note – the note at which they cruise through the day. Sometimes I find notes that open the heart or just get people really high. However, what we're looking for is the one where the person goes into the most peace and stillness. That note that most feels like **home.**

Once you have found the note, there are many options to use it to help you come back home. First, you can simply tone the note with any of the vowel sounds. This is especially effective for helping the note to re-emerge within your being. You can also buy a crystal bowl or tuning fork in your key. You can also listen to songs in your key. We have a few of our songs in every key, so we can send you a song in your key if you like. Just email me at David@SoundHealingCenter.com. I listen to a song in my key just about every day. It is especially effective in the mornings, or whenever I feel a bit "whacked" out, anxious or ungrounded.

Ultimately, the most effective technique of all is to get on a sound table with a song in your key. Then the frequency is vibrating intensely through your whole system, helping to bring you back home.

The truth is that any consistent frequency will essentially resonate your own root frequency. When a consistent tone is resonated within you, your root frequency is naturally triggered. Since your system knows all frequencies, it recognizes the tone as creating a musical interval. In fact, it isn't as important to find your own frequency, as it is to simply have a consistent frequency vibrating. The one underlying power of sound and music is that it gets your own frequency humming again. However, any type of consistent drone (any music that stays on one note the whole song) will be more conducive to resonating your frequency. The trick is to find drone music that is the right combination of calming versus activating so as to not make you bored or too agitated.

**Of course, if the consistent frequency or song
is in the key of your Soul
it is even more powerful.**

We have had huge success healing many symptoms at our Sound Healing Therapy Center with this technique. One woman was contemplating suicide and within two weeks of listening to a song in her key, she was completely transformed back into a state of peace. The stories are endless. It has helped with anxiety and a huge range of physical issues. When you are at peace without resistance many physical issues seem to resolve on their own.

It is so nice to know where home is
and know how to return at anytime.

Your Soul Timbre

As previously mentioned in our discussion about auras, Alice Bailey talks about each part of our system having a particular frequency or ray. As mentioned, there is the Soul frequency, which is the same from lifetime to lifetime, but there are also frequencies for your physical body, mental body, emotional body and spiritual body. If this is the case, then your whole system is a combination of 5 main notes. You can think of it as the Soul note being the fundamental and the other 4 notes being harmonics. Therefore, your whole system would be a specific sound (timbre or harmonic structure).

It follows that finding and resonating your own specific timbre would help bring you back to your natural healthy self, resonating perfect harmony within and without.

However, just perhaps, your Soul is more than one frequency. In fact, many people believe that our Soul carries all the information from all our past lives. Based on this supposition, then where is all the information carried? One frequency does not carry the information. I tend to believe that you have your core frequency, and there are harmonics that carry all the information from all your past lives. Harmonics at the quantum level are outside the realm of time.

Your Soul Song

*"People say that the Soul, on hearing the song of Creation,
entered the body, but in reality the Soul itself was the song."
- Hafiz (1320-1390)*

I was talking to an acupuncturist about how each acupuncture point is a frequency. Therefore, when energy runs through a meridian it is actually playing a song! It is moving from one frequency to the next, one acupuncture point to the next. She then said, "Yes...that is your Soul Song."

It made me think, that the movement of energy throughout the body is simply playing a song of all the frequencies of the symphony that we are. Our Soul Song is the song that is being played throughout our body 24/7.

Many people (including us) teach classes on how to find your Soul Song. To illustrate the importance, I recently received the following article in my email box.

> When a woman in a certain African tribe knows she is pregnant, she goes out into the wilderness with a few friends and together they pray and meditate until they hear the song of the child. They recognize that every Soul has its own vibration that expresses its unique flavor and purpose. When the women attune to the song, they sing it out loud. Then they return to the tribe and teach it to everyone else.
>
> When the child is born, the community gathers and sings the child's song to him or her. Later, when the child enters education, the village gathers and chants the child's song. When the child passes through the initiation to adulthood, the people again come together and sing. At the time of marriage, the person hears his or her song too.
>
> Finally, when the Soul is about to pass from this world, the family and friends gather at the person's bed, just as they did at their birth, and they sing the person to the next life.
>
> To the African tribe there is one other occasion upon which the villagers sing to the child. If at any time during his or her life the person commits a crime or aberrant social act, the individual is called to the center of the village where the people in the community form a circle around the person and sing the Soul Song.
>
> The tribe recognizes that the correction for antisocial behavior is not punishment; it is love and the remembrance of identity. When you recognize your own song, you have no desire or need to do anything that would hurt another.
>
> A friend is someone who knows your song and sings it to you when you have forgotten it. Those who love you are not fooled by mistakes you have made or dark images you hold about yourself. They remember your beauty when you feel ugly; your wholeness when you are broken; your innocence when you feel guilty; and your purpose when you are confused.
>
> You may not have grown up in an African tribe that sings your song to you at crucial life transitions, but life is always reminding you when you are in tune with yourself and when you are not. When you feel good, what you are doing matches your song, and when you feel awful, it doesn't. In the end, we shall all recognize our song and sing it well.
>
> - Liora www.twinflame1111.com

Who knows for sure whether your Soul is a frequency, timbre or song, or simply energy. Whatever part of this information resonates with you, take it and use it as you like.

Chapter 47 – Connecting to Spirit and Source with Sound

"Listening is nothing less than our 'royal route' to the Divine."
- Dr. Alfred A. Tomatis (1920-2001)

"Music is the mediator between the life of the senses and the life of the spirit."
- Beethoven (1770-1827)

"Sound is the force of creation, the true whole.
Music then, becomes the voice of the great cosmic oneness
and therefore the optimal way to reach this final state of healing."
- Hazrat Inayat Khan (1882-1927)

Sound and music are powerful avenues for connecting us to the higher energies of what many call Spirit, Source, or God. Even if you already know how to connect to Spirit, the right sounds and music can enhance that connection and make it even stronger. Certain frequencies might do it, but more commonly certain sounds (timbres) or certain passages in a song (musical intervals and rhythms) are effective. You can also connect energetically with intention. When you get all 4 levels of frequency, timbres, music and energy going in tandem, whole worlds of unfathomable healing power and levels of consciousness that we have never imagined can open before us. Yet once again – "The more ways you lead a horse to water, the more chance that it will drink."

I see Source or God, as one in the same and will use the terms synonymously. For the purposes of discussion, we describe Source as All There Is. Source is everything in the Universe and it is also inside of us at many different levels. In fact, we are a hologram of Source, so the complete essence of God is within us – but it is also all around us. We are not separate from Source – we are Source.

When you look at the nature of Source or God from a frequency perspective, it seems to have a few obvious characteristics.

1. Source is consistent.
It seems that the energy of God is as consistent and peaceful as it gets. Therefore, based on the laws of resonance, whenever we resonate a consistent sound, we are also leading back to that unfathomable (but perceivable) consistency of Source. Throughout the book we have explained many ways to instill this consistency.

2. Source is alive and a flowing energy.
When enveloped in Source energy we enter a flowing energy that is not stagnant. It is alive and vibrant. It is 100% activating and 100% calming at the same time.

3. Source is not just one frequency – It is all frequencies.

I always think of the frequency of God or Source as being all frequencies in the Universe. In fact, when people explain the experience of being one with Source and everything in the Universe they report perceiving not one frequency in particular, but all the frequencies in the Universe simultaneously.

The ultimate goal is to get to this place where we all are one. We may be able to intellectualize the concept of oneness but very few have actually experienced such a state. People who have accessed this state report that their lives are forever changed. In a state of oneness there is only peace and love. It is a place where we are in touch with all frequencies in the Universe at the same time – as though we are all frequencies in the Universe. In truth, we are!

Portals to Oneness

You can get entrained to Source by just connecting to it, but most people don't have a clue how to do this. Sometimes it just happens spontaneously. Sometimes it happens when people go through a trauma. Some report having experienced it on drugs. Some have had the experience in Church. Commonly people report such an experience after having had a near death experience.

There are many techniques that use the full range of sounds and energy in the hierarchy of sound to bring us back to Source.

1. Osmosis (Resonance and Entrainment)

Just like Love, I would say that the #1 way to be entrained into a state of Oneness with Source is to be entrained by the energy of a person who is in that natural state. Many go and sit with Spiritual leaders in order to get there by osmosis. But, for some, this just doesn't work.

2. Long Term Sounding

Ecstatic states are also a portal to oneness. Ecstasy with sound is commonly achieved by simply listening to or creating sound for long periods of time. As mentioned, 8 minutes is often the minimum amount of time it takes to get into the "zone." When I was in Egypt it took a minimum of around 30 minutes of toning before the ceiling opened up in the temples. It is said that to achieve ecstasy with a mantra, you need to repeat it 108 times. Some say for 40 days. Retreats in India even have people tone sounds for days on end.

3. Setting Intention

Simply set your Intention to go into that primordial place of oneness we are in when we are born.

4. Using Particular Sounds, Timbres or Music

If you believe a certain frequency will bring you there, it very well might. Many use their Soul note to access Source. When at peace we often sink into our natural connection.

Sometimes a particular sound can do it. Perhaps the sound of a particular Tibetan bowl, tingsha or bell might simply transport you. A certain sound that comes through somone's voice (including your own) might just trigger a return to wholeness.

Certain music can do it. I must admit, that I have even been transported to a place of serious oneness surrounded by white light during a Pink Floyd concert. I have felt it often at Kirtan concerts, and at concerts with Deva Premal or Snatam Kaur.

The great thing is that once you find a particular sound "trigger" or "anchor" you can often use it to access the bliss.

5. Using Colors or Visuals
For some certain colors or combinations of colors can do it. For others, just looking at certain sacred geometry structures such as the flower of life

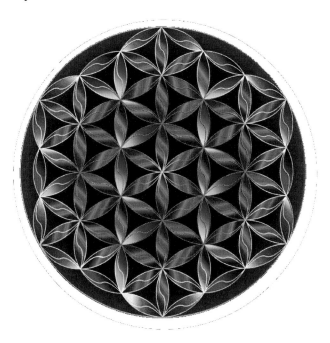

Flower of Life

might take them into the state. Even more powerful can be an animation, simple or psychedelic. For many, the most powerful trigger of all is nature. It might be as simple as a walk through a green field or forest. Even nature videos can work.

Some people have even entered this peaceful state while focusing on mathematical patterns of nature and Source – such as the Fibonacci sequence, the Golden Mean, or simply focusing on the mathematical beauty of the harmonic structure of sound (mathematical multiples).

6. Using Theta
As previously discussed in the Section on Brainwave Entrainment (Section IX) theta can

be a portal to the Universe. Simply listening to binaural beats or rhythms that put you into theta can take you out – and in at the same time. Again, this is the goal of the modality of "Theta Healing."

7. Tuning into More than One Thing or Sound at a Time

One of the most powerful portals into oneness and Source (particularly for beginners) is to tune into more than one thing at a time – simultaneously. As mentioned, this also brings you into a theta state.

For example, when you tune into sparkles on the ocean, it is easy to get lost in the waves of sunlight moving across the sparkles. At this point you have disappeared. You are simply the experience. This also commonly happens when listening to sounds and music. You disappear and become the experience. You can simply de-focus your mind and listen to all sounds at once versus listening to the details of any one sound in the mix.

Another way to experience this portal is to tune into all of the chakras at once as in our Chakra Guided Meditation. Tuning into 7 frequencies simultaneously will make you disappear, so that you are only the experience of the energy flowing between the chakras.

Another technique is to tune into all frequencies of the Universe simultaneously. You simply become all of the sounds of the Universe by adding them bit by bit until you are all the frequencies of the Universe, which is the truth of what you are anyway. In fact, we all are the complete spectrum of the frequencies of the Universe...so this is where we are all one. Some call this sound "The Cosmic OM." To merge with the Cosmic OM is a profound experience.

Once again, the best chance of re-connecting to Source is to do all 7 of the techniques above. Because (as if you haven't gotten it already), the more ways that you lead a horse to water; the more chances the horse will become One with the Universe and All That Is.

**When you truly enter the portal of Oneness with All,
you normally return with a clear perspective that
this illusion of separation we all live with
is just plain silly.**

SECTION XI – Synthesis, Holograms and Daily Life

In this section we look at ways to use the information, techniques and skills from the rest of the book in unique combinations to achieve even more powerful effects and changes in our lives.

Chapter 48 – The Ultimate Three-Step Healing Process

Over years of doing different types of treatments and interviewing natural healers I have discovered a three-step process that seems to be the most powerful. This process can be done on yourself or on another, and also works with other healing modalities.

Step 1 – Resonate Bliss
The first step is to use sound or music to bring a person into as high a state of bliss as possible. Of course, this will be dependent on the individual's current state of mind. However, since Spirit is not far from the surface in any of us, most of us can go pretty high with even basic techniques and procedures. If someone is extremely depressed, you may not get as far, but you are still harmonizing whatever is going on.

This might be as simple as toning, "OM." It might involve playing a crystal bowl with the intention of asking for help from higher sources. It might be as simple as listening to a song that you love, or getting on a sound table and being vibrated into bliss.

Whatever technique you use, do it is as long as is comfortable. Some might do just a minute. Others might do as long as a half hour in a serious healing session.

**The main point is
to access as much Spiritual energy and Peace as possible,
in order to be able to use this energy
in the next stage of the process.**

This step is much the same as the process we described for resolving conflicts between couples. You make sound together simply to connect.

Step 2 – Weeding
The second step is to gently work on whatever you or the person you are working with has going on – whether it be physical, mental, emotional or Spiritual issues. Now that you have done the first step, use any Source energy to enliven the process, and use the peace and stillness to bring even more consistency.

This part of the process might be about breaking up blockages, stuck energy or even something like a tumor. It might also include transforming an issue. This might include

328

releasing a stuck emotion or even transforming cancer cells. It might also consist of simply bringing people into a high state of bliss including Gratitude, Compassion, Love, Joy, a connection to their Soul, or a connection to Source and Oneness.

Of course, you can use any of the techniques explained in the book, other techniques you might have learned elsewhere, or you might even just come up with your own techniques as you go. Don't be afraid to trust your own intuition and intention.

The key to making this process work well is accessing higher powers of grace from the 1st step, versus simply *working hard* to do the healing. Releasing and healing need not always be a difficult process. The more grace you bring to the process, the more effective it normally is.

Step 3 – Resonate Higher Bliss
Now that you have healed or harmonized the issue, resonate as much love and light as possible. The ultimate goal is to create your own powerful resonant field of love and light, so you get used to being in the zone all the time. Then, it becomes more and more natural to come back home to your Soul connected to Source – with Universal Love flowing through your heart.

Now that you have done the work, do an exercise to bring in as much love and light as possible to fill in the dark areas that you just cleared out. Tone, play a bowl, go on a hike in the sun, resonate with your Soul, use the sound techniques in the book to open your heart, connect to Source and resonate that place of bliss where you are one with the Universe. Then, don't forget to resonate gratitude! You might even make the sound of gratitude.

You can also think of this part as a celebration. Celebrate even the slightest healing that occurred in the second stage. Often when even just one simple stuck emotion or deep issue is released it is much easier to use sound or music to fill a person up with love or Spirit.

**Resonate Bliss Love and Light
in order to contribute
to a Stronger Resonant Field on the Planet**

Then, you just might think about how you might share this energy. Perhaps you know of someone else in need.

Chapter 49 – Using Sound to Deal with Challenges and Conflicts

10 Ways to Handle Challenges and Conflicts in
Relationships, Health, Wealth, World Changes, and Hypersensitivity to Sounds.

Challenges and conflicts are the #1 cause of us losing track of our own stable, peaceful vibration. This chapter looks at 10 ways to handle challenges and conflicts. These include the big 3: relationship, health and wealth challenges. It also includes any anger, fear or anxiety over world changes – whether caused by greedy people or natural disasters such as global warming, storms, tornadoes, earthquakes, hurricanes, solar flares, or pole shifts where we might lose our consciousness completely. These techniques are also extremely effective for dealing with loud or annoying sounds around us – especially for those of you that are hypersensitive to sound.

It seems that the last bastion of raising our consciousness is to simply not be reactive to any situation – even down to the point of "hmph." Many spiritual leaders say that "suffering" is simply our resistance to a situation. In fact, some spiritual seekers often put themselves through much pain by meditating for lengthy periods in uncomfortable positions and places (like caves) and they do not suffer. They do not suffer, because there is zero resistance in them. A different person in the same situation might be completely miserable.

This is the first step – no reaction, no judgment. The next step is to resonate your own frequency so that you are not entrained by any so-called negative frequencies around you. Even more advanced is to bring a positive vibrational energy to the situation. Not only are you not reacting, you are actively helping the situation. Ultimately, the most advanced level is to see all as a part of your self. In a place of Oneness nothing is ever a big deal.

In the class we offer on this subject, we actually play a really annoying synthesizer sound to represent the challenge or conflict – and no one is ever annoyed by the sound! Eventually, not only are people not annoyed by the sound, they actually go into a state of bliss the moment the sound begins. Imagine – having no fear or anxiety whatsoever over any upcoming challenge or conflict because you know you now have the tools to actually go into a state of bliss in the midst of the challenge.

Instead of using an annoying sound to represent our challenges and conflicts, simply take a minute and write down all of the challenges and conflicts you have in your life now – including health, wealth, relationships, world changes, or even annoying sounds. Go ahead and write them all down – we'll wait until you are done.

You don't want to resonate trouble by focusing on potential problems. However, you do want to be ready for them in case they show up.

Now…let's begin.

1. Allowing and Acceptance

The opposite of resistance is allowing. Simply letting it be with no reaction. This is really about having no judgment. The second that we determine that something is good or bad, suffering follows. If we label a situation "bad," then find we can't get away from it, it is a bummer. According to Buddhism, even if we label something "good," it is stressful when we don't have it, because we desire to be around it; and, it is stressful when we lose it.

The question is, "What are things, if they are not good and bad? What is at the basis of reality where things just are?" The answer is, "Everything is vibration." When we see things as vibration – they just are. We can see things from a variety of levels – Frequency, Timbre, Musical Flow, or Energetic Flow (sound familiar). It is what it is. Interesting, huh? Ahhhhh... so it is.

If you were to come up with a sound for the energy of allowing, what might it sound like? For me, it is mostly just silence. It might also be something like an "Ahhhh."

Go into the energy of allowing now.

Think about all of your challenges and conflicts and ask to bring the energy of allowing to them. Can you allow them to be? – no resistance, no reaction. They are what they are. The vibration is what it is.

The next 3 techniques are mostly about resonating your own natural state of peace, or creating your peace with sound and energy so that the outside dissonance doesn't affect you.

2. Being present in the vibrations and rhythms in your body

In this technique you go into a complete state of presence where you are a point of awareness. Again, in this place there is no judgment. You are simply present with what is.

Being present in your body is one of the best ways to get off the roller coaster of outside entrainment. Tune into the coherent frequencies in your body. Feel your body. That is, feel the frequencies and vibrations in your body. There are 70 trillion cells in your body. Even if you are experiencing pain, there are always more cells that are humming happily, than there are in pain. Feel the frequencies and vibrations of everything around you: sights, sounds, smells, touch including temperature and clothing, and perhaps tastes. Notice your breath, including its rate. Notice your heart beating. Notice gravity pulling you to the center of the earth.

All of these vibrations are completely coherent and peaceful, in relation to the challenge and the conflict.

Now think about all of your challenges and conflicts and simply notice how your body feels and how the feelings simply pass on through when they are met with no resistance. Also just notice the rhythm and quality of the energy of the conflict. What might this so-

331

called negative energy sound like? Then just let it be what it is. Just be present with its song – regardless of its quality.

Next time you are in the fire of a challenge, simply tune into your body and be present with whatever is happening. No resistance; no suffering.

3. Toning
Sometimes certain challenges are just too much for our body. Certain sounds are just too loud. Being present in my body isn't enough, it seems. The next technique of toning brings a coherent frequency into your body. Even if you are in pain, toning will replace the pain.

Simply make the sound of "OM," "AH," or any other vowel sound. Make it out loud with quite a bit of volume. This technique brings that consistent vibration inside your body at a physical level. It is especially effective for any physical ailment or pain in the body. It is also especially helpful for relieving any type of worry, anxiety or fear. In fact, it is good for about any situation – except when you are in a conflict with someone right in front of you. Toning in their face will probably not help resolve the conflict.

In these cases you might try toning silently to yourself. Try it now. Do an "OM" silently in your head. This is also especially helpful when in any public place, such as a business or party.

Consistency is the essence of peace. And as previously mentioned, vowel sounds are consistent, coherent sounds. They bring that consistency into every cell of your body, including your mind. They even resonate the consistency of your Soul, Spirit and Source.

Again, you are simply creating a frequency in yourself that overcomes the discordant frequency around you, or inside of you in the case of pain or anxiety.

4. Toning your Root/Soul Frequency
Even though at this point you may not know what note your home note is, it is nice to know that there is a frequency inside of you where you are completely at home. If you believe that we have a Soul, your Soul is the most peaceful place within you. Your Soul is never affected by anything that ever goes on. It is the ultimate peace and stillness, and it is totally connected to Source.

So, even if you can't find the note inside you, you can still go to this place of peace that is your Soul or home note.

Simply, listen for a note that feels like home. If you are able to do a frequency sweep in your head, sweep up and down until you find a note that feels like home (don't worry about whether it is right or wrong – it doesn't really matter as long as it feels good). It generally is the lowest note that feels like home (versus a high note). If you can't imagine a frequency sweep in your head, then do it out loud, until you find a note that

332

feels like you have come home, and are at rest.

Then, tone this note with the intention of going to that place of peace that is your Soul. Again, it will completely overcome any other frequency of a challenge or conflict.

I have to say…once you do find your Soul note for sure, it is amazingly powerful for returning yourself to peace and clarity when you tone it. It is worthwhile to get a bowl or tuning fork in your key to help remind you. There are even smartphone apps in the iPhone that tell you what note you are toning (it's just a guitar tuner app). Listening to songs in your key will help you to get to know the frequency.

It can take quite awhile to be able to access this note at will, especially when in the midst of a bit of chaos. Even musicians can find it difficult at first to access the note on their own. However, once you get it down, it's like having the most powerful tool in the world inside you – a tool that is capable of overcoming the chaotic energy of any challenge or conflict.

The key to each of the previous techniques is to simply get off the roller coaster of so-called negative vibrations around you. You are no longer on the ride being entrained. You have created a new second vibration, or found it inside yourself – one that is resonating peace, stillness and equanimity. You resonate the peaceful vibration instead of the chaotic one.

The following techniques are about bringing a positive coherence <u>to</u> the so-called negative frequency. Even if it doesn't harmonize, change or affect the negative vibration (which it actually often does), it leaves you in a blissful state of coherence – both sound-wise and energy-wise.

5. Sing Along
This technique is especially good at dealing with annoying and irritating sounds.

First, if you have a sound that is just making you crazy or making your skin crawl, the first step is to get rid of the resistance. Make it your friend. The worse you "label" the sound, the more you suffer.

The worse you "label" the sound, the more you suffer.

Then, just sing along with it. Next time you hear a siren, howl like a wolf with it. Get a rhythm going with your voice to match the jackhammer. Make a song out of a hurtful feeling. Match the sound of the motorcycle. Find the note of that annoying fan and tone along with it. Play, play, play with it. Make it your friend.

I've had people do the same with tinnitus (ringing in the ears). Instead of suffering, try and sing along with it (at a lower octave, because it is normally higher than your voice can go).

You can even do the same with a pain in your body. Play with sounds until you find a sound that matches or dances around the energy of the pain. Make it your friend – stop the suffering.

Play with the sound of any fear you might be in. Be silly with it.

Some people like to mimic the sound of a person's critical tone (not in front of them though). Play with it. Don't do it in a demeaning way where you are above them. Just play with the energy of it, until the resistance subsides.

6. Welcoming
Imagine what the sound of "Welcoming" might sound like. Say, someone comes to your door…now make the sound of welcoming. It is a sweet sound. It is an inviting sound.

To be clear, welcoming is not lying down and letting the world roll over you. You still set boundaries (some of us might even "Occupy Wall Street"). However, you welcome the challenge or conflict instead of getting stressed about it. Welcoming is akin to accepting what is. Then you can bring a positive frequency to the conditions and get on with solving the problems. You might still need to take action to deal with the issue, but you can even welcome that.

So we welcome the radiation coming from Japan. We welcome the nuclear power plant melting down. To get upset and angry only hurts your own physical body even more. We welcome the pain. We welcome the conflict, no matter how intense.

You see?

Now, focus on your own challenges and
bring the energy of welcoming to them.

Notice how all the tension around the issue immediately dissipates. Now make the sound of welcoming while focusing on your own personal challenges and conflicts. Whenever you make the sound of an energy it creates a much stronger resonate field – and the sound resonates through your body physically!

7. Gratitude
Gratitude, Oh, Gratitude…one of the most powerful sounds there is.

As in welcoming, when you can be grateful for a conflict or challenge, it completely transforms your energy around it. Again, you don't want to invoke a challenge or conflict. But, you can invoke gratitude once you're facing it.

But, how can we be grateful for challenges and conflicts that we would rather avoid? First, of course, we can always be grateful for a challenge because it makes us stronger. It makes us more prepared for similar challenges in the future. It also gives us an opportunity to grow. However, on a more basic level, challenges and conflicts create movement; they are activating. Just like a dissonant chord, they bring gifts of energy.

Also, difficulties sometimes bring major changes. For example, how can we be grateful for the nuclear plant meltdown at Fukushima? It has resulted in many nuclear power plants not being built or finished around the world. It has also resulted in more regulations for power plants around the world. And, most importantly it opened the collective heart. When the tsunami happened and the radiation started pouring out, the heart of everyone on the planet went out to those who had died or been hurt. But also, people's hearts opened to the serious possibility of our planet actually being made uninhabitable. Our built-in natural response of compassion to human suffering was triggered.

You never know how you might end up being grateful for a so-called negative event. Years ago, I had a chief financial officer steal over a $1,000,000 from my school, and it caused the school to go under. After a couple of years of anger therapy...... I put together a play called "Compassion" based on this guy who ripped me off. It is a major Cirque style play with IMAX 3D and speakers in every seat of the auditorium. And now we are getting funded to create an installation and take it on tour around the world. So now, I can go back to this guy and say, "Thank you!"

Some say we can even be grateful for the horrible destruction that Hitler created, as destructive forces commonly break down solidified structures that are holding us back from moving forward to more light and connection. Many agree that World War II actually brought the planet together more so than ever – again as the collective heart opened for the millions who were killed.

**You just never know
what higher plan might be involved
with any negative situation.**

Finally, the Dalai Lama says that when someone hurts you (so to speak), they are actually hurting themselves by creating karma for themselves. And...they are giving you an opportunity to learn compassion. He says that you don't learn compassion by studying how to do it. You learn it through practice. So whenever you feel someone has hurt you they are providing you with an opportunity to learn and practice compassion, then you can be grateful to them.

**They are actually
sacrificing themselves for you.**

Therefore, we can be grateful to them.

If you can't figure out how to find gratitude for a person or situation, then you can simply revert to gratitude for all the things we have. The key is to simply be in a higher emotion that is healthy for you and helps to create a stronger resonant field on the planet.

There are so many things to be grateful for. If you haven't made a gratitude list now is a great time to do it. Here's a good list to get you underway.

Gratitude for:

Life
This breath
Loved ones
Family
Babies
For every thing that someone has done out of simple caring...particularly things that are given freely without expectation of any return.
The health I have
Love
Goosebumps and chills
Beauty
Happiness
Joy
Home
Hot and cold running water in my home
And, OMG, a hot shower in my home
My car
This body
Gratitude for the heart
Feelings...for all the senses – touch, smell, sight, hearing
Doggies
Kitties
All animals in the world
Nature
The planet and all the stars – the sun in particular
Frequencies
All the things we may not like
All the people that have hurt you
Every frustration, aggravation, irritation, disturbance, annoyance, nuisance, disappointment, dissatisfaction, anger, resentment, pain, fear, and suffering
Gratitude for everything
For no reason at all
Gratitude for being able to experience gratitude
Gratitude for others being grateful

Now...feel all of this gratitude in your body. Let it surround you like a bubble. And, feel it through every cell in your body. Also, at the same time, think about all the gratitude on the planet. There are 400,000 babies born everyday, so there are probably at least 600,000 people in gratitude on the planet right now. I would say there are probably millions. So, tune into not only all the things you are grateful for, but also all of the gratitude on the planet. Then again, if gratitude had a sound, imagine what it would be.

Then make the sound out loud…

Now, focus on all of your challenges and conflicts
with both the energy and sound of gratitude.

If you need help, search for our "Sound of Gratitude" on Youtube.

It has a large group of people toning the energy of gratitude with 100% focus, including visuals of all the things we can be grateful for.

8. Compassion

Compassion is a close relative of Unconditional Love. When I created the play "Compassion," I studied all the ways to invoke compassion.

First, we have a built-in natural compassionate response to other's pain. If we see someone suffering in front of us, compassion naturally wells up within us. Although for some, TV and the level of homelessness has desensitized us to other's suffering.

The tricky part is to have compassion for those who have hurt us. There are several techniques that people use.

• I often ask myself, "Why might they have done what they have done?" The answer I find is that they have been entrained into craziness and confusion by society – often by parents, family or friends – but especially by television. It has become the norm to be mean, to call someone an asshole, to get angry and upset over the smallest act of inconsideration. I tell myself, "They know not what they do."

Also, people are commonly just tired, worn out, hungry or stressed. I know that I am not nearly as nice and considerate when I haven't had enough sleep, when I'm really hungry or stressed over some situation. Sadly, my capacity for kindness becomes diminished. I often think of this when someone is inconsiderate. I would say that there are very few "mean" people – most people are simply trying to survive and make it through.

• See the person as a baby. Imagine George Bush as a sweet little baby totally connected to Spirit. Or even more intense, imagine Hitler as this cute little baby that is 100% a part of Source. This often helps me when I need to bring up compassion.

• Imagine what it would be like if you got upset or acted out with vengeance. You would be simply creating an incoherent sound vibration – hurting yourself and adding to that negative resonant field on the planet. "Eye for eye, and what do you get? A whole world that is eyeless."

• The Dalai Lama talks about a mental process to evoke compassion. You see the other as also not wanting suffering – just like you. You also see them as desiring happiness – just like you. In this respect you can connect to them and see how you are just the same.

337

• Ultimately, to take it to the highest level – is to go to a place of Oneness where you are truly one with everyone. When you leave the craziness of separation that we live in, and see them as part of yourself, compassion naturally comes through. I am you, you are me. Often a sense of peace or stillness happens – often with a bit of sadness in it. This is the ultimate level of compassion.

Now, go into the energy of compassion. The Dalai Lama is one of our best mentors in this regard. There used to be 3,000 ashrams in Tibet. There are now three. And the Dalai Lama continues to hold compassion for the people in the Chinese government. When asked what he would say to a Chinese soldier who has killed hundreds of Tibetans, he said he would go over to him and hold him for all the pain he is feeling.

I also heard an interview on NPR with two guys – one from Palestine and one from Israel. Both men's entire families had been killed – wives and children – and they got together and went to schools throughout Palestine and Israel. They stood in front of the students and said (paraphrased), "If anyone has reason for anger and revenge, it is us. Our families are gone. But we have come here to tell you that forgiveness and compassion are the only answer. Otherwise, there will be more and more people suffering like us."

The essence of compassion is the energy of the Buddhist Goddess Quan Yin (which, interesting enough, is said to be centered in a city in China).

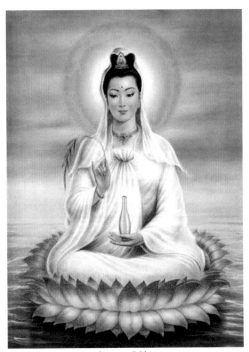

Quan Yin

Now, feel the energy of compassion, not only in yourself, but also tap into the powerful energy of compassion on the planet.

Listen for a sound that resonates this energy of compassion,
and make it out loud now.

Now, bring this energy and sound of compassion to all your conflicts and challenges – and to all of those who have hurt you (so to speak).

And now, bring that energy of compassion to yourself, to transform feelings of not being good enough in some way…or for that part of you that has come up with the illusion that you are not good enough. Also, bring up compassion for anything you feel you might have done to hurt others, or yourself.

9. Unconditional Love
To bring love to a conflict or challenge is one of the sweetest ways you can help yourself and possibly even transform a whole situation.

We went into detail on how to open your heart with sound in Chapter 45.

Bring love into your heart now. If you know how to connect to Universal Divine Love, do it now.

Now, make the sound of this love.

And, focus this loving energy on each of your challenges and conflicts.

Ahhhhhhh…what a wonderful feeling.

10. Oneness with All
When you see the situation and the people involved as sacred then the whole situation transforms. Again, we go to a sound of peace, sometimes with a tinge of sadness.

As discussed in Chapter 47, when you see the other as a part of you, then you begin to look at how you can help yourself as a whole. Also, when you see the vastness of all the frequencies in the Universe that you are a part of, then this one little issue becomes less than miniscule. Also, you see the darkness as part of the whole of the Universe. It is no longer bad; it is part of the beauty of All That Is. Perfect in every way.

If you like, go back to page 330 and use the techniques we described to access this place of Oneness once again.

Then, focus on all your conflicts and challenges.

From this perspective, they are no longer conflicts and challenges.

You now have a wonderful toolkit to deal with any conflict or challenge in your life: To be able to hold your own frequency and not be affected by others around you, and to be able to help transform yourself, and ultimately everyone else on the planet.

Different people will resonate with different techniques in this list of ten. And, you will find that different techniques work better for different situations. Sometimes gratitude is the deal, other times compassion, maybe love, or maybe just simply toning in your head might be all that is needed. Use whichever one resonates with you for whatever situation you come across. Here is a chart that might be helpful, but is by no means definitive.

1. Allowing and Acceptance – Good for just about anything. Whenever you get rid of resistance and judgment, suffering ceases. Perceive the world as it is – Frequencies, Timbres, Music and Energy.

2. Being Present and in Your Body – Especially good when you are avoiding a situation or it is so intense that you feel out of your body.

3. Toning – Toning out loud is especially good when around noise or loud sounds, or when in pain because the frequency of the sound in your body keeps out the external sounds. I find that toning silently is really good in public places, or when in the midst of a situation where I'm completely overwhelmed.

4. Toning Your Root/Soul Frequency – Once you learn the note of your own resonant frequency, this note can completely transform your whole system into a place of complete stillness. Until then, having an instrument or a song in your key can be really helpful. This is especially good for disruptive noises or just about any conflict.

5. Singing Along – Ideal for noises and loud sounds and pain, although if you make fun of any situation (without being disrespectful) it helps lighten things up.

6. Welcoming – A little more sophisticated technique than allowing; therefore, good for about anything. When you can be happy in any situation you have more capacity for every challenge.

7. Gratitude – Good for most situations, although some people find it difficult to figure out how to be grateful when someone has hurt them. It is also sometimes hard to be grateful for catastrophes. This is especially good for any wealth issues. In fact, for any issue, it is good for you to simply count your blessings.

8. Compassion – This one is ideal for when people hurt you, or especially when you hurt yourself.

9. Unconditional Love – This one is nice for most situations since you don't have to have a reason. It is especially good for those who do things out of ignorance or pain. It is also good for any health issues, or even for wealth issues.

10. Oneness with All – Every situation could benefit from this energy. It is especially effective for any relationship challenges, and might also be the best for catastrophes or world changes.

It's always best to assess each situation and intuitively do whichever technique feels the most appropriate at the time.

Again, having done these techniques, you see that not only can you overcome being upset by any issue in your life – whether it is health, wealth, relationships, world changes, or wily sounds – you can also use the situation to go to a really high state of consciousness.

At one point during this class, one woman said, "Can you keep playing those weird synthesizer sounds – so I can continue in this state of bliss." Just imagine approaching any conflict or challenge in your life with a sense of glee – because now you get to go into a really wonderful high state of consciousness.

Just imagine.

Chapter 50 – Living with Sound – Using Sound in Your Life Daily

"Oh music!
Thou who bringest the receding waves of eternity
nearer to the weary heart of man as he stands upon the shores and longs to cross over!
Art thou the evening breeze of life, or the morning air of the future one?"
- Jean Paul (1763-1825)

Now that you have a whole new perspective on how sound affects us physically, mentally, emotionally, and spiritually – where do you begin to implement these concepts and techniques into your daily life? Of course, if you have a particular illness, pain, emotional trauma or psychological issue you are dealing with, you probably have already gravitated to one or more of the techniques explained in the book.

However, if you take it a bit further and incorporate some of these vibrational techniques into a daily or weekly practice, then you are doing health maintenance. Actually, it is more than just maintenance, it is actually working towards raising your vibration (whatever that means to you) so that you live a healthier, happier and more fulfilled life.

There is a full range of techniques for using sound throughout the day – from really simple and basic techniques to a fully expanded Sound Healing practice.

Seeing It All as Vibration
Again, the goal is to perceive everything as sound and music – ultimately, frequencies, timbres, musical intervals, chords, rhythms, musical flow, and energetic flow.

When we see everything as vibration there is no judgment, it is simply the frequency that it is! If a vibration is supporting our health, we can merge with it. If not, we center in our own sound or bring a higher vibration to it.

When we enter the world of vibration – sound, light, color, geometry and the quantum, and learn the tools at our disposal for resonance and entrainment, we regain our power – a power that does not overwhelm or hurt others. Through the laws of resonance outlined in detail in Chapter 19, we are able to make conscious changes in our world. We look for and find the resonant frequency of everything around us – and inside of us. We then look at the different ways to use a strong resonant field to overcome a weaker one. We also see that we can seriously transform any cell or state of consciousness with really powerful resonant fields. We regain our birthright – empowered and in harmony with nature and Spirit.

Coming Home Every Day
It seems that the ultimate goal is to establish a center of peace on the inside that you can

return to at any time; and, cultivate a smooth sense of flexibility and flow on the outside.

It is so important to be able to come home to a place of rest and peace everyday. We have discussed many ways to do this with a wide range of sound tools. Simply play a crystal or Tibetan bowl, use tuning forks, or spend some time toning, chanting or doing mantras.

The key is to honor the frequency in the silence as the sound fades out slowly.

The other part of life is to develop more and more of a sense of flow in your life. The essence of health is flow – both musical and energetic flow. Pay close attention to things that are flowing freely. Watch things in nature, watch other people that seem to be in the flow, notice the quality of flow in music, and most importantly pay attention to the quality of the flow within your own system at all levels – physically, mentally, emotionally and spiritually. If you see anything impeding the natural flow within, figure out where the problems are and pull out your sound tool box and go to work – or rather, go to play!

Creating a Daily Practice

At the end of each semester at our Sound Institute we ask our students to come up with a sound practice they would like to do and one they will commit to doing every day. Over the years, we have collected over 100 techniques. Choose the ones that resonate with you and create your own practice.

Many of these practices can be done for a minute or two, 10 minutes, or 20 minutes or more. Schedule how long you want to do each practice every day. At the minimum you might just do 5 minutes in a day. Or you might do 5 minutes when you wakeup and 5 minutes before you go to sleep. Or, even add another 5 minutes in the middle of the day. If you can, double the time or add a bit more time each day. Don't stress yourself out. Do what feels right for you.

Voice Work

1. Tone any vowel sound of your choice. I especially like to tone in the car. Tone your home note if you know what it is, or play with different pitches to see if you can find it.
2. Tone or sing your signature or Soul Song.
3. Sing a chant. You can choose one, or you can make one up.
4. Chant a mantra.
5. Do overtone singing for at least 8 minutes a day.
6. Tone how you are feeling.
7. Tone stuck emotions. You might even plan a longer session once a week or once a month to do some serious work on releasing some deep emotional issues or negative subconscious beliefs.
8. Tone to your plants and animals.
9. Do a sound chakra treatment (preferably in the morning).
10. Go to a Kirtan concert (call and response).

11. Tone the ideal day.
12. Sing "Light" language - Like gibberish with an intention of love and light.
13. Practice singing the musical intervals.
14. Make a new song every week.
15. Tone in resonant spaces such as caves, tunnels and churches.

Listening
16. Listen to any of your favorite Sound Healing, New Age, Meditative, or Relaxation music.
17. Listen to a CD in your Root/Soul frequency. I often put mine on repeat while I work.
18. Go for a sound walk and listen to all of the nature sounds around you. Also listen for the sound of all of the plants and trees.
19. Listen to binaural beats to entrain your brain.
20. Get on a sound table once a day or one or two times per week.

Playing
21. Play an instrument – a crystal bowl, Tibetan bowl, or anything you might have. It is especially nice to improvise and pay close attention to how the sounds are affecting you. Sing or tone along with the instrument.

Treatments
22. Do a Sound Healing treatment on someone.
23. Practice Voice and Sound Healing on others.
24. Do a Tuning Fork treatment on the chakras.

Energy
25. Connect to a higher emotion daily – Compassion, Gratitude, Joy, Unconditional Love – and make the sound of the emotion too.
26. Do a meditation on Being One with Everyone and the Universe.
27. Send sound to various organs and parts of the body. Send the sound of love to each organ.
28. Channel higher beings or guides. Let them come through your voice.
29. Bring female and male energy from both above and below and balance you.

**Doing sound everyday
can and will
transform your life!**